Percutaneous and Minimally Invasive Foot Surgery

Cyrille Cazeau • Yves Stiglitz
Editors

Percutaneous and Minimally Invasive Foot Surgery

Springer

Editors
Cyrille Cazeau
Clinique Victor Hugo
Paris, France

Yves Stiglitz
Clinique Victor Hugo
Paris, France

ISBN 978-3-030-98790-9 ISBN 978-3-030-98791-6 (eBook)
https://doi.org/10.1007/978-3-030-98791-6

Translation from the French language edition: "Chirurgie Mini-Invasive Percutanée Du Pied - 2ème édition" by Cyrille Cazeau and Yves Stiglitz, © Sauramps Medical, Montpellier, France, 2015. Published by Sauramps Medical. All Rights Reserved.

This Springer imprint is published by the registered company Springer Nature Switzerland AG
The registered company address is: Gewerbestrasse 11, 6330 Cham, Switzerland

Foreword 1

We measure the success of a literary work by its critical acclaim and how many copies are sold. But in the scientific world, since our books are not promoted through advertising, it can be measured simply by the quality of its content and the fact that the initial edition has sold out. This is the case here.

As readers and authors, we are grateful for the second edition of the book *Minimally Invasive and Percutaneous Surgery of the Foot.*

For an author, there is nothing more frustrating than to realize—not long after the first edition has been published—that certain important points were not developed sufficiently, not to mention that elements one feels very strongly about were not included. These regrets are not eternal; the next edition solves all this. Since the first edition was published in 2009, considerable progress has been made in the theory and practice of percutaneous and minimally invasive foot surgery. This progress is captured in the second edition. Various chapters have been expanded, refined, and updated while new ones have been added to bring us closer to evolutionary reality, or should we say *revolutionary*?

In some ways, percutaneous and minimally invasive surgery is a revolution. It has overtaken our way of working, in a constructive and irreversible manner. Since the differences between surgery with a very small incision and percutaneous surgery are often difficult to discern, both in the immediate postoperative course and the outcomes, it is logical to group these two procedures within the same book.

It is important to understand that—and this is one of the qualities of books that Cyrille Cazeau is involved in—minimally invasive and percutaneous procedures are derived from traditional open surgery and use many of the same principles. We are not being catapulted into an entirely different world. The experience and knowledge of pioneering, highly respected surgeons is an important aspect that is highlighted in these books, especially the second edition. Thus we are far from adopting a doctrinaire approach. This book provides detailed explanations and will help surgeons justify and carry out these procedures.

Nevertheless, and especially for percutaneous surgery, these techniques have resulted in very different protocols, postoperative course, and management. Thus immediate weight bearing on the operated foot is no longer banned, it is encouraged! Similarly, postoperative dressings have taken on a vital role in preserving the correction.

On the other hand, in a more general way, the patient is always right. By this I mean the answer lies in the patient's foot—or more specifically the forefoot—which is requesting n certain outcome, not a certain surgical procedure. For example, I want the spontaneous shortening after a metatarsal osteotomy to be as close to correct as possible, aided by soft tissue release if needed. One of the reasons good results are achieved with percutaneous osteotomy is that the burr is thicker than a saw blade and the distal fragment will be allowed to shorten as much as it needs to. Nevertheless, we surgeons still direct the procedures, especially for lateral displacements, and definitely for rotation.

One of the new developments—or at least something that is being performed more often—is securing these osteotomies with fixation devices once the correct positioning has been achieved. This allows the patient to recover more quickly and, more importantly, ensures the desired outcome. It also brings us closer to the advantages of open surgery. This progress is highlighted in the second edition.

Thank you to Cyrille Cazeau who coordinated and combined the various elements of this book. The lessons he provides in his introduction and cautionary note must not be forgotten, and his all-encompassing view of minimally invasive foot surgery must not be ignored. This comes from a man who has an open mind and is proficient in domains extending well beyond foot surgery: from human biometrics (where Cyrille is the secretary of the French society) to his biomechanics studies and his tireless use of various aids and media. Together, these make Cyrille Cazeau a leading surgeon and researcher. The way in which he organized these two editions of *Minimally Invasive and Percutaneous Surgery of the Foot* is quite remarkable, which you will see for yourself when you read this book. We are all grateful to Joanne Archambault, PhD, and Dr. Yves Stiglitz for translating this second edition into English and to Springer for publishing it.

Le Bouscat, France Samuel Barouk

Foreword 2

Since 1990, when Louis Samuel Barouk visited Lowell Scott Weil, Sr. in Chicago, there has been a great collaboration between the French Foot and Ankle surgeons and the Weil Family. Dr. Barouk took the techniques that he learned from Dr. Weil, Sr. and popularized them throughout France, Europe, and the world. There has been a longstanding respect and friendship between the surgeons of France and our family. I first met Cyrille Cazeau in Paris in May 2018. We enjoyed a wonderful meal together (it was Paris) and shared thoughts about forefoot surgery. We quickly realized how much we enjoyed each other's company, and it was my great honor to spend the next day with Cyrille in his operating theater. There I saw his thoughtfulness, skill, and consideration for forefoot surgery. It is no surprise that he would create such a comprehensive text on current trends in forefoot surgery. As I have stepped into my father's shoes and carried forward our wonderful rapport with the French foot and ankle surgeons, Cyrille and I have deepened our relationship and I am proud to call him a friend and honored to write this on behalf of his work.

Weil Foot & Ankle Institute
Mount Prospect, IL, USA

Lowell Weil Jr

Contents

1 Introduction

Cyrille Cazeau

1.1 Emergence of Percutaneous Surgery

Forefoot surgery has undergone a radical transformation over the past 20 years in France. Technical procedures on tendons, ligaments, and joint capsules have been broadened to include the bones themselves. Before 1980, percutaneous procedures were done only on soft tissues. The mechanical goal was retention of the distended structures on the convex side of the deformity while lengthening or transecting the retracted ones on the concave side. The most commonly used were the McBride and Petersen procedures. The only case in which the bone was to be touched was when sacrificing a joint or resecting a bone, like the proximal phalanx base of the hallux (Keller) or during complex, stiffening bone procedures (Schnepp, etc.).

From a pathophysiology viewpoint, the medial bump associated with hallux valgus is mainly related to the angle between the first metatarsal (M1) (metatarsus varus) and the proximal phalanx of the hallux (P1), which can occur in combination with pronation and elevation. Trying to forcefully correct these by tensioning the soft tissues is doomed to fail. Patrice Diebold was the first surgeon in France to popularize the mechanical principles of M1 realignment osteotomy (Fig. 1.1). In the 1980s, he came back from a fellowship in the USA with the ability to perform a V-shaped distal epiphyseal-metaphyseal osteotomy on M1 called the chevron osteotomy. This procedure closely followed the introduction of phalangeal osteotomy procedures.

Next, in the early 1990s, Samuel Barouk brought an M1 diaphyseal osteotomy to France called the Scarf (Fig. 1.2). His talents as a surgeon, combined with this tireless communication work, resulted in wide diffusion of the M1 osteotomy concept in France and made such that the scarf osteotomy became the gold standard for correcting hallux valgus.

Whether we talk about a diaphyseal, distal metaphyseal, or proximal metaphyseal osteotomy, these techniques all pertain to the bone itself. They emerge from an understanding of the deformity and how to correct it in all three anatomical planes. A preoperative strategy can be established based on specific biomechanical parameters, precise calculation of metatarsal lengths, and the amount of correction needed. By decomposing the deformity into all three anatomical planes, the true nature of the deformity is captured, which makes it easier to understand its geometry and define which correction to perform.

C. Cazeau (✉)
Clinique Victor Hugo, Paris, France

C. Cazeau, Y. Stiglitz (eds.), *Percutaneous and Minimally Invasive Foot Surgery*,
https://doi.org/10.1007/978-3-030-98791-6_1

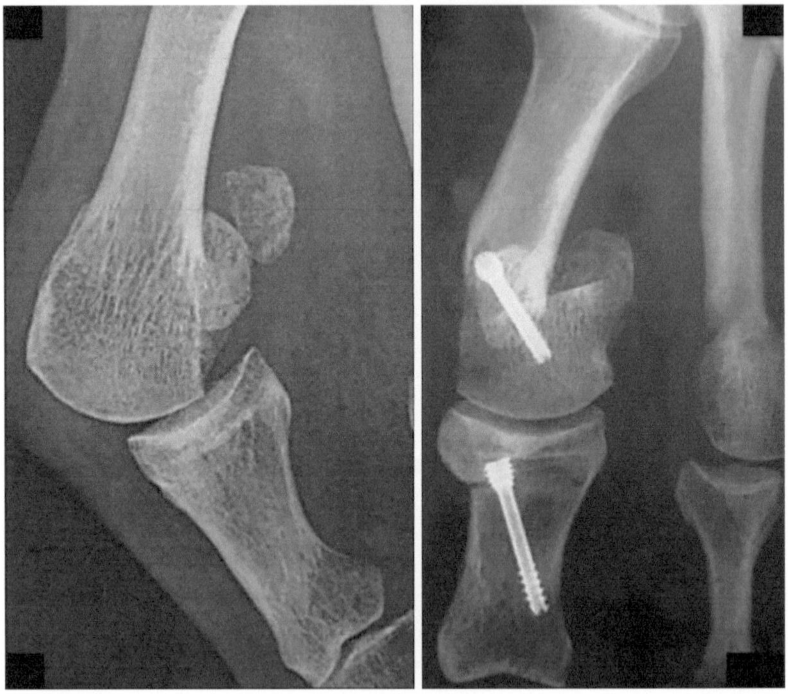

Fig. 1.1 M1 realignment chevron osteotomy. © Cyrille Cazeau 2015. All Rights Reserved

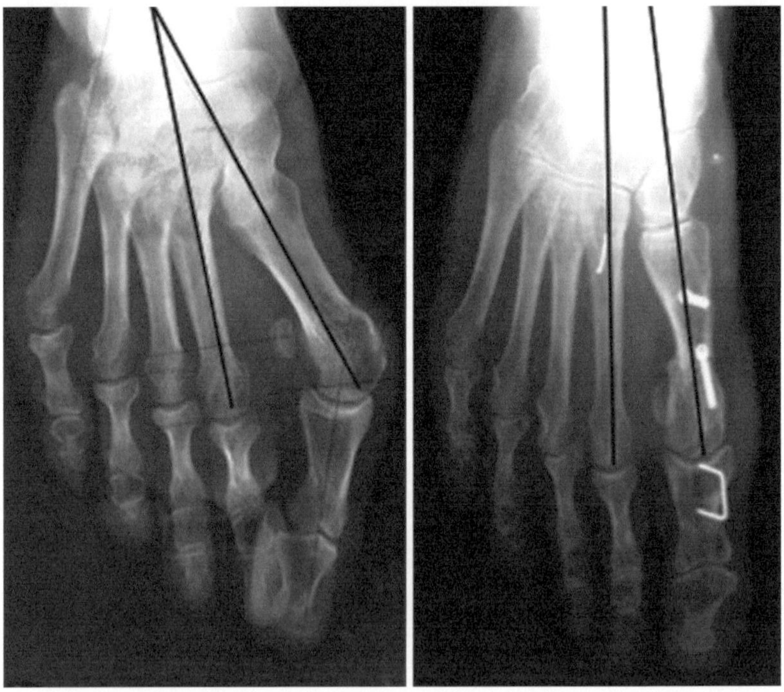

Fig. 1.2 Scarf osteotomy. © Cyrille Cazeau 2015. All Rights Reserved

1.2 What Is Percutaneous Surgery?

Like conventional open surgery, percutaneous surgery consists of carrying out soft tissue procedures and osteotomies, but instead they are done through a cutaneous slit using small scalpel blade (Beaver) and motorized burrs. The procedures are monitored intraoperatively with fluoroscopy. Originally, no bone fixation was used; the osteotomies were held by solid dressings until bone union occurred, then by small custom-made silicone toe wedges. Percutaneous bone fixation can always be added to improve stability and allow immediate mobilization. However, percutaneous surgery is challenging to carry out because of the lack of direct visual monitoring other than fluoroscopy and the required precise manual skills that differ greatly from conventional surgery. Whether it represents simply an evolution of standard surgery or is a completely different concept will be debated later on. It requires specific training with experts during theoretical courses and cadaver workshops such as the ones offered by the GRECMIP (French research group on foot and ankle minimally invasive surgery), which pioneered percutaneous forefoot surgery in France.

1.3 History of this Revolution

This technique was first used in the USA by podiatrists in the 1940s. However, it was quickly abandoned because the early results were disappointing. Dr. Stephen Isham—who was both a physician and podiatrist—was instrumental in re-establishing the credibility of this type of surgery, which he taught in a rigorous manner. It appeared in Europe about 20 years ago thanks to Dr. Mariano de Prado, who worked in Murcia, Spain. His collaboration with Spanish anatomist Pau Golano helped to establish the surgical and anatomical bases that were essential to performing these procedures safely. Percutaneous surgery was introduced to France in 2002 by a surgical team in Bordeaux, who subsequently established the GRECMIP.

1.4 Growth of Percutaneous Surgery in France

Unlike in Spain where—under the impetus of Mariano de Prado—percutaneous surgery solved nearly all foot problems, its introduction in France was purposely and carefully limited by GRECMIP members. Initially, the conditions treated were limited to hallux valgus (HV), lateral metatarsal pain (or metatarsalgia), and toe deformities. Very promising results were presented in 2007 during the First International Conference of Minimally Invasive Foot and Ankle Surgery held in Arcachon, France. The indications and correction possibilities progressively expanded after this. One example is M1 osteotomy. At the start, only a distal Reverdin-Isham osteotomy was being performed, mainly to correct the distal metatarsal articular angle (DMAA). Now, procedures on M1 include percutaneous chevron osteotomy, metatarsophalangeal and cuneometatarsal fusion along with basal osteotomies. Furthermore, some surgeons now add percutaneous bone fixation.

The aim of this book is to present only the techniques that we feel are reliable as they make up the bulk of our daily practice. We did not include techniques that we feel that need to be evaluated further before they are disseminated to the public.

1.5 Integrating Percutaneous Surgery into your Practice

The integration can be done gradually and à la carte. Surgeons can incorporate the techniques, alone or in combination, in their surgical arsenal: at the start, performing percutaneous procedures on the soft tissues and then attempting easy osteotomy techniques such as lateral metatarsal shortening. They can then mix the techniques as they wish, for example, by continuing to perform open procedures on M1 and doing everything else percutaneously. One could even continue to perform a basal M1 osteotomy as an open procedure by combining it with percutaneous DMAA correction using the Reverdin-Isham osteotomy.

Each surgeon can modify his/her habits without it being a seismic change. But it goes without saying that development of these new techniques is an intrusion that has led us to question how we practice. Some surgeons have doubts about the possibilities of percutaneous surgery.

In cases where they consider it not suitable, they can at least reduce their extensive open approaches to minimally invasive ones. Since the first edition of this book was published, the goalposts have already shifted, such that proponents of open techniques now perform the same procedures through minimally invasive approaches (see Chap. 12).

1.6 Simple Technical Evolution or Radically Different Concept?

The aim of the debate is not to compare these new techniques to conventional surgery, prove that one is superior to the other or support the myth of a fight to death between the *Ancients* and *Moderns*. The various factions have an ongoing dialogue because they agree on the underlying goal: functional anatomy must be restored to eliminate pain and reestablish physiological gait patterns.

Minimally invasive surgery is making inroads in all subspecialties of orthopedic surgery, and the foot is no exception. The patient will only benefit, as it theoretically provides faster recovery for many reasons, not just because the scars are smaller.

1.6.1 Technical Evolution in Conventional Surgery

Certain percutaneous procedures correct a deformity using the same geometric principles as conventional surgery. The varus induced percutaneously in the proximal phalanx of the hallux is the same as the one produced through an open procedure—only the technique differs. In both cases, a medial closing wedge osteotomy is done, as described by Akin (Fig. 1.3). The oste-

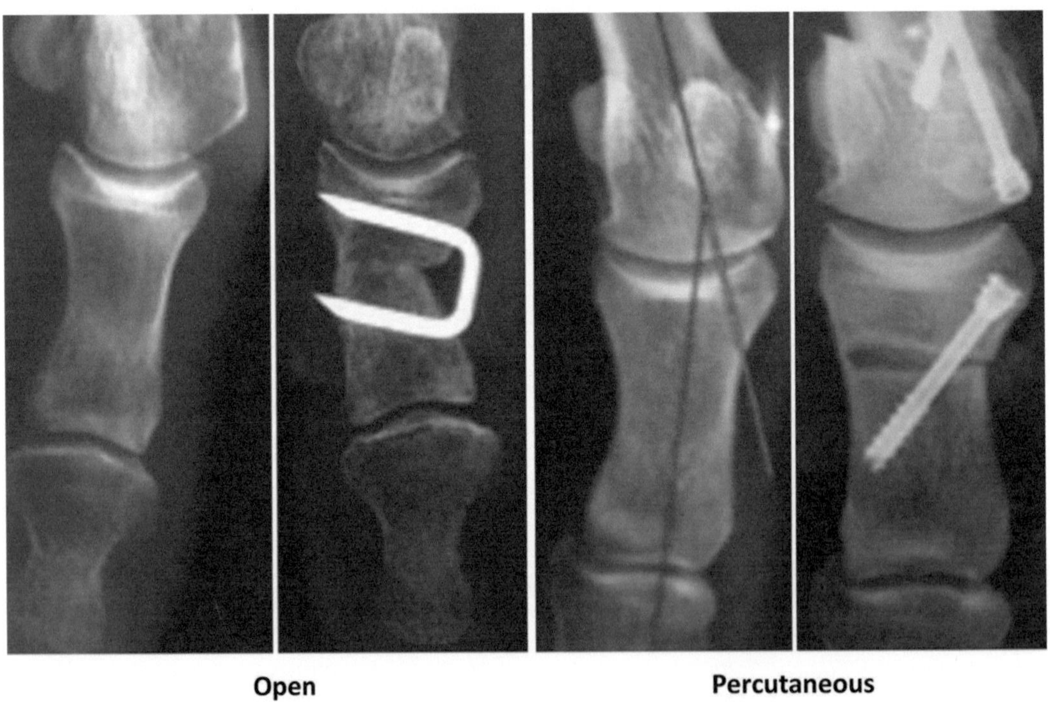

Fig. 1.3 Akin medial closing wedge osteotomy. © Cyrille Cazeau 2015. All Rights Reserved

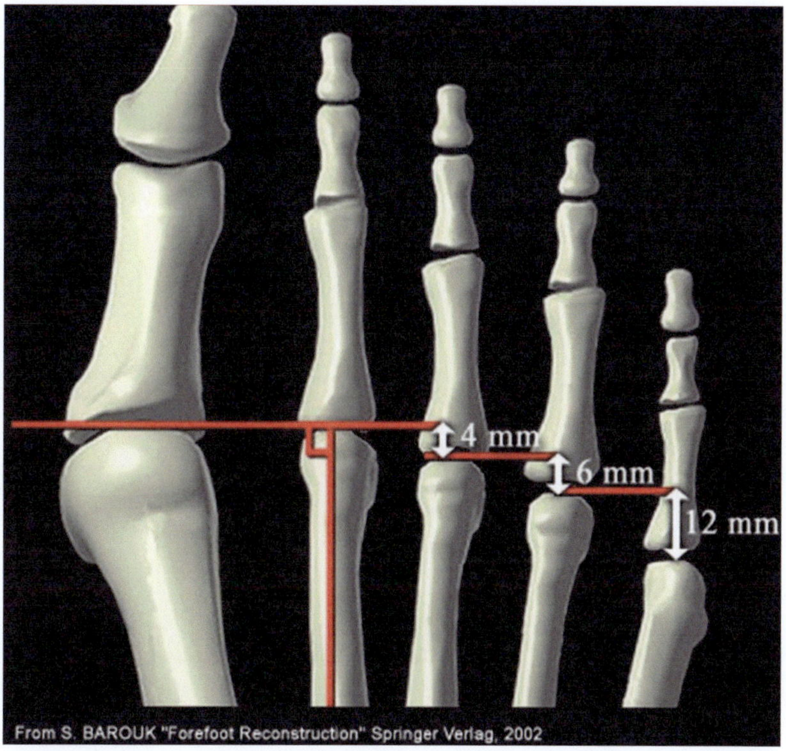

Fig. 1.4 Harmonious lateral metatarsal lengths. Reproduced with permission from Barouk L.S. (2003) Eight Principles of Forefoot Reconstruction. In: Forefoot Reconstruction. Springer, Paris. https://doi.org/10.1007/978-2-8178-0780-54. © Cyrille Cazeau 2015. All Rights Reserved

otomy done percutaneously with a wedge burr is the same one done open with an oscillating saw. In our early cases, no bone fixation was used, as the hallux was held in the correct position by the dressing and then a silicone insert. Later on, some surgeons added percutaneous fixation. This is now standard practice. While these variation may have significant symbolic importance in the eyes of patients and even certain surgeons, theoretically, correcting the deformity is based on the exact same principles: a medial closing wedge osteotomy is performed to induce varus. This makes it a technical variant that does not bring conventional principles into question.

1.6.2 Different Concept

This might be the opposite to conventional surgery. As an example, we can use metatarsalgia due to load transfer, secondary to first ray insufficiency. We will comply with the biomechanical specifications no matter which technique is used, namely, the need for shortening and lowering of the metatarsal heads; however, the strategy is completely opposite. During conventional procedures, surgeons take exact measurements of each metatarsal's shortening and then perform Weil osteotomies to adjust and set the metatarsals so they match Maestro's metatarsal parabola. Full weight-bearing is delayed until bone healing has been achieved. The preoperative planning requires precise calculations, as described by Samuel Barouk (Fig. 1.4). We do not want to debate whether this arithmetic exercise is justified or whether the single-plane projection of metatarsal angles and lengths makes the metatarsal parabola reliable. Instead we want to emphasize that percutaneous surgery, through distal metatarsal minimally invasive osteotomies (DMMO), does not rely solely on preoperative calculations. The 45° cut releases the heads, which settle harmoniously without fixation where the retraction forces and weight-bearing loads require it. Self-adjustment upon weight-bearing is a substitute both for preoperative planning and unloading the forefoot. It is fascinating to observe that the resulting length of each metatarsal is often the same as the one targeted during preoperative planning (Figs. 1.5 and 1.6).

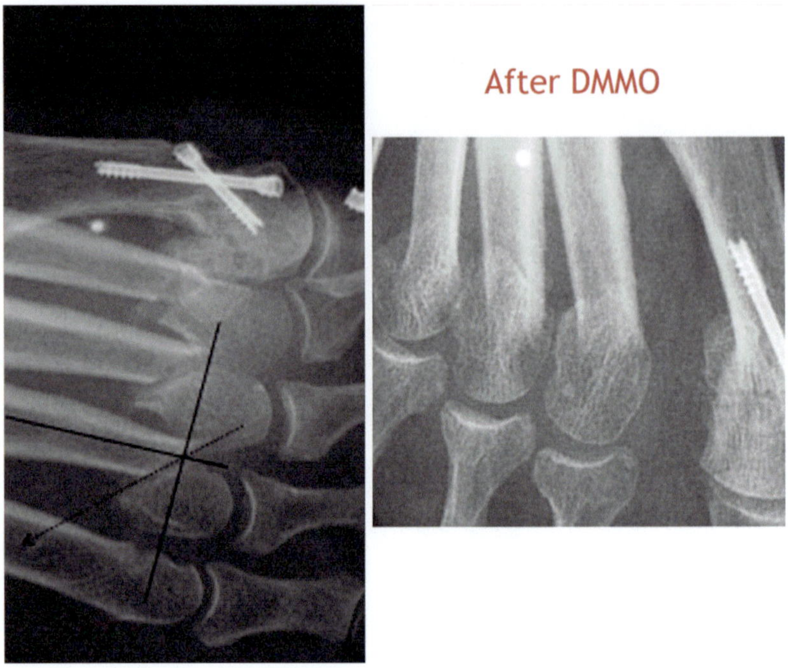

Fig. 1.5 Radiographs of metatarsals after DMMO. © Cyrille Cazeau 2015. All Rights Reserved

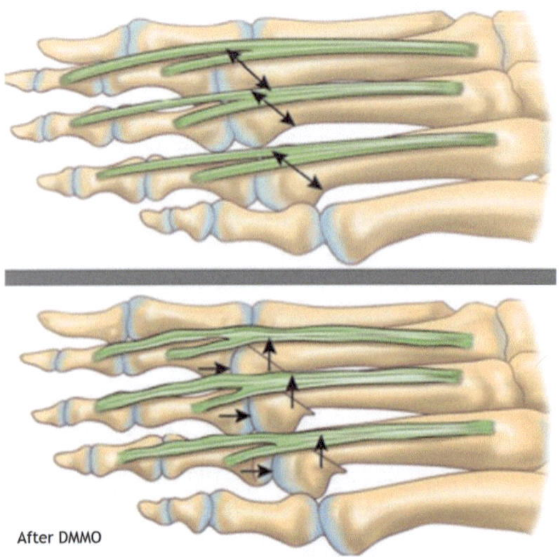

Fig. 1.6 Configuration of metatarsals before and after DMMO. © Cyrille Cazeau 2015. All Rights Reserved

1.7 Biomechanical Translation of this New Concept

Let's considered a simplified system consisting of two blocks, separated by the future DMMO cut (Fig. 1.6). The proximal block corresponds to the posterior portion of the forefoot up to the osteotomy cut. The second block, immediately distal to it, consists of the metatarsal head and neck and the metatarsophalangeal joint and the toe. The muscle, tendon, and fascia elements attached beyond the future osteotomy cut exert a resultant traction force directed posteriorly. The bone elements apply the same amount of force but in the opposite direction; these forces form an action-reaction couple according to Newton's third law.

These elements are considered as a rope. The tension on this rope is the force applied to the fixed elements located at its end, represented by the distal bone/joint block. This tension is an energy reserve that will be restored during the reverse shortening operation. This is the potential energy related to the fact that the distal bone/joint block is placed in the tensile load field. When the resultant of the tensile forces equals zero after the osteotomy, the block is in translational equilibrium. Thus the sum of forces that act on it is zero, because the automatic shortening of the heads post-osteotomy helps to remove the previous tension on the rope. This is the advantage of allowing self-adjustment because the block's displacement along the osteotomy plane will stop once the tension returns to zero. We are now in stable equilibrium, where the potential energy is the least. The associated plantar weight-bearing exerts a vertical ascending force that ensures the block's posterior displacement will be accompanied by its elevation. Pain relief is likely related to the removal of tensile forces and/or removal of plantar compression on the heads. In most cases, postoperative radiographs show the metatarsal heads are aligned relative to each other in a pattern that differs little from the metatarsal parabola (Fig. 1.5).

The principle of self-correction sometimes applies to a chevron osteotomy: the metatarsal head's automatic lateral displacement occurs once the second cut is completed, without even having to press on the head (push-pull maneuver).

The conventional preoperative planning process, which aims to achieve perfection relative to a standard model (metatarsal parabola), has been shown to be effective empirically despite the posterior-anterior radiographic views not taking into account the metatarsals' angles and lengths.

The static model of stable equilibrium through percutaneous surgery results in the same anatomical outcome and immediate pain relief. Full and immediate weight-bearing using a stiff-soled postoperative shoe is not just an option offered to patient but a requirement that is crucial to the success of these techniques. It is a direct extension of the procedure.

This is a far cry from heel-only weight-bearing, which mechanically precludes any forefoot loading at all. This is a notable conceptual difference with conventional surgery: the operated forefoot must be loaded. This strategy leads to faster recovery, contributes to bone union, stimulates the contraction of intrinsic muscles, and improves arterial and venous circulation. These osteotomies have actually changed our strategy for neck fractures in the middle metatarsals.

This reasoning, which describes metatarsal shortening, similarly applies to the removal of tensile forces that produce varus in the horizontal plane exerted on the base of the hallux, or even correction of lateral ray deformities in the vertical plane. Elimination of the resulting tensile force can also be achieved by transecting the application point of these ropes, as evidenced by tenotomies.

The primary goal is not to bring into question the mechanical logic of this procedure, but to make us think about the consequences of transecting retracted structures. The results of extensive tenotomies at the toes is something to consider.

> **Words of Wisdom**
> Percutaneous surgery cannot be summarized by its semantic definition. It has a heuristic function in various fields: pain management, immediate weight-bearing, surgeon's technical expertise, greater role of dressings, and technological and anatomical innovation.

An analysis of patient needs, in terms of recovery speed, is the central axis among which all the percutaneous options are laid out. The aim is to quickly achieve autonomy for work-related and day-to-day activities. The obvious potential added value is faster functional recovery and fewer complications, although this must be confirmed in prospective studies.

1.7.1 Absence of Pain

The elimination of pain is in part related to the surgical technique itself, given the planned mechanical soft tissues release, small size of the incisions, and absence of extensive approaches. In addition, the possibility of outpatient surgery or short hospital stays has coincided with the introduction of improved regional anesthesia techniques (popliteal block, distal foot block, perimetatarsal conduction block) and better postoperative analgesia.

1.7.2 Immediate Full-Plantar Weight-Bearing

Here again, percutaneous surgery has raised the bar. The generation of L. S. Barouk and P. Diebold helped to disseminate the concept of osteotomy, which was a major transgression in the eyes of their elders. We certainly could not ask them to take the risk of allowing immediate full-plantar weight-bearing. Forefoot unloading (heel contact) shoes were their one and only option. All the other surgeons followed their lead. Surgeons who are proponents of the percutaneous strategy were trained at the time when the osteotomy had become a common concept and was no longer technical wizardry. Under these conditions, the stable mechanical nature of these osteotomies, with or without fixation, in combination with a postoperative shoe with rigid rocker-bottom sole that simulates the gait pattern, has allowed immediate full-plantar weight-bearing. This confidence in the possibility of weight-bearing is in fact a requirement, which allows the self-adjustment that is essential after DMMO—and not to mention, the added value in terms of venous circulation, arterial microvascularization, and stimulation of intrinsic foot muscles. It is very surprising from an intellectual viewpoint that the ongoing efforts in orthopedic surgery to provide immediate mechanical stability to constructs (e.g., femoral neck fractures) had not yet been applied to the foot.

1.7.3 Surgeon's Technical Expertise

Percutaneous surgery cannot be dissociated from the invention of novel, precise manual skills on the surgeon's part. These are difficult to carry out as they are performed in a working space created by limited tissue release. This is in contrast with arthroscopy, which has a natural working space—the joint.

During percutaneous surgery, a surgeon must use both hands simultaneously when executing maneuvers (Fig. 1.7), not only to hold tools (pen-shaped tools with foot pedal control) but also to gather proprioceptive information that acts as a constant guide. Our teachers told us that a tibial osteotomy could not be done by a deaf surgeon—such is the importance of the noise the saw blade makes, which becomes metallic on the bone cortices. Percutaneous surgery is like a surgery of proprioception (admittedly aided by systematic fluoroscopy use early on and then during tricky maneuvers).

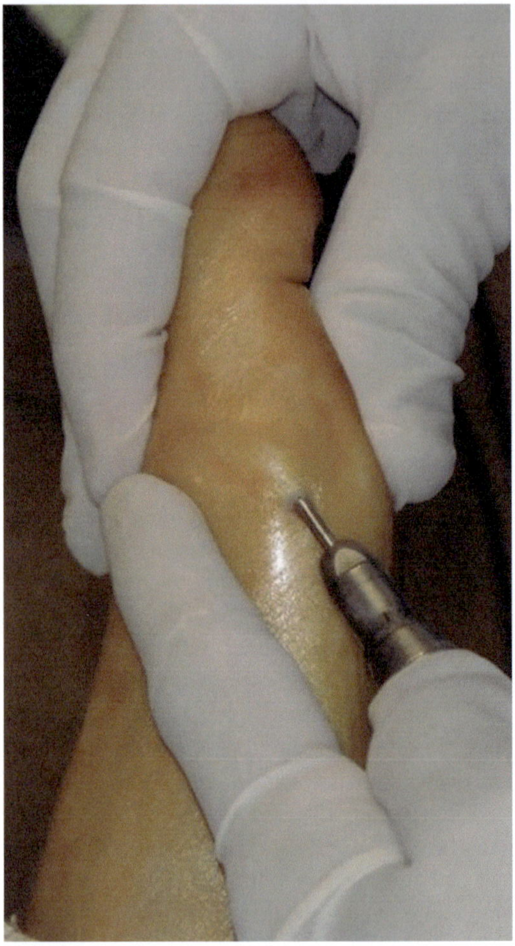

Fig. 1.7 Both hands used during percutaneous surgery.

1.7.4 Technological Innovation

Technological innovation has resulted in the development of tools, specifically burrs, identical to those used in otorhinolaryngology, that are used to ream and especially cut through bone, instead of using standard oscillating saws. The various shapes described in the chapter 6 on instrumentation each have specific uses. But cutting by rotation creates two problems: slipping and uncontrolled maneuvers due to the initial rotation speed and bone necrosis due to the high rotation speed. The solution was to combine slower rotation speeds with higher torque motors; these are available as speed limiters or are integrated into the console for powered surgical instruments. It is unthinkable and dangerous to want to start doing percutaneous surgery of the forefoot without having the specific tools needed (burrs, powered surgical instruments, fluoroscopy system).

1.7.5 New Roles of Dressings

The status of postoperative dressings has been elevated considerably in the context of percutaneous surgery. Beyond simply ensuring the surgical site remains sterile, it provides immobilization after an osteotomy without fixation (see Chap. 34).

It also helps to modify the bone alignment postoperatively using silicone wedges custom-made for the patient. It often contributes to relieving pain and preventing edema by providing a firm hold on the toes. It provides psychological isolation of the operated structure and, thanks to its volume, can act as a sock when the patient is at home, before venturing outdoors.

1.7.6 New Anatomical Work

The destiny of anatomists and surgeons diverged a few generations ago. It turns out that percutaneous surgery led to requests for novel (and challenging) anatomical studies in which the goal was to define micro-approaches that do not damage critical structures. One has to acknowledge the remarkable scientific and artistic works of Pau Golanó, an anatomist in Spain, which underpin the concepts and precise surgical skills required in percutaneous surgery. We also take this opportunity to honor the memory of Pau, who died suddenly in 2014.

1.8 Conclusion

In some ways, percutaneous and minimally invasive surgery of the foot can be considered a more refined technical evolution of conventional open surgery. The second aspect is more original and constitutes a new concept.

No one will dispute that percutaneous surgery has driven surgical practices to become less invasive, whether for the choice of approach, invention of novel surgical skills, possibility of true weight bearing, management of pain, anatomical research, or individualized geometric adjustments. Keeping this in mind, the term *percutaneous* must be considered as an ellipse encompassing a much larger system.

We acknowledge the founding members of GRECMIP—Doctors C. De Lavigne, S. Guillo and O. Laffenêtre—who promoted this surgery in France. The international reputation of this learned society has greatly increased since 2009, and many of its members have contributed to this book.

Foot and Ankle Anatomy: An Interview with Pau Golano

2

Cyrille Cazeau

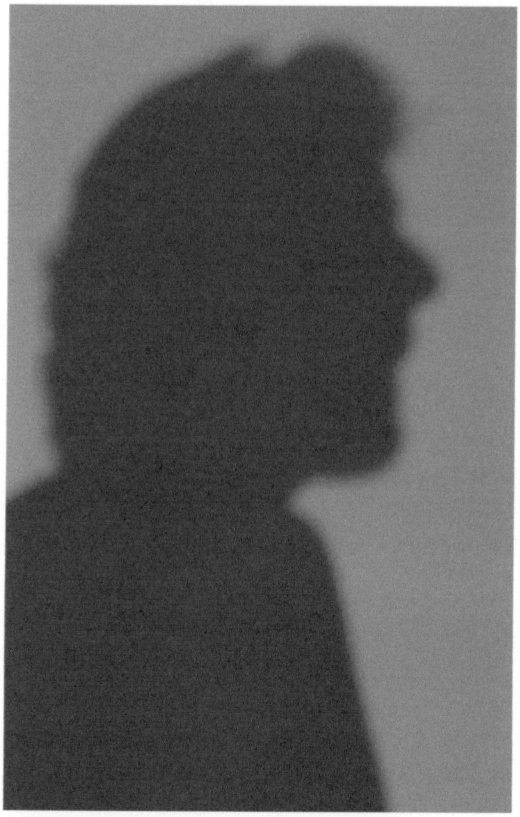

Foot and Ankle Anatomy: An Interview with Pau Golano.

Paeu Golanó died suddenly on July 23, 2014. By the age of 49, he was already internationally renowned and left us with unique work, both scientifically and artistically. We were lucky enough to interact with him regularly during GRECMIP meetings and to learn about his unique career path during an interview that I performed for the publicatione *Maîtrise Orthopédique* in May 2012. I miss him because he was one of the rare colleagues who had a sufficiently open mind to be curious about cross-disciplinary scientific domains.

May his legacy cast an eternal glow on our mini-incisions.

Pau Golanó received his medical and surgery degrees in Spain. Early on, he was interested in anatomy and started out as an assistant. He climbed the rungs of the academic ladder to become a Professor at the University of Barcelona. But this conventionality hides the most significant thing about him—he was a revolutionary. In fact, the unique way in which he approached his specialty resulted in him being ostracized in anatomical circles but admired in the international surgical community. In fact, 80% of his work was published in surgical journals, and his impact factor

C. Cazeau (✉)
Clinique Victor Hugo, Paris, France

C. Cazeau, Y. Stiglitz (eds.), *Percutaneous and Minimally Invasive Foot Surgery*,
https://doi.org/10.1007/978-3-030-98791-6_2

was much higher than that of his anatomy colleagues.

But he was not enamored with anatomical specimens the first time he encountered them. The memories that he brings up are shared by many of us. At that time, the cadavers had blackish flesh saturated with foul-smelling embalming fluids, and their tissues had strange textures ranging from intact to deteriorated. Lying on crumpled sheets or a bed of wood chips, they were highlighted by pale neon lights. His artistic sensitivity (he loved to photograph animals), his frustration with seeing meticulously prepared anatomical specimens being spoiled after an afternoon of manipulations, and his frequent contact with surgeons led him to see anatomy in a different light.

His work environment resembled an operating suite. The specimens that emerged from it were photographed like models and were worthy of being placed in a museum. This summarizes his style.

But let's not ignore the substance. Golanó said the aim of his work was to help develop new surgical techniques; for this reason, he had ongoing collaborations with surgeons and radiologists. He did not perform anatomy with the goal of advancing anatomy; instead, he saw it as a tool for implementing new surgical practices. Irrespective of the specialty, surgery has shifted toward minimally invasive approaches. We are just starting to understand how precious his work is to us in this context.

The techniques presented in this book are done through a cutaneous dot widened no more than a minimally invasive approach. The lack of direct view makes it harder to avoid critical anatomical structures, whether using a miniature beaver blade or motorized burrs. Golanó systematically dissected the small anatomical areas that we cross, precisely described the structures to avoid, and contributed to defining the exact skin penetration points and trajectories to take.

He sought to overcome the emerging problems associated with these innovations and largely contributed to simplifying their implementation. He even changed how dissections were done: he placed the specimen in the standard surgical position because he knew that modifying the joint angle alters the topography of the anatomical structures in questions. We can all picture the classical example of a hand flexor tendon transection due to a knife wound; it is visible with the fingers flexed, but undetectable when the fingers are extended as it has shifted distally. He prepared videos showing the dynamic movement of anatomical structures as a joint moves through its range of motion. Lastly, he compared MRI or CT scan slices with his own anatomical slices, which enriched each modality mutually.

The images presented here (Figs. 2.1, 2.2, 2.3, 2.4, 2.5 and 2.6) are not intended to be an exhaus-

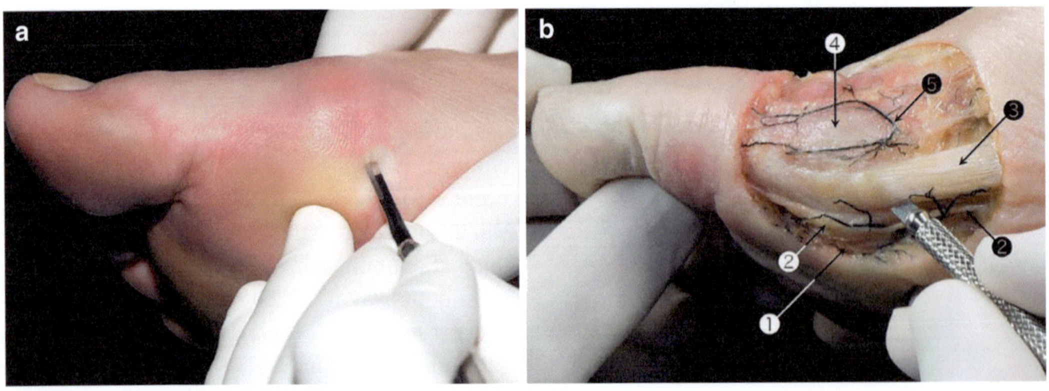

Fig. 2.1 (**a**) Medial approach located at the proximal and slightly dorsal portion of the medial sesamoid, at the posterior and inferior portion of the first metatarsal. It is used for exostectomy and for the Reverdin-Isham osteotomy. (**b**) Anatomical relationships: (1) Medial sesamoid, (2) Medial digital nerve, (3) Tendon of abductor hallucis muscle, (4) Joint capsule, (5) Arteries arising from first plantar metatarsal artery and medial plantar artery.

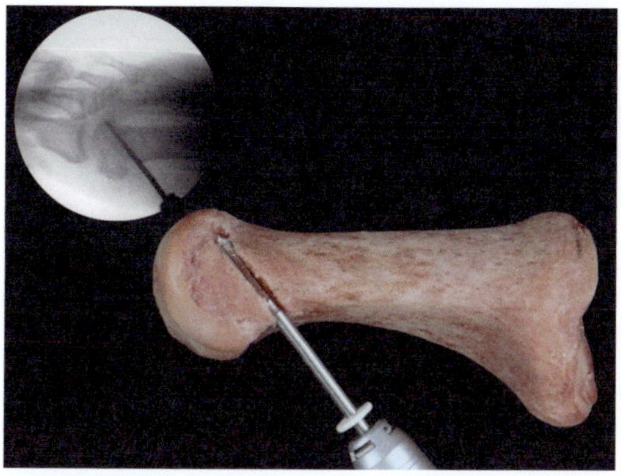

Fig. 2.2 Anatomical and radiological correlation of the Reverdin-Isham osteotomy. © Paulo Golano 2015. All Rights Reserved

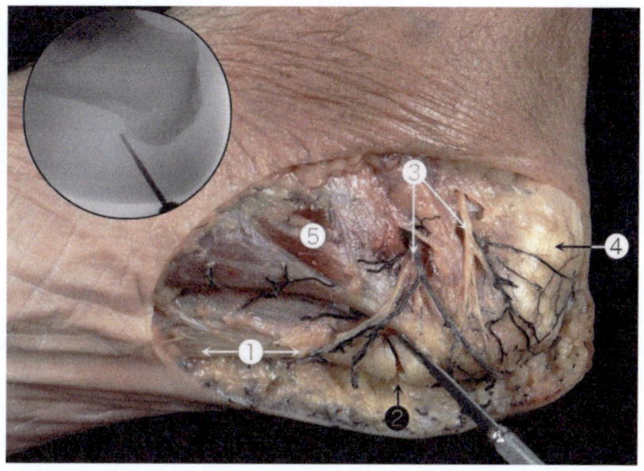

Fig. 2.3 Anatomical relationships for percutaneous fasciotomy. (1) Plantar fascia, (2) Transected plantar fascia, (3) Branches of medial calcaneal nerve, (4) Achilles tendon, (5) Abductor hallucis muscle. © Paulo Golano 2015. All Rights Reserved

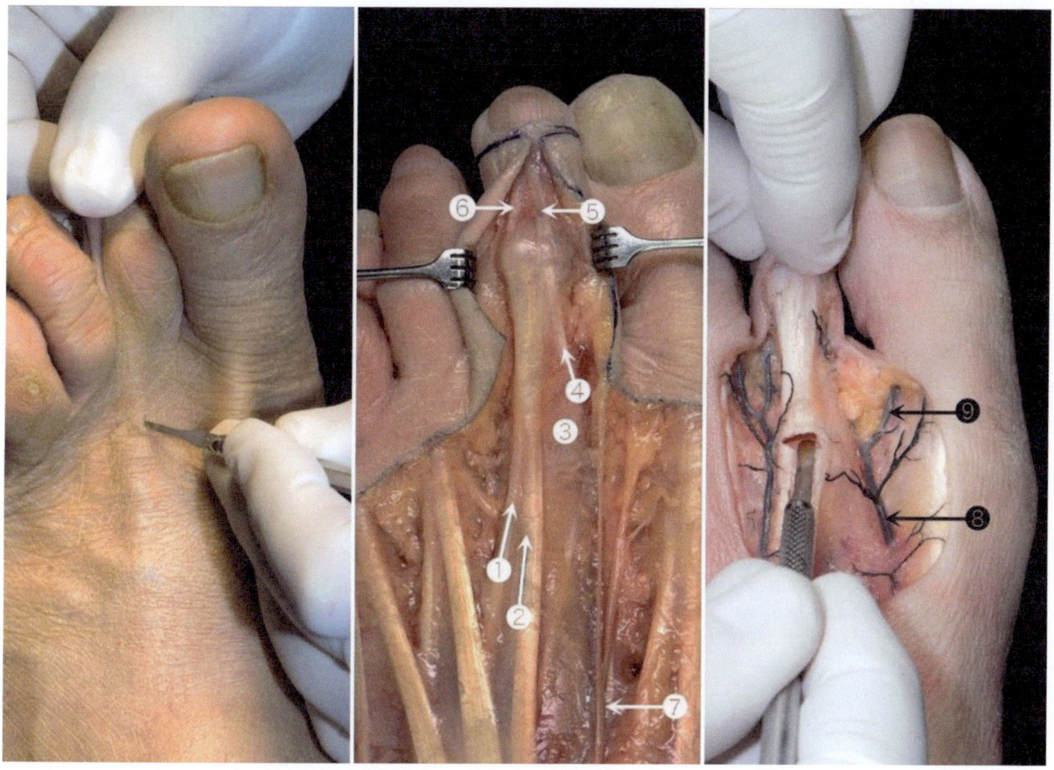

Fig. 2.4 Tenotomy of the toe extensors is a very common surgical procedure for treating deformities. The incision must be parallel to the tendons and neurovascular structures at the metatarsophalangeal joint where the extensor mechanism forms an expansion, the "extensor wing." (1) Extensor digitorum brevis tendon, (2) Extensor digitorum longus tendon, (3) Extensor sling, (4) Expansion of lumbrical muscle for extensor mechanism, (5) Medial slip, (6) Lateral slip, (7) Deep peroneal nerve (medial branch), (8) First dorsal metatarsal artery, (9) Digital dorsal artery to the lateral side of the hallux. © Paulo Golano 2015. All Rights Reserved

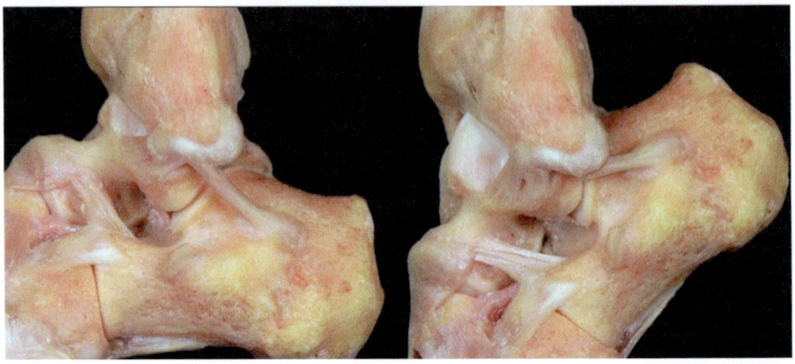

Fig. 2.5 Medial view of the lateral collateral ligaments of the talocrural or ankle joint during the stance phase (left) and in plantar flexion (right).

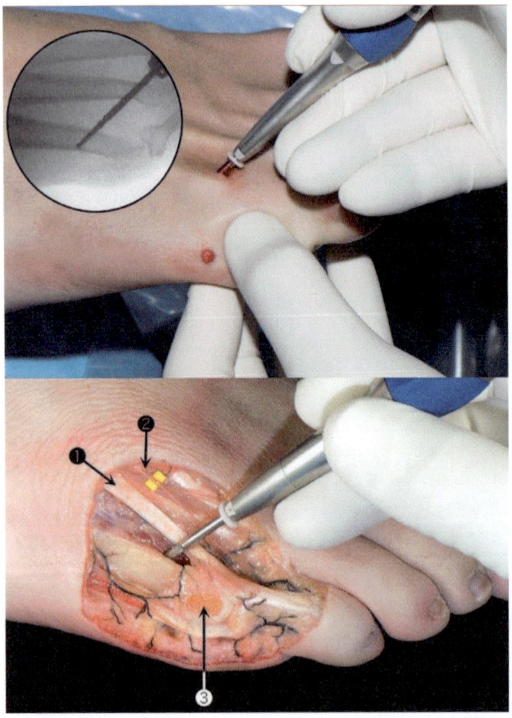

Fig. 2.6 Anatomical relationships for osteotomy of the fifth metatarsal used to treat bunionette. (1) Extensor digitorum longus tendon, (2) Branches of the superficial peroneal nerve, (3) Exostectomy.

tive anatomical atlas, but to give examples of how they contribute to certain procedures. For more images, we invite you to consult the two main textbooks that he co-authored [1, 2].

References

1. de Prado M, Ripoll PL, Golanó P. Cirugía percutánea del pie. Barcelona: Elsevier; 2003.
2. de Prado M, Ripoll PL, Golanó P. Minimally invasive foot surgery. Barcelona: About Your Health Publishers; 2009.

3 Instrumentation and Devices

Olivier Laffenêtre

Forefoot surgery, whether minimally invasive or percutaneous, requires specific instrumentation and devices. From the time when the academic version of percutaneous surgery without fixation was taught by S. Isham and M. de Prado, the focus has greatly shifted toward hybrid surgery, which mixes conventional and percutaneous procedures. Changes have also occurred in bone fixation, as specific instruments and hardware for minimally invasive surgery have been introduced recently.

More generally, specific fundamental manual instruments are common to all procedures, which can be combined and performed *à la carte*.

3.1 Scalpels

The scalpel is used to make the mini-incisions. We recommend using a beaver handle with suitable blades:

- Type 376400 which makes an incision about 3 mm in width in the same axis as the handle.
- Havel's® MIS blades, which are best suited to small incisions (1 mm) on the lateral rays and toes.

3.2 Elevators

Elevators are used to create a working space by separating the soft tissue from the bone; this allows bone procedures (resection, osteotomy) to be done without damaging neighboring critical structures (tendons, neurovascular bundles). An elevator is less aggressive and thicker for the working space at the M1 head; the more aggressively designed raspatory is reserved for the proximal phalanx. We recommend these specific instruments (Fig. 3.1) instead of a dural elevator or Muller or Morel-Fatio miniature rasps.

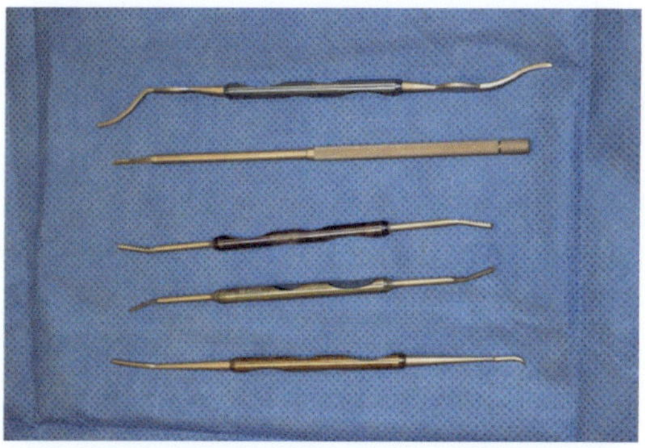

Fig. 3.1 Rasps and elevators specific to percutaneous surgery. © Olivier Laffenêtre 2015. All Rights Reserved

O. Laffenêtre (✉)
Institut de la Cheville et du Pied, Paris, France

C. Cazeau, Y. Stiglitz (eds.), *Percutaneous and Minimally Invasive Foot Surgery*, https://doi.org/10.1007/978-3-030-98791-6_3

3.3 Rasps

Specific rasps have been designed to extract bone debris (not rasp the bone) after any bone resection procedure. They are available in different sizes and angles (Fig. 3.1).

3.4 Powered Surgical Tool

The powered surgical tool is the fundamental element of this chapter. Without the appropriate powered handpiece, percutaneous procedures become extremely dangerous, even in the hands of an expert. The surgical handpiece must have the same axis of rotation as the burr and have a high torque capacity. The rotation speed should be controlled by a foot pedal and must be on the slow side (maximum of 10,000–15,000 rpm) (Fig. 3.2). Some manufacturers offer specific torque reducers, while others offer this function automatically through the console. No matter what, insufficient torque makes slow-speed work impossible. When the speed is too fast, the risk of superficial and skin burns, or even deeper bone burns, increases.

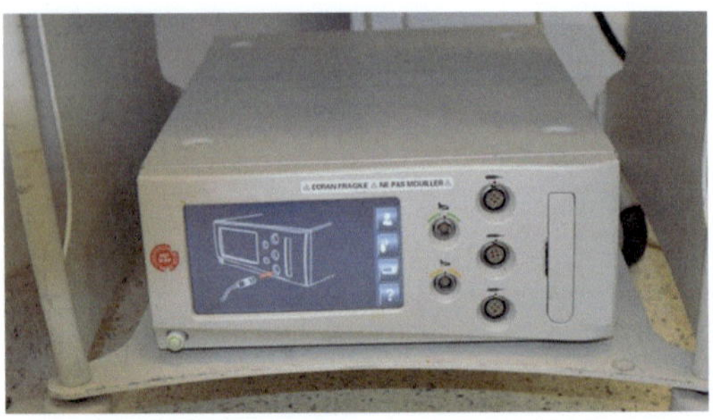

Fig. 3.2 Powered surgical handpiece specific to minimally invasive surgery that has precise speed adjustment and torque reducer.

3.5 Burrs

Burrs are essential to the practice of percutaneous surgery. They are specifically designed to carry out an osteotomy or bone resection without damaging the soft tissues. Depending on the situation, they can contribute to extracting the bone debris after an osteotomy (Fig. 3.3):

- Triangular or wedge shape burrs are used for bone resection.
- Long or short Shannon burrs (of different widths) are used for standard osteotomies, while more triangular burrs are used for large osteotomies.
- Specific burrs are available for certain techniques or procedures such as basal metatarsal osteotomy with automatic lowering effects (burrs with wider end; burrs to perform chevron osteotomies).

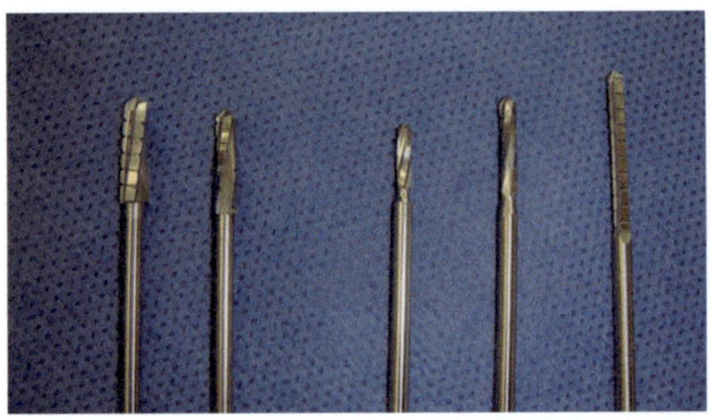

Fig. 3.3 Rasps and elevators specific to percutaneous surgery.

3.6 Fluoroscopy

In general, several of the steps during percutaneous or hybrid surgery should be verified with fluoroscopy. We recommend using a mini-C-arm as the radiation exposure is significantly less (dose reduced 10–100 times relative to a standard fluoroscopy unit) (Figs. 3.4 and 3.5). Its small size and great maneuverability make it easy to use and well-suited to minimally invasive surgery of the foot.

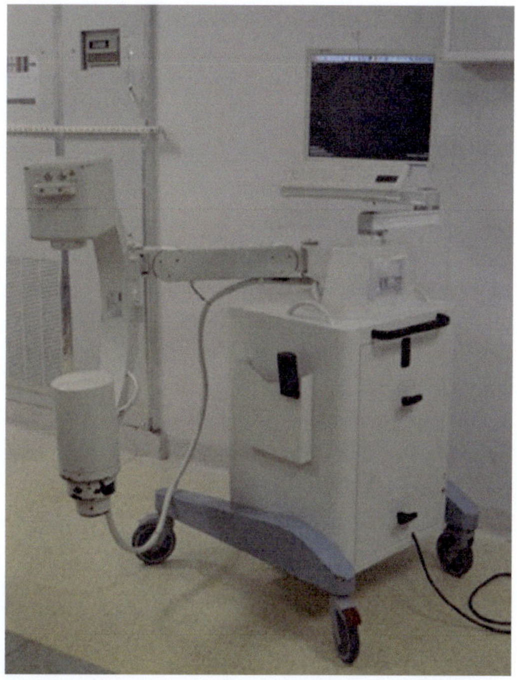

Fig. 3.4 Mini-C-arm fluoroscopy used in percutaneous surgery.

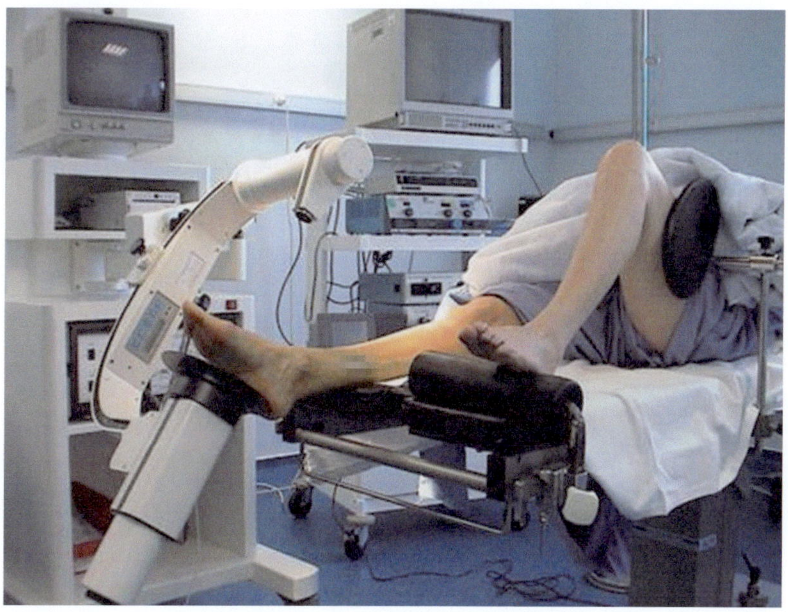

Fig. 3.5 Intraoperative use of a mini-C-arm.

3.7 Specialized Instruments

Certain procedures such as percutaneous chevron osteotomy require specialized instrumentation. Likewise, certain instruments (retractors, etc.) have been designed to make a certain procedure easier to perform and more reproducible.

The recent trend toward fixation of certain distal or proximal metatarsal or phalangeal osteotomies means that specific fixation devices have been introduced for this purpose, such as pin-like compressive screws, self-tapping screws with and without compression, or screws made of different materials (titanium, stainless steel, and even bioresorbable) (Fig. 3.6).

3.8 Materials for Postoperative Course

This chapter would be incomplete if we did not review the materials needed to ensure the postoperative course is uneventful. Indeed, the dressing applied by the surgeon in the operating room is an essential step of the procedure. One criticism of percutaneous or minimally invasive surgery is the tedious requirement of using complicated dressings, which must be redone and monitored regularly. This complicates the postoperative course and eliminates one of the benefits of this surgery! While it is true that rigor is the master key of the follow-up period,

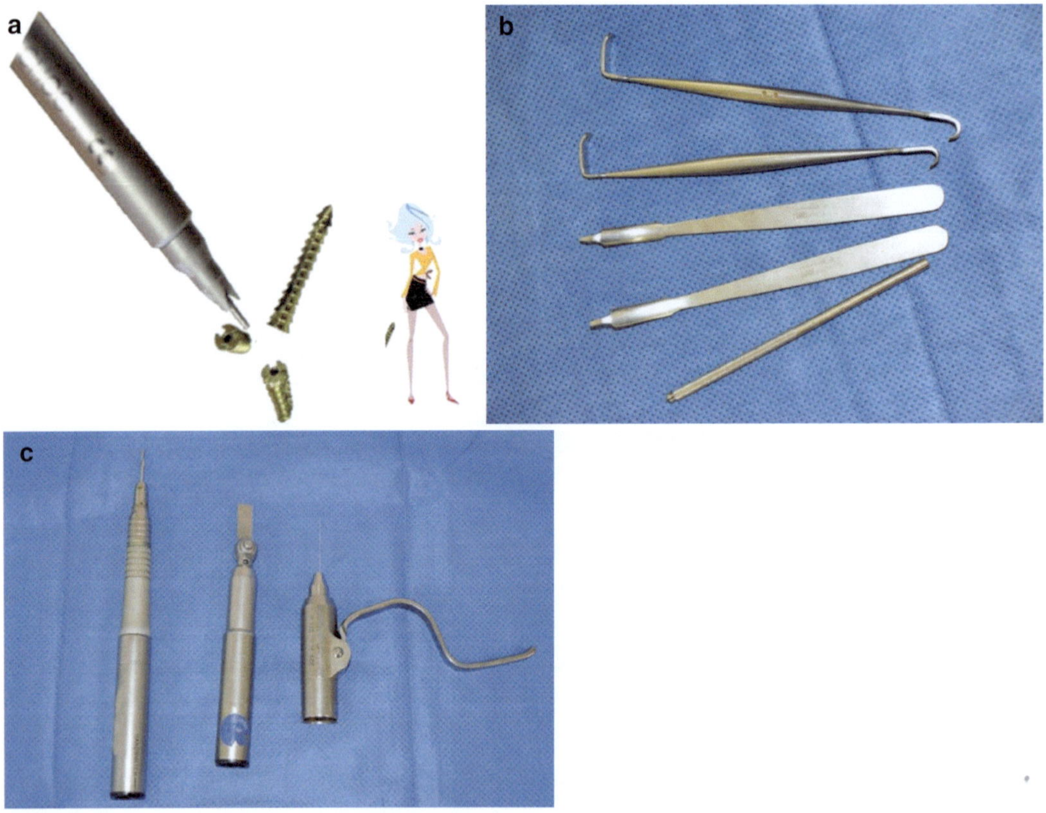

Fig. 3.6 (**a**) Specialized screw for minimally invasive surgery. (**b, c**) Instrumentation and materials used in specific procedures.

each surgeon will eventually settle on his own formula and timing. Every operating suite has gauze, bandages, and sticky elastic bands. However, certain formats are preferable to others, and radiopaque markers must not be placed in the gauze as this will interfere with the radiological follow-up. For the first dressing, cohesive strips are essential for the lateral rays and small toes, along with silicone elastomers to make toe orthotics that hold various osteotomies or complex lesser toe treatments. Preshaped devices are also commercially available.

Editors' Point of View

Instruments such as elevators are used to create a safe working space; however, the tissue disruption can cause hematomas, pain, and edema. Unless they are essential to the procedure, it is best to avoid using them (e.g., dorsal side of P1 during Akin osteotomy or for DMMO). A fluoroscopy system should be available in the operating room in the case problems arise. Nevertheless, the goal of the learning curve is to master the procedure to the point where fluoroscopy is not needed. The criteria for success are described in each chapter.

Geometric Fundamentals of the Hallux Valgus and Surgical Options

4

Yves Stiglitz and Cyrille Cazeau

4.1 Introduction

By definition, the term *hallux valgus* designates a clinical deformity in which the hallux is deviated in valgus. But despite this designation, the big toe is only partially responsible for the deformity in most patients. The first metatarsal (M1) is most often involved in the architectural abnormalities:

- Metatarsus varus (M1–M2 angle)
- Metatarsus elevatus
- Excessive M1 length (index-plus foot)
- In certain cases, external rotation of the articular surface (DMAA or DM2A)

To a lesser extent, the hallux can be the site of the following:

- Pronation, which is partly due to M1.
- Interphalangeal valgus, i.e., loss of parallelism between the MTP1 and IP joints, with the latter being deviated laterally.

  For each patient, the clinical presentation can combine some or all of these basic deformities into a specific deformity that will be treated surgically.

  Various options are available from standard ones to more recent ones, including percutaneous techniques that are put forward by the surgeon as often as requested by the patient. The claimed simplicity of their execution and their postoperative course must not conceal the fact that the long-term clinical outcomes depend on the intraoperative procedures and their ability to bring the appropriate correction in the three anatomical planes. If one or more of these basic deformities is not corrected or purposely ignored because the surgeon wants to use a certain (sexy) technique, the risk of failure increases.

The technique should be selected only *after* the preoperative planning, and this plan must be followed exactly.

A medial closing wedge osteotomy of the proximal phalanx (P1) (Akin osteotomy) is a simple way to meet the objectives associated with the hallux. The basic geometric reasoning used during planning is straightforward. It consists of inducing varus by medial subtraction and potentially eliminating the pronation by derotation.

But it is different at M1 where the deformities must be corrected in all three planes. The surgeon should aim to achieve optimal postoperative positioning of the M1 head, keeping in mind that any displacement in one plane may have implications for the other planes. This can be achieved by performing an osteotomy, the details of which are not the primary purpose of this chapter.

Y. Stiglitz (✉) · C. Cazeau
Clinique Victor Hugo, Paris, France

C. Cazeau, Y. Stiglitz (eds.), *Percutaneous and Minimally Invasive Foot Surgery*,
https://doi.org/10.1007/978-3-030-98791-6_4

Nevertheless, the technique chosen must be one that can achieve all the specifications defined preoperatively.

The aim of this chapter is to describe the geometry of the basic correction to be made in each dimension and especially to understand the relative implications of one dimension on another.

4.2 Geometry

To achieve the ideal postoperative position, the M1 head must be shifted during the procedure, which we call *translation*. This translation is the complex three-dimensional resultant of three basic displacements: lateralization, shortening, and lowering.

From a geometric point of view, a simple trigonometry formula is used to calculate translation: $T = \sqrt{A^2 + L^2 + R^2}$, where T is translation, A is lowering, L is lateralization, and R is shortening.

The surgeon defines the amount of lowering, lateralization, and shortening that has to be carried out during the preoperative planning stage. These three parameters are the surgical specifications referred to earlier on.

4.2.1 Planning on AP View

In this plane (Fig. 4.1), the displacement of the M1 head aims to correct the M1–M2 angle (metatarsus varus) and to potentially shorten M1.

Geometrically, lateralization is achieved by the following relationship:

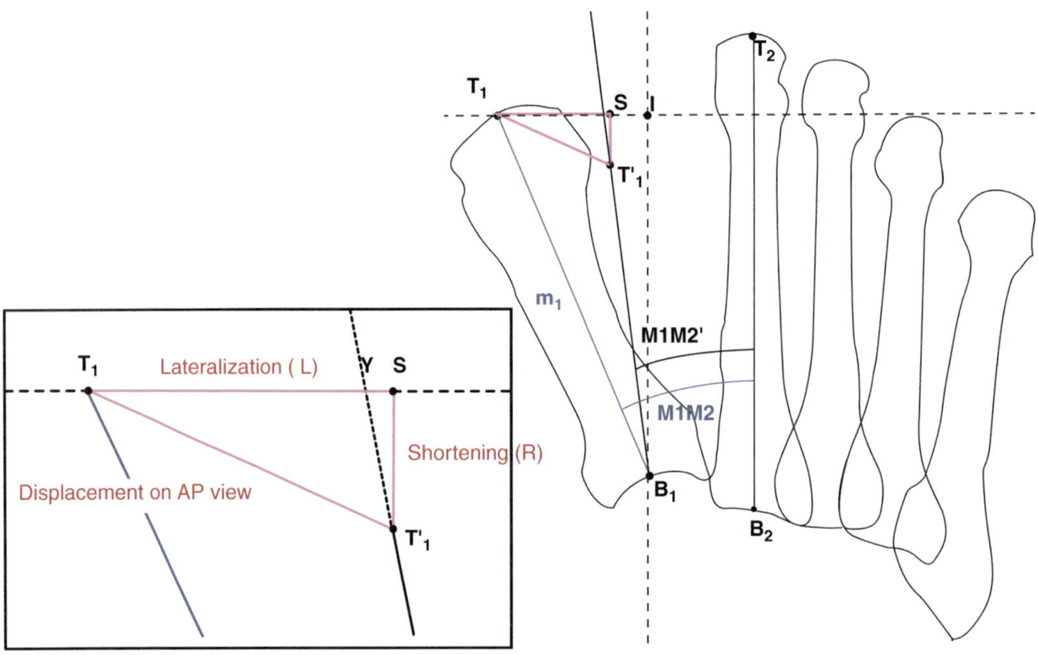

Fig. 4.1 Geometric diagram of an AP radiograph of the forefoot. T_1: center of articular surface of first metatarsal head before osteotomy; T'_1: center of articular surface of first metatarsal head after osteotomy; B_1: center of articular surface of first metatarsal base; M1: length of first metatarsal; T_2: center of articular surface of second metatarsal head; B_2: center of articular surface of second metatarsal base; I: intersection between a line parallel to B_2T_2 passing through B_1, and a line perpendicular to B_2T_2 passing through T_1; S: intersection between T_1I and a line parallel to B_2T_2 passing through T'_1; Y: intersection between the lines $B_1T'_1$ and T_1I; angle M1M2: angle formed between the lines B_1T_1 and B_2T_2; angle M1M2′: angle formed between the lines $B_1T'_1$ and B_2T_2.

$$L = m_1 \cdot \frac{\sin \Delta}{\cos\left(M_1 M_2'\right)} + R \cdot \tan\left(M_1 M_2'\right) \text{where} \Delta = \left(M_1 M_2\right) - \left(M_1 M_2'\right)$$

4.2.2 Planning on Lateral View

In this plane (Fig. 4.2), two basic displacements are shown: shortening and lowering, with shortening being identical to the one previously defined on the AP view.

Given the angulation of M1 on the lateral view, any shortening also induces elevation. This means that compensatory lowering must be planned to neutralize the elevation induced.

The surgeon can also decide, based on the clinical presentation, to add supplementary lowering, e.g., to reload the first ray in the case of load transfer to the lateral rays. This adds to the realignment effect that helps to restore the useful length of M1, by increasing the cosine of the M1–M2 angle. In total, the sum of the compensatory and supplementary lowering results in:

$$A = R \cdot \sin(\text{Ground} - \text{M1}) + A_{\text{suppl}}.$$

4.2.3 Planning in Frontal Plane

In this plane, the displacement of the end of M1 can be decomposed into lowering and lateralization, as defined above (Figs. 4.1 and 4.2). Thus no additional calculations are needed to take these parameters into account.

4.3 Surgical Application

For a given patient, preoperative planning requires that the desired lateralization, shortening, and lowering of the M1 be defined. The surgical step then consists of translating these

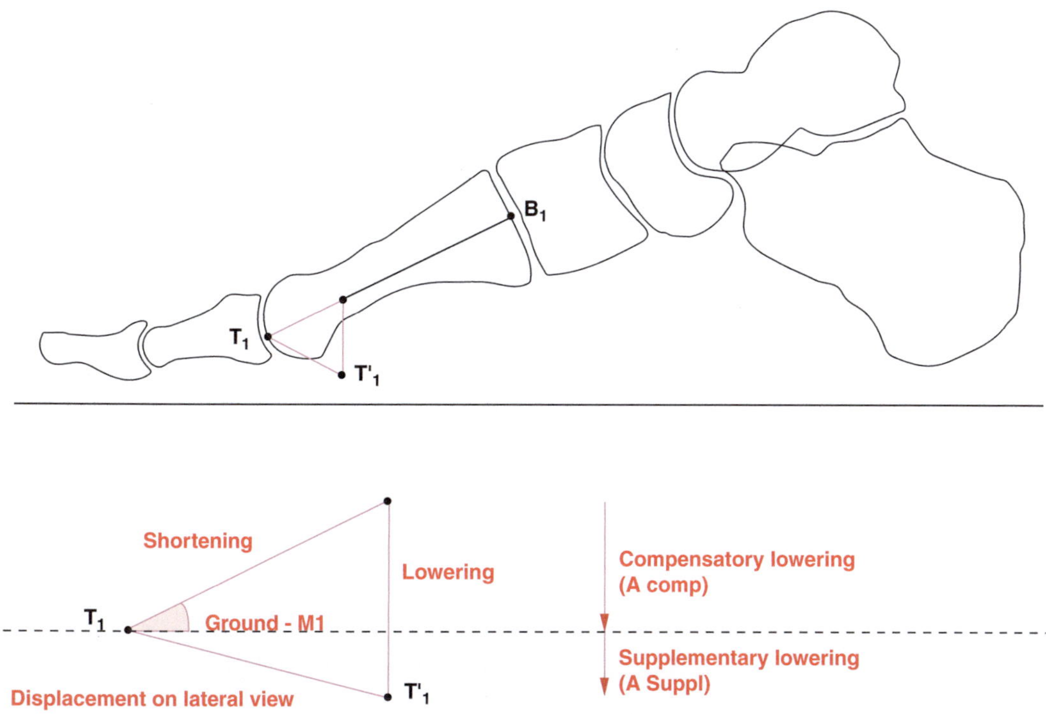

Fig. 4.2 Geometric diagram of a lateral radiograph of the forefoot. $\mathbf{T_1}$: center of articular surface of first metatarsal head before osteotomy; $\mathbf{T'_1}$: center of articular surface of the first metatarsal head after osteotomy; $\mathbf{B_1}$: center of articular surface of first metatarsal base.

objectives into the orientation of the osteotomy cuts. For the following example, we will apply these principles to a chevron osteotomy. It is understood that this planning process can (and should) be used for any M1 osteotomy.

4.3.1 Geometric Characterization of the Chevron Osteotomy

The distal chevron epiphyseal-metaphyseal osteotomy (Fig. 4.3) is characterized by two cuts made at 60° to each other on a lateral view and joined at the center of the M1 head: a nearly horizontal inferior cut and a nearly vertical superior cut.

4.3.2 Superior Cut

The superior cut is made medial to lateral and potentially distal to proximal if any shortening is desired. Thus this cut controls shortening and lateralization, which are linked by the saw's orientation on the bone during the osteotomy. To complete this geometric reasoning, if α designates the angle formed by the blade and a line perpendicular to the M2 axis (Fig. 4.4), we can write $\tan \alpha = R/L$.

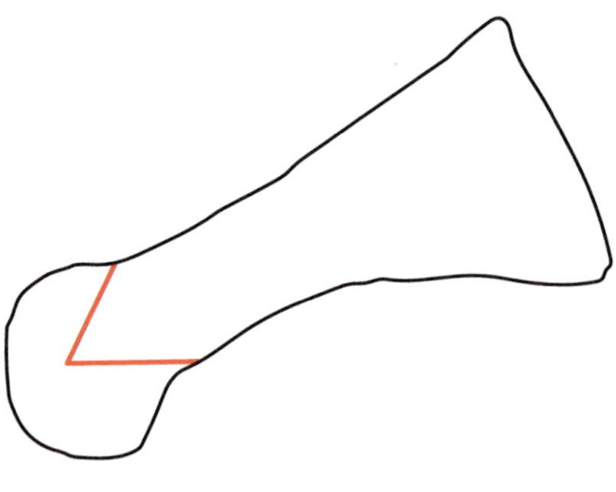

Fig. 4.3 Drawing of a chevron osteotomy. © Yves Stiglitz 2015. All Rights Reserved

4.3.3 Inferior Cut

The inferior cut is made medial to lateral, potentially incorporating a plantar direction if lowering is desired. Here again, the lateralization-lowering couple is related by the saw blade's orientation during the osteotomy. As previously, the formula $\tan \beta = A/L$ is valid (where β is the angle between the saw and the sole of the foot).

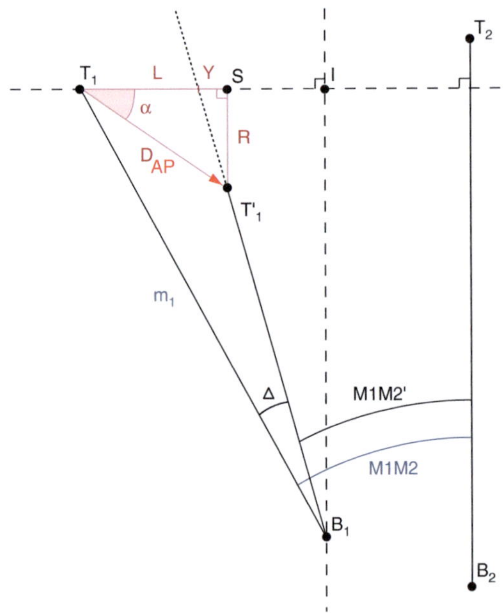

Fig. 4.4 Geometric effect of the superior chevron cut. This is the same drawing as Fig. 4.1. T_1: center of articular surface of first metatarsal head before osteotomy; T'_1: center of articular surface of first metatarsal head after osteotomy; B_1: center of articular surface of first metatarsal base; M1: length of first metatarsal; T_2: center of articular surface of second metatarsal head; B_2: center of articular surface of second metatarsal base; I: intersection between a line parallel to B_2T_2 passing through B_1, and a line perpendicular to B_2T_2 passing through T_1; S: intersection between T_1I and a line parallel to B_2T_2 passing through T'_1; Y: intersection between the lines $B_1T'_1$ and T_1I; angle M1M2: angle formed between the lines B_1T_1 and B_2T_2; angle M1M2′: angle formed between the lines $B_1T'_1$ and B_2T_2. L lateralization, R shortening, D_{AP} AP view displacement, Angle α angle formed by the axis of the saw blade and a line perpendicular to the M2 axis, Angle Δ angle formed by the lines B_1T_1 and $B_1T'_1$. © Yves Stiglitz 2015. All Rights Reserved

4.3.4 Relative Displacement of Bone Segments

Once the osteotomies have been made in accordance with the planning, the corrections are achieved by translating the M1 head along the two cut planes. Geometrically, the translation T combines the basic displacements mentioned previously in the three anatomical planes. We can also show the formula mentioned above:

$$T = \sqrt{A^2 + L^2 + R^2}$$

Overall, the chevron technique is controlled by three parameters:

- α angle,
- β angle,
- Translation T.

4.4 Practical Consequences

The aim of this geometry exercise is to highlight the relationships between the bone cuts made and the corrections achieved, in all three anatomical planes. The osteotomy cuts should always be planned while taking into account the consequences induced in the other dimensions. Figure 4.5 shows the shortening effect related to the lateral and posterior orientation of the chevron osteotomy cut. Figure 4.6 shows the potential lowering of the M1 head due to the downward and lateral orientation of the inferior osteotomy cut. In particular, there is a clear link between the planned shortening and the elevatus of M1, and consequently, the need for compensatory lowering to counter it.

Certain cases of metatarsalgia can be attributed to load transfer because the first ray is function-

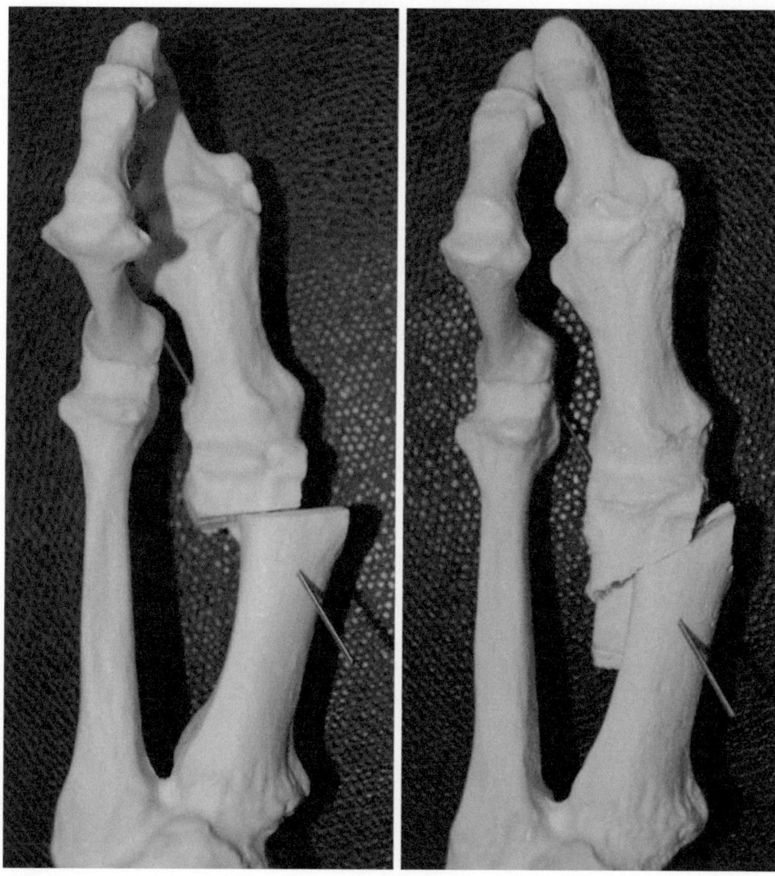

Fig. 4.5 Shortening due lateral and posterior orientation of chevron osteotomy cut. © Yves Stiglitz 2015. All Rights Reserved

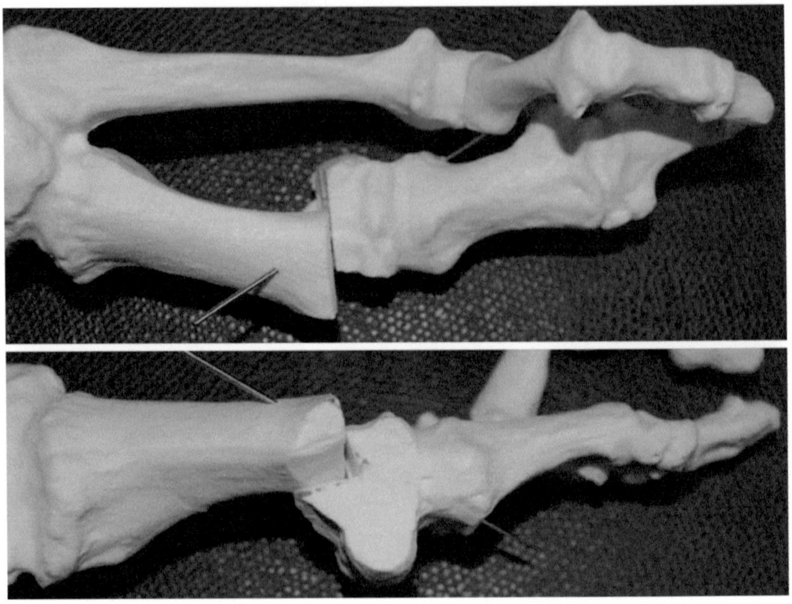

Fig. 4.6 Lowering of M1 head due to downward and lateral orientation of inferior osteotomy cut. © Yves Stiglitz 2015. All Rights Reserved

ally insufficient. This is the case of hallux valgus with a metatarsus elevatus component; this is also the reason iatrogenic pain may occur after hallux valgus surgery. Thus it is essential to understand the geometry of the bone cuts and their three-dimensional effects in order to make them as accurate as possible, and especially to prevent the development of postoperative metatarsalgia.

Given that this is a book on minimally invasive and percutaneous surgery of the foot, one question immediately comes to mind when reading this chapter: *Will the procedures described in the following chapters be able to solve this planning problem and implement the planned corrections exactly?*

The planning step is an indispensable theoretical exercise conducted before any technical manipulation. It is the product of reasoning, fed by the clinical findings and meticulous radiographic analysis.

The chosen procedure is acceptable if it can meet two essential prerequisites:

- It can theoretically meet the surgical specifications.
- Its technical execution has been mastered by the surgeon.

As with any procedure, minimally invasive and percutaneous procedures are subjected to these conditions. Thus it is incumbent on the surgeon to select a procedure that he/she has mastered and that is very likely to achieve the planned corrections.

4.5 Conclusion

Hallux valgus surgery involves complex three-dimensional geometric principles. Preoperative planning is key to obeying them. The type of osteotomy should be selected only after the preoperative plan has been completed. The plan should be followed exactly, including when performing minimally invasive and percutaneous osteotomies.

Editors' Point of View

While it is difficult to carry out intraoperative corrections that are as precise as the ones described in this chapter, the concept outlined here will give surgeons a better understanding how a procedure performed in a given plane impacts not only that plane but the other planes. A cutting guide based on these concepts is being developed.

Principles of Mechanical Stability for the Surgical Correction of Forefoot Deformities

5

Cyrille Cazeau and Yves Stiglitz

5.1 Introduction

Independent of the technique used and the surgeon's preferences, surgical correction of a forefoot deformity must abide by mechanical principles that are essential for healing. Geometric correction of deformities and immediate stability of the construct must be achieved and the surgical indications respected.

Percutaneous and minimally invasive surgery are a recent trend, with the primary advantage being fast functional recovery for the patient. However, this does mean it is exempt from these rules. This chapter is focused on the possibilities of immediate stability, before any bone healing, to allow the foot to find itself in the usual functional context as quickly as possible. This is the subject of ongoing research, both in the context of trauma surgery and elective surgery. This can be achieved in a myriad of ways; thus, the techniques presented here only serve as examples of these principles.

5.2 Complying with Standard Criteria

As with conventional surgery, the following three points must always be followed:

- Have the right reasons for operating (i.e., the correct indications) and verify that the expected outcomes is consisted with the one the patient hopes to achieve.
- Perform an architectural correction of the bone axes in all three anatomical planes to improve mechanical function.
- If possible, achieve immediate mechanical stability to allow true full weight-bearing (Fig. 5.1a) (i.e., full weight-bearing in shoe with rigid convex sole that simulates gait) and toe movement, even before the biological process of bone healing is completed. When only the heel is loaded, the operated forefoot area is unweighted (Fig. 5.1b).

While all this can be achieved with percutaneous and minimally invasive techniques, they must be implemented correctly to replace some of the more unstable conventional techniques.

C. Cazeau (✉) · Y. Stiglitz
Clinique Victor Hugo, Paris, France

C. Cazeau, Y. Stiglitz (eds.), *Percutaneous and Minimally Invasive Foot Surgery*,
https://doi.org/10.1007/978-3-030-98791-6_5

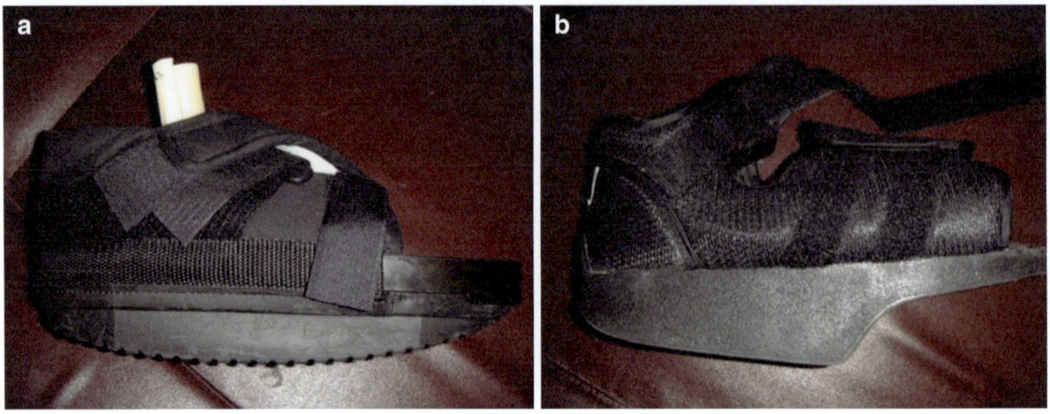

Fig. 5.1 Postoperative shoes: True full weight-bearing with convex sole (**a**). Unweighted forefoot heel contact shoe (**b**). © Cyrille Cazeau 2015. All Rights Reserved)

5.3 Surgical Indication

A reminder that the surgical indication should be based solely on pain, discomfort while wearing shoes, and considerable hindrance during activities of daily living, requests to improve appearance or to prevent further deterioration should not be considered.

5.4 Architectural Correction

Our understanding of forefoot biomechanics has greatly improved since the 1990s, an era in which L.S. Barouk and P. Diebold brought the osteotomy concept to France as the only means to reorient a bone in the three anatomical planes. This was no longer the infamous *bunion shaving* procedure, where a simple exostectomy was combined with soft tissue techniques like the McBride procedure. An osteotomy involves bone cuts that geometrically lower, shorten, and modify the orientation of the articular surfaces, based on an analysis of the deformity.

The most basic criteria to meet is the metatarsus varus, defined by the intermetatarsal angle (M1–M2). Several techniques exist, depending on the location of the procedure, which can be at the base of the metatarsal (Fig. 5.2a), diaphysis (Fig. 5.2b), or distal epiphysis-metaphysis (Fig. 5.2c). The type of approach can in fact vary. The standard approach is an open one, like the one used by proponents of the scarf osteotomy. The minimally invasive approach is reduced to 2 to 3 cm. A percutaneous approach means the opening is reduced to 2 mm. This is independent of whether the intermetatarsal angle is corrected or not (Fig. 5.2).

Functional insufficiency of the first ray can be accompanied by load transfer metatarsalgia at the lateral rays. In this scenario, the M1 head will need to be lowered (Fig. 5.3) along with being realigned. From a physics point of view, the insole-making and surgery abide by the same principles. Insoles bring the ground to the bone by applying a support under the M1 head, while surgery brings the bone to the ground through realignment and lowering. The first ray may also need to be shortened (Fig. 5.4) to release an arthritic metatarsophalangeal joint.

It may be useful to induce rotation in the frontal plane in order to correct excessive pronation of the first ray (Fig. 5.5a). It may also be necessary to induce rotation in the horizontal plane to reduce abnormal lateral deviation of the distal metatarsal articular surface (Fig. 5.5b).

Lastly, the valgus of the hallux is corrected by a closing wedge osteotomy (Fig. 5.6), defined by the metatarsophalangeal (MP1) angle. Stability is ensured by preserving a lateral bone wall to act as

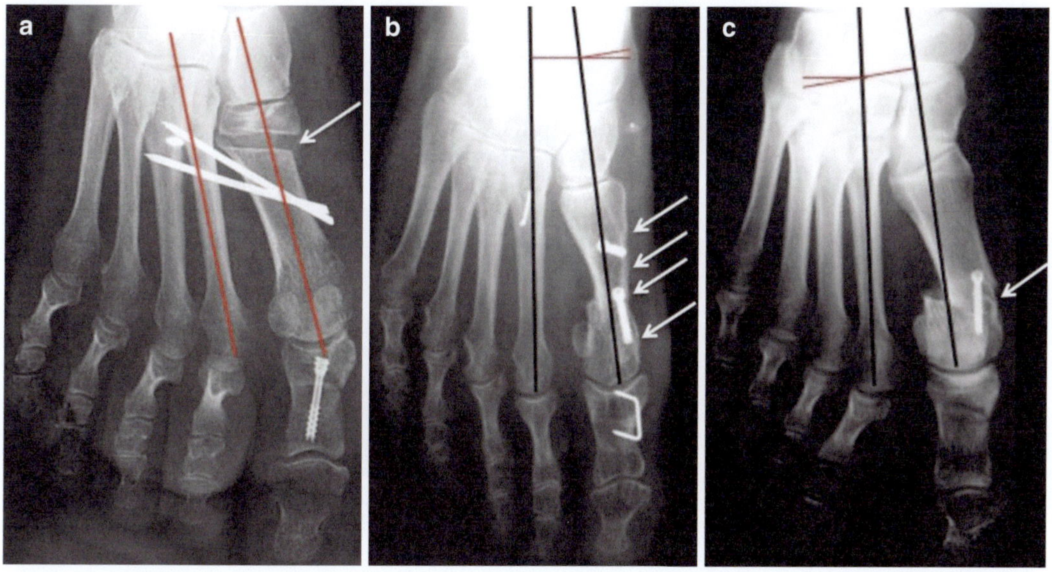

Fig. 5.2 Potential locations for M1 osteotomies: metatarsal base: percutaneous (**a**), diaphysis: open (**b**), and distal epiphysis-metaphysis: minimally invasive (**c**). © Cyrille Cazeau 2015. All Rights Reserved

Fig. 5.3 Effect of lowering the M1 head (3/4 view). © Cyrille Cazeau 2015. All Rights Reserved

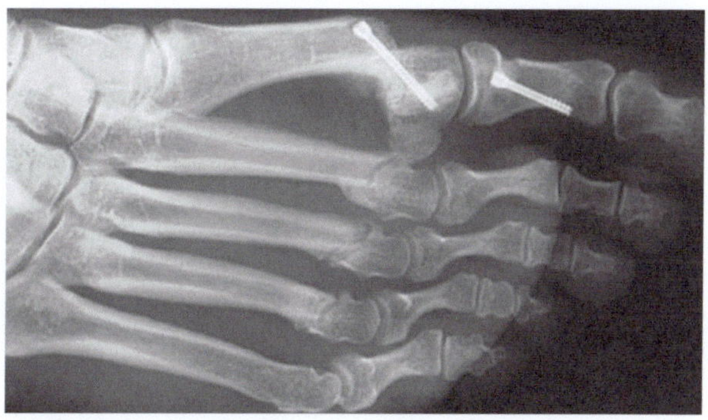

Fig. 5.4 A cut along the red dotted line will result in M1 shortening. © Cyrille Cazeau 2015. All Rights Reserved

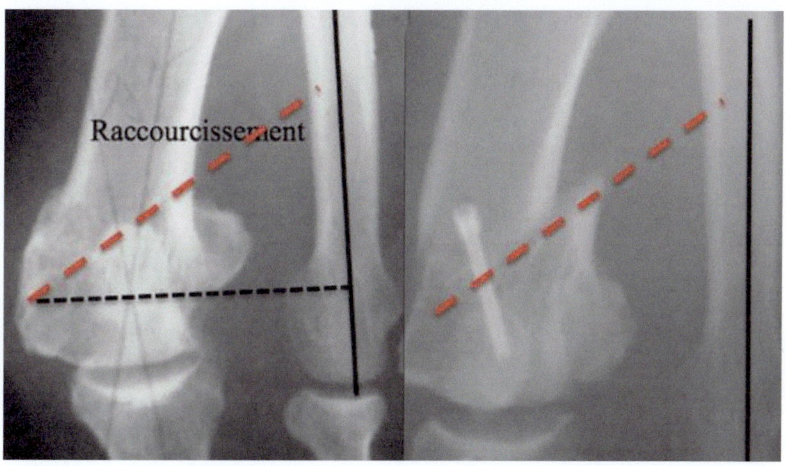

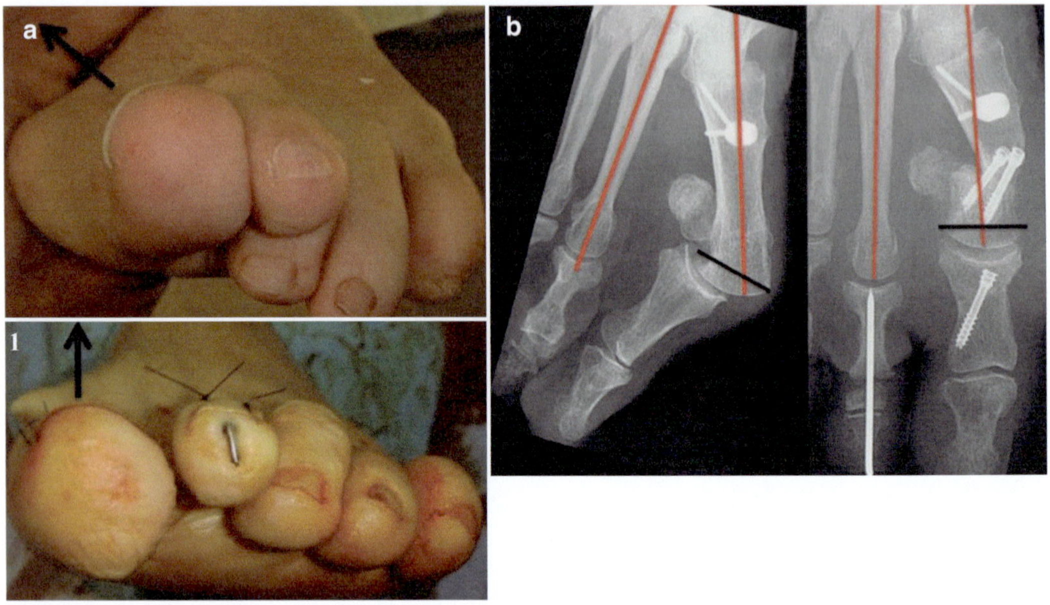

Fig. 5.5 Correction of pronation of first ray (**a**). Reduction of distal metatarsal articular angle (DMAA) (**b**).

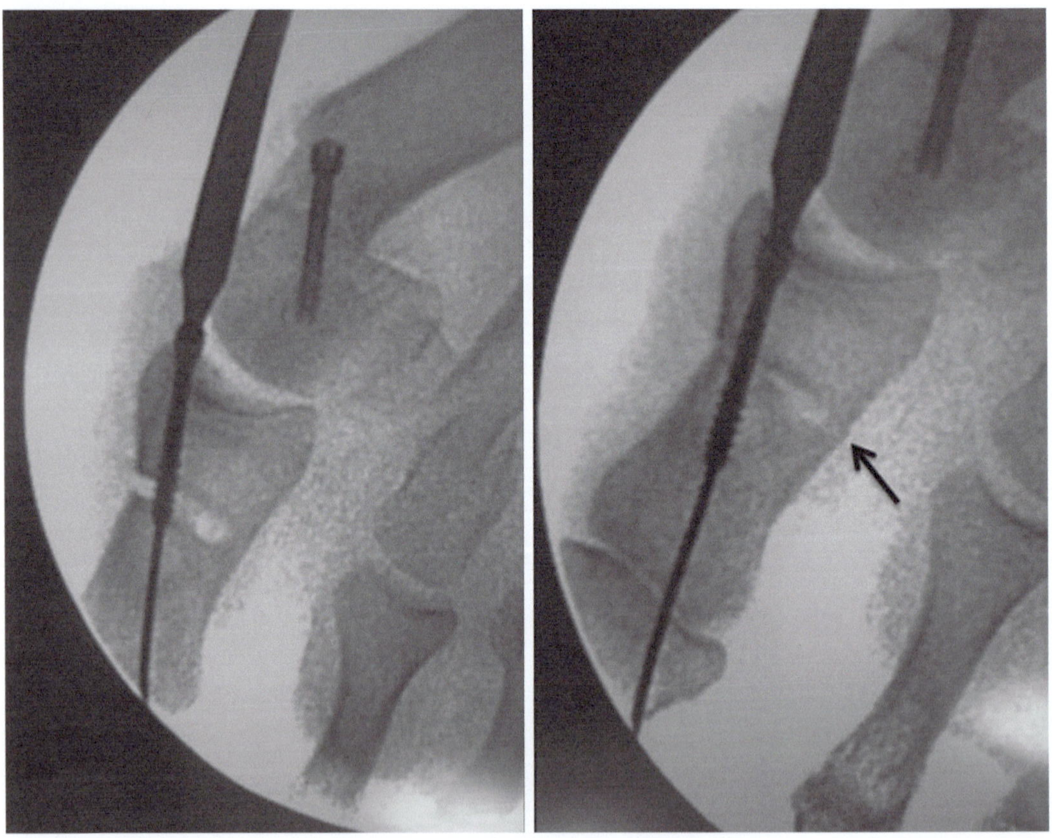

Fig. 5.6 Hallux valgus is correct by closing wedge osteotomy.

a hinge, having a good match and good compression of the osteotomy surfaces, along with the fixation method.

For the lateral rays, it is sometimes necessary to perform a distal metatarsal minimally invasive osteotomy (DMMO) to combat the load transfer metatarsalgia. Under these conditions, the shape of the anterior transverse arch must be preserved, whether the procedure is done open or percutaneously. Spontaneous regression of the plantar hyperkeratosis is evidence that the load transfer has been eliminated (Fig. 5.7).

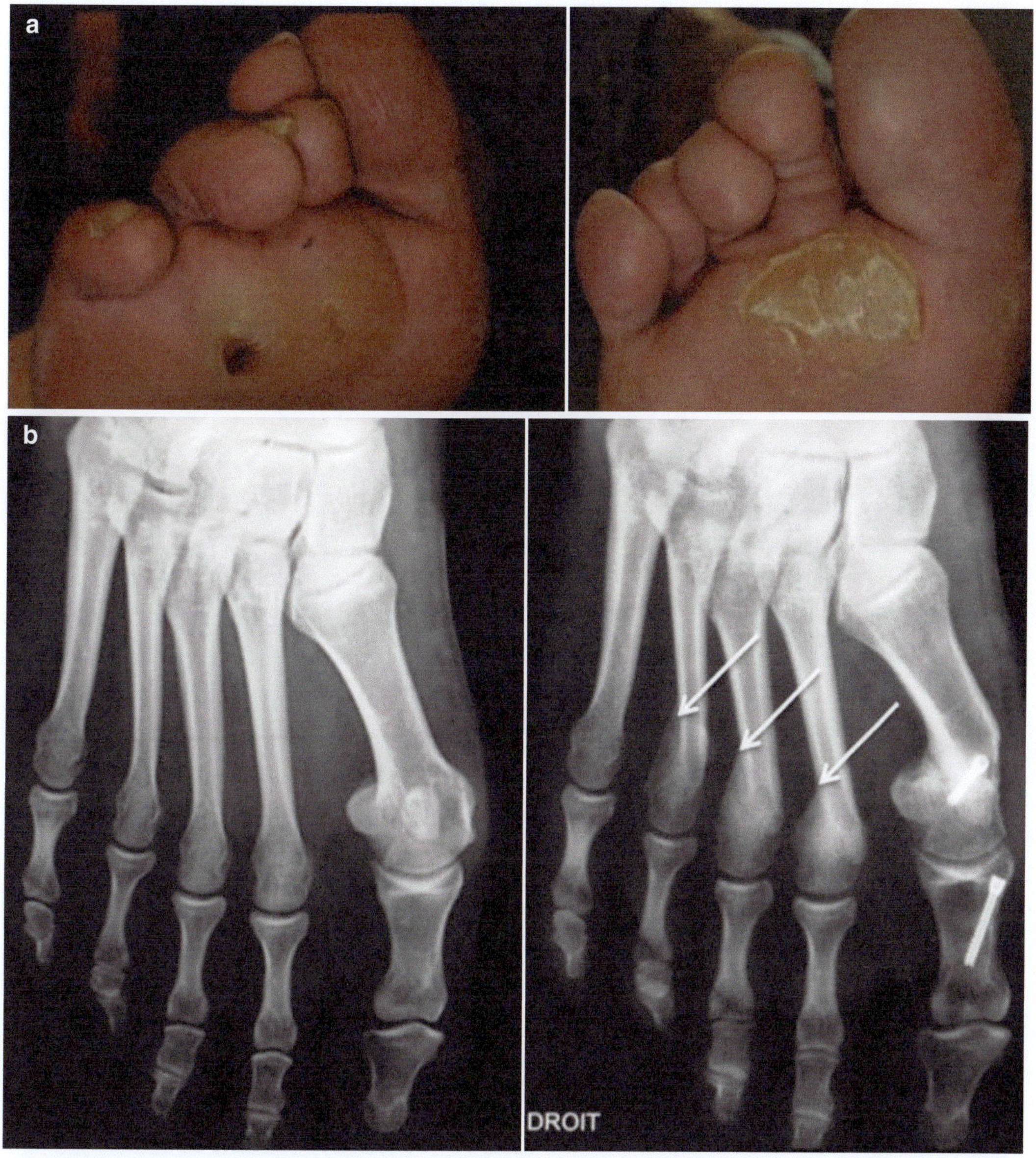

Fig. 5.7 Regression of plantar callus as a proof of load transfer elimination (**a**). Load transfer corrected by DMMO and first ray realignment (**b**).

5.5 Immediate Mechanical Stability

Progress in orthopedic surgery has typically involved reducing the size of the approach and transitioning to internal fixation, which was precarious early on, but ultimately could allow immediate use. One well-documented historical example is fixation of femoral neck fractures. The morbidity and mortality were unbearable in an era when early return to activities was impossible. The type of screw used in foot surgery is not innovative; it was introduced 20 years ago. But it is now available in smaller 2-mm and 3-mm diameters. The screw's head is threaded, which allows it is stay inside the bone and eliminates the need for hardware removal. The differential threads allow for compression as the distal part of the screw advances more quickly into the bone. Its titanium composition means that is does not set off airport security scanners and has no MRI signal.

Stability is a complex concept (Fig. 5.8), which depends on the geometric fit between bones, the location of the bone cuts, and the fixation, whether or not the osteotomy was done percutaneously. The metaphyseal location in strong cancellous bone, the crossing point of the cuts near the center of rotation, the geometric fit with a 60° angle between the two mini-chevron cuts all contribute to stability, in addition to the fixation method. The stress peaks in finite element analysis models are at their lowest.

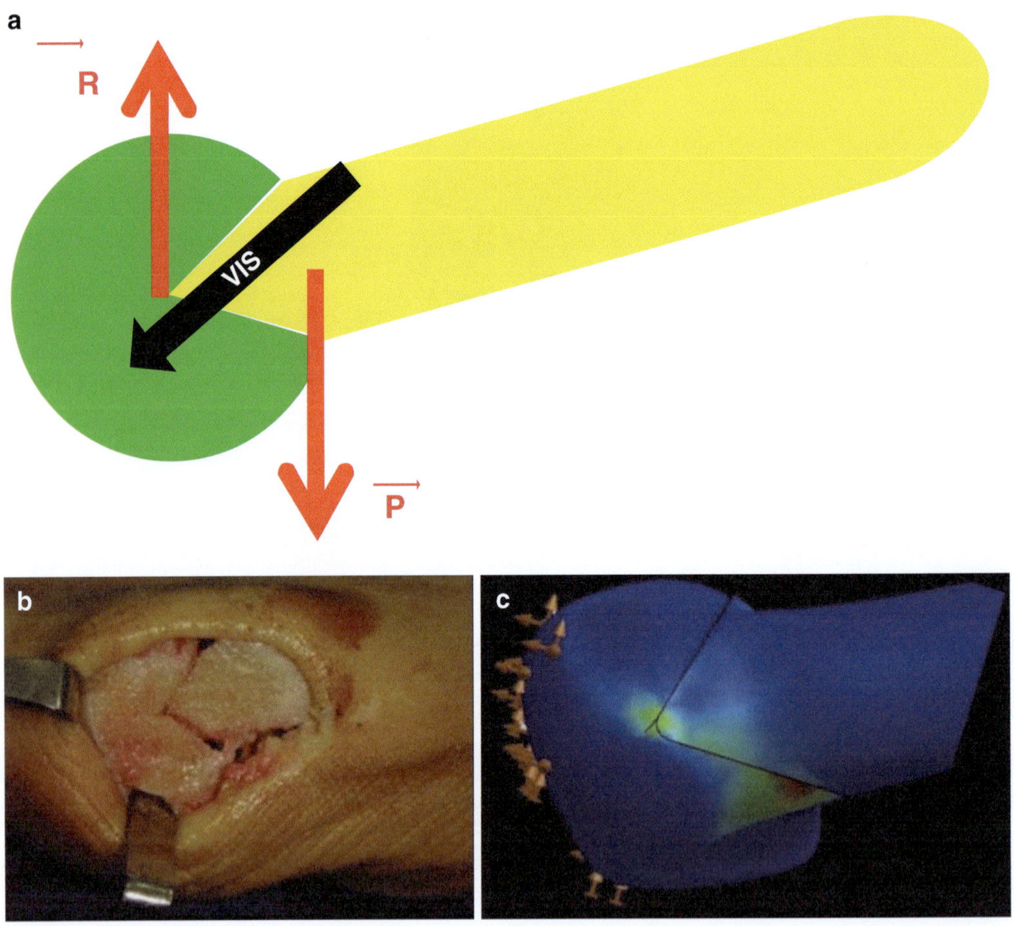

Fig. 5.8 Chevron osteotomy: forces involved around the cuts (**a**), intraoperative view (**b**), and finite element model (**c**).

During a minimally invasive chevron osteotomy, the geometry of the bone cuts combined with the fixation method allows immediate weightbearing, which is mechanically stable even before the bone heals (Fig. 5.9a). However, this strategy is not suitable in every case. For example, in an insulin-dependent diabetic patient, fixation was not used because the patient's diabetes was poorly controlled (Fig. 5.9b). While the geometry of the cuts is the same in both cases, the diabetic patient is only allowed to put weight on their heel since screw fixation was not done. Even when a large displacement chevron osteotomy is required, complying with the above-mentioned criteria allows immediate full weight-bearing and the early development of a bone callus (Fig. 5.10).

We want to emphasize that the *new technique* concept does equal *no screw*, despite the patients' fantasies that associate this concept with the presumed benign nature of the procedures.

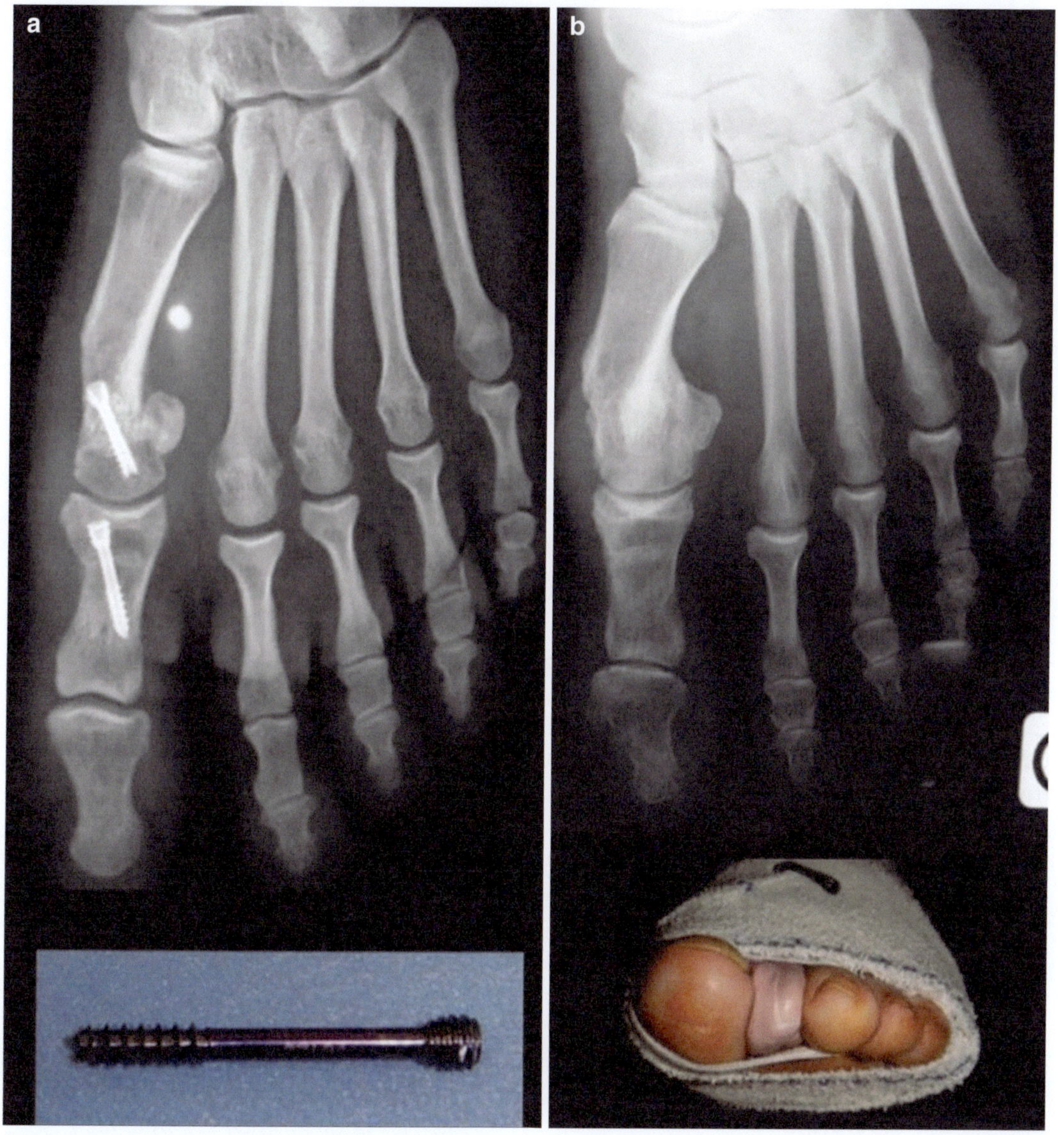

Fig. 5.9 Screw fixation used with chevron osteotomy that allows immediate full weight-bearing (**a**). When screw fixation is not feasible, only heel-contact weight-bearing is allowed, and the screw is replaced by an external fixation device (**b**).

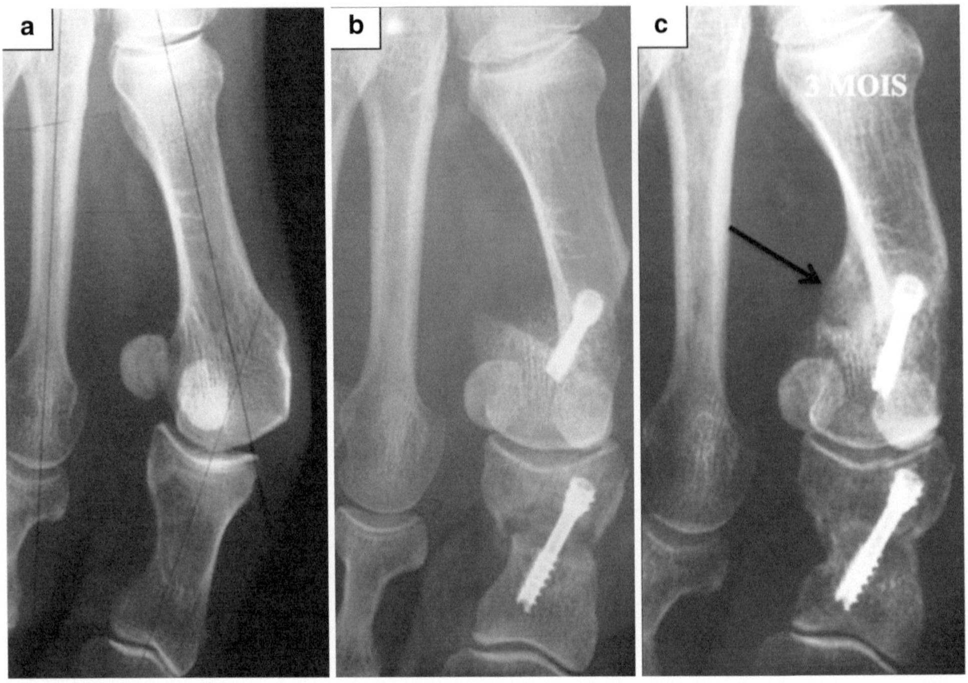

Fig. 5.10 A large displacement chevron allows immediate weight-bearing thanks to the geometry of the cuts and the bone fixation; preoperative (**a**), immediate postoperative (**b**), and 3 months postoperative with the black arrow pointing to a visible callus (**c**).

5.6 Psychological Considerations

Mechanical stability is essential but not sufficient to allow patients to fully bear weight on their operated foot immediately postoperative. Since patients know their foot bones have just been cut, shifted, and screwed, the psychological aspect of their recovery is crucial. There must be no pain from the time the patient leaves the surgery ward to when healing has been achieved. In fact, pain is a phenomenon that evolved to protect us from danger or injury; thus, it is interpreted as a sign of weakness and will lead to refusal to bear weight. Furthermore, small, carefully laid out scars are external evidence of the good work done internally, through a transitivity argument.

5.7 Conclusion

Thus the surgeon must choose the optimal techniques that will correct the observed deformities in the three anatomical planes, allow immediate use of the operated foot, and minimize the damaging nature of the surgical approaches. The mechanically stable character of the proposed corrections before the bone has healed must allow immediate weight-bearing on the foot in its normal functional context. The recovery rate is an essential factor. This is where minimally invasive and percutaneous techniques come into play.

Editors' Point of View

It is obvious that placing a structure that has been altered surgically back into its normal functional context will lead to faster recovery. This idea is explained in the chapter 9 on the impact of gravity. Under these conditions, a surgeon must keep these principles in mind when selecting the best technique and aim beyond simply correcting deformities.

Gravity and Growth

6

Cyrille Cazeau

6.1 Introduction

About 400 million years ago, the first forms of life on Earth were plants. Originally aquatic, they colonized continents and subsequently were subjected to mechanical forces much stronger than in water. They adapted in such a way that roots grew into the soil and aerial elements grew in the other direction. Under these conditions, wood must be sufficiently rigid to withstand failure while also being flexible enough to absorb plastic and elastic energy. Phylogeny and ontogenesis can explain their adaptation to this new environment [1] in which the stresses greatly affected growth and morphology. The common thread between the plant and animal kingdoms is gravity. Present from the origins of life, it is unavoidable, constant, with fixed direction that is both an unchanging reference and a physical restriction factor [2].

Bone tissue has a predominant role in this terrestrial acclimation; its development can be considered as a reaction to gravity (it quickly goes away in microgravity situations). However, this acclimation is not limited to bone and happens in most of the organism's tissues, as far as they are impacted by the resistance to gravity, either directly (muscles, lungs) or indirectly through fluid mechanics (hearth, circulatory system).

C. Cazeau (✉)
Clinique Victor Hugo, Paris, France

The entire animal kingdom is affected—both vertebrates and invertebrates—as evidenced by the universal presence of mechanoreceptors, with fish being the only exception. *Within a living organism, all tissues are affected.*

Other living organisms are not subjected to gravity because of their miniscule mass (Foraminifera). Subjected to forces of superficial tension, viscosity, Brownian motion, and electric charges, they escape the above description due to their symmetry and polarity [3].

Here, we will try to draw analogies between the plant and animal kingdoms in terms of gravity's mechanisms of action. According to Aristotle, "the search for relationships between apparently independent things and the search for similarities between dissimilar things in the eyes of mortals."

6.2 Mechanoreceptors: The Starting Point

6.2.1 Bone Cellular Organization

There are three main types of cells in the bone [4]: osteoblast, osteoclast, and osteocyte (Fig. 6.1).

The first two are involved in bone remodeling that contributes to ongoing maintenance by replacing the old bone with a new bone. Osteoclasts are activated to degrade the bone, and then osteoblasts make extracellular matrix (collagen) which is mineralized by the intermediary of various hormones. The osteoblast dies in a pre-

C. Cazeau, Y. Stiglitz (eds.), *Percutaneous and Minimally Invasive Foot Surgery*,
https://doi.org/10.1007/978-3-030-98791-6_6

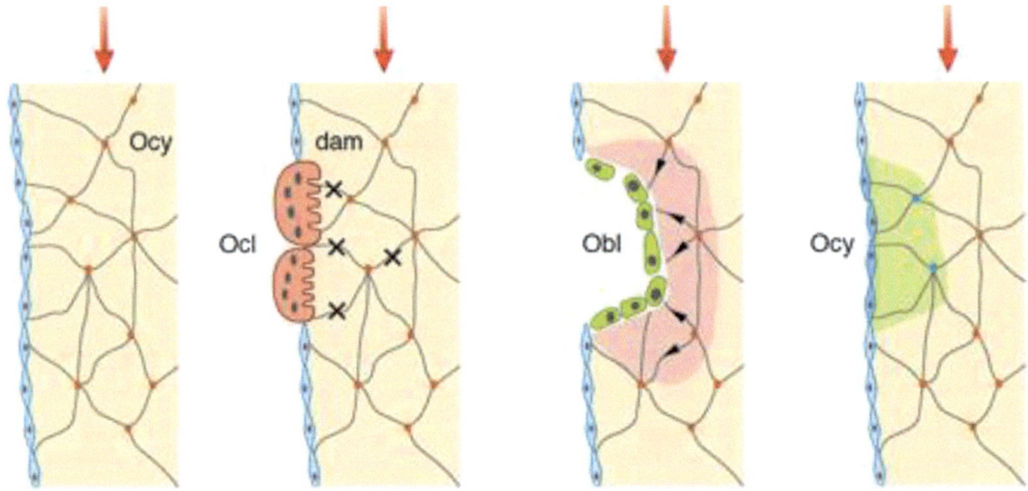

Fig. 6.1 Three types of bone cells. Ocy osteocyte, Ocl osteoclast, and Obl osteoblast. Dam *damage*—these are micro-injuries caused by mechanical stresses due to a vertical force. © Cyrille Cazeau 2015. All Rights Reserved

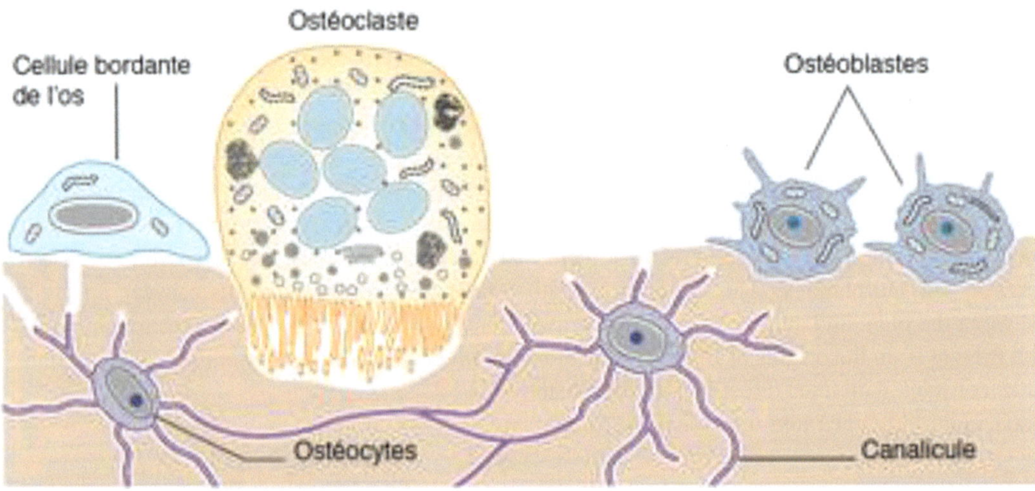

Fig. 6.2 Osteocytes communicate through their dendritic connections in the lacuno-canalicular network. © Cyrille Cazeau 2015. All Rights Reserved

programmed manner and lets itself get encased in the bone matrix that it built; it them becomes the third player, the osteocyte.

Its cell body is located in the bone lacuna surrounded by extracellular matrix. Its dendrites extend out and connect it to its neighbors (Fig. 6.2).

These dendritic processes are sensitive to mechanical forces, while the ciliated cell surface is sensitive to the movement of extracellular fluids. Together they can detect stresses and deformations in shear, stretching, and pressure changes. Thus, they play a central role in maintaining the balance between bone formation and resorption [6, 60].

6.2.2 Intracellular Transmission: Cytoskeleton and Extracellular Matrix

6.2.2.1 In Animals that Have a Bony Skeleton

The cytoskeleton and extracellular matrix function as follows. The dendritic network is activated by the cytoskeleton. It consists of actin (resistance to tension), microtubules (extremely high compression resistance), and intermediate filaments that provide stability (Fig. 6.3).

The mechanical load perceived by the mechanoreceptors is transmitted to the cytoskeleton, which then deforms and triggers biochemical reactions. The position and shape of the microtubules and filaments are then modified based on the forces of gravity [5, 6], whereas microgravity destroys them. The cytoskeleton can be compared to a model known in the architectural world as "tensegrity" [7]: a three-dimensional structure consisting of tensional and compressional elements configured to resemble a trellis in space (Fig. 6.4a, b).

It is the sum of forces applied to the cellular skeleton that solidly holds the shape of each ele-

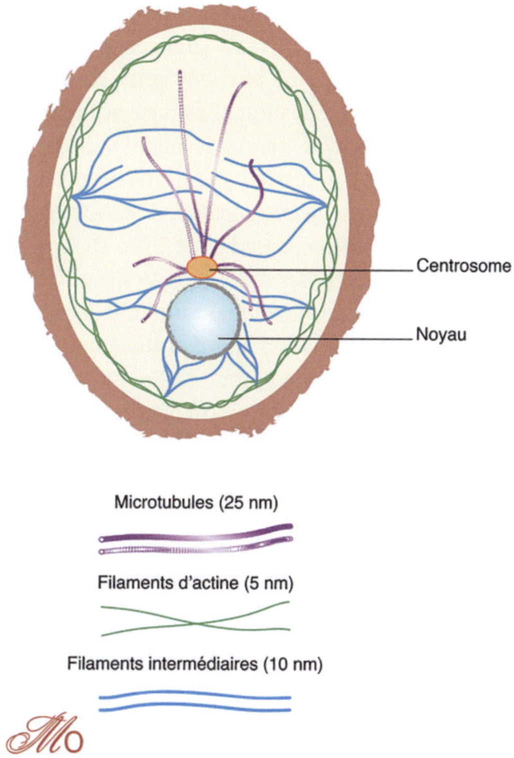

Fig. 6.3 Cells contain three types of fibers that make up its cytoskeleton, whose role is to relay external forces into the cell. © Cyrille Cazeau 2015. All Rights Reserved

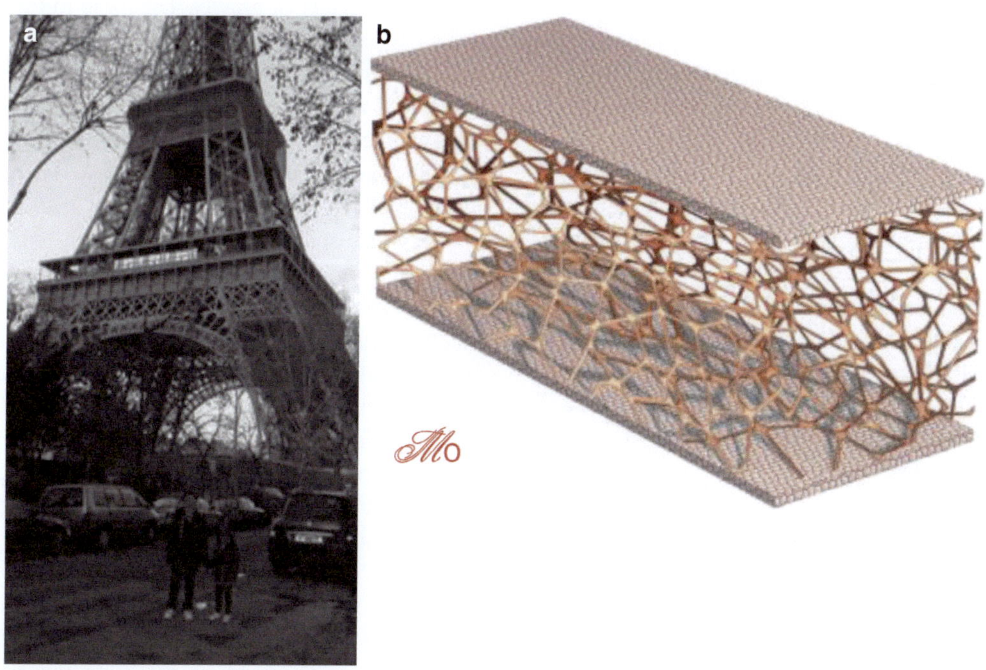

Fig. 6.4 (**a**, **b**) Trellis model illustrating the tensegrity structure concept, which explains the distribution of forces and self-stability. © Cyrille Cazeau 2015. All Rights Reserved

ment, and then of the entire unit. Thus, it is likely that all cells are sensitive to changes in gravity, by the intermediary of this tensegrity structure, not by the direct activation of a single receptor.

The extracellular matrix is mainly made of collagen fibers that resist traction, and other components such as hydroxyapatite, a substrate of bone mineralization. Based on in vitro studies, it appears that osteocytes react more to shear forces in the extracellular interstitial fluid than to direct mechanical deformation and that the extracellular matrix acts as an amplifier of the mechanical signals transmitted to the cytoskeleton.

6.2.2.2 In Plants

Plants also have a cytoskeleton and extracellular matrix, although it will not be described here. The cellular tissues have high mechanical properties, such as turgescent, hydrostatic, or wood tissues.

6.2.3 Summary

We can find similarities between the plant and animal kingdoms: mechanical loading is perceived by the cell membrane by the intermediary of mechanoreceptors, transmitted by the extracellular matrix to the intracellular cytoskeleton according to the tensegrity model, which is translated by alterations to exocytosis and endocytosis processes, and results in the assembly of molecules and polymers that play a part in combating gravity. This tensegrity concept explains the "individual" internal relay of external forces. It is defined in the architectural world as "the ability of a structure to self-stabilize by the interplay of tension and compression forces that are distributed and balanced out."

6.3 Translation by Physical Elements

6.3.1 Physical Properties

6.3.1.1 Young's Modulus (*E*)

This is a constant property of a material that relates its deformation to the effect of physical stress. The stress applied (sigma = σ), either in compression or tension, is the relationship between an applied force (F) and the area (A) of the material's cross-section, in units of pressure (MPa).

$$\sigma = \frac{F}{A}$$

The deformation of a material ε is its observed lengthening or shortening (L) expressed relative to its initial length (L_0).

$$\varepsilon = \frac{L - L_0}{L_0}$$

The two values are related:

$$ð = E \times \varepsilon$$

The higher the Young's modulus (E), the stronger the material, and the less it will deform for a given stress. When a bone increases its cortical thickness by mineralization, it also increases its ability to withstand deformation. The same applies to a branch making lignin.

6.3.1.2 Second Moment of Area (SMA) (I_z)

This is a *geometric* property of an area (I_z) that reflects how its points are distributed relative to an arbitrary axis (I_z, horizontal here) that passes through the center of gravity. The basic formulas are show in Fig. 6.5, with the SI units being meters to the fourth power (m^4). The higher an object's SMA, the more the resistance attributed to its geometry is high, independent of its Young's modulus, i.e., independent of the material it is made up of.

The SMA of a full cylindrical beam is similar to that of a hollow cylinder. The difference is that the hollow cylinder does not require anywhere as much material to be created. In this way, the geometry of bones resembles that of the exoskeleton of arthropods (crustacean, insects, and others, Fig. 6.6) and that of plants. In certain groups such as bamboo and other Gramineae, the hollow tube structure is obvious [13]. For trees, its morphology can be likened to a combination of hollow tubes. The central portion of each tube is composed of aligned cells organized in conductive vessels and/or peripheral fibers, depending on the group. These fibers make up the rigid

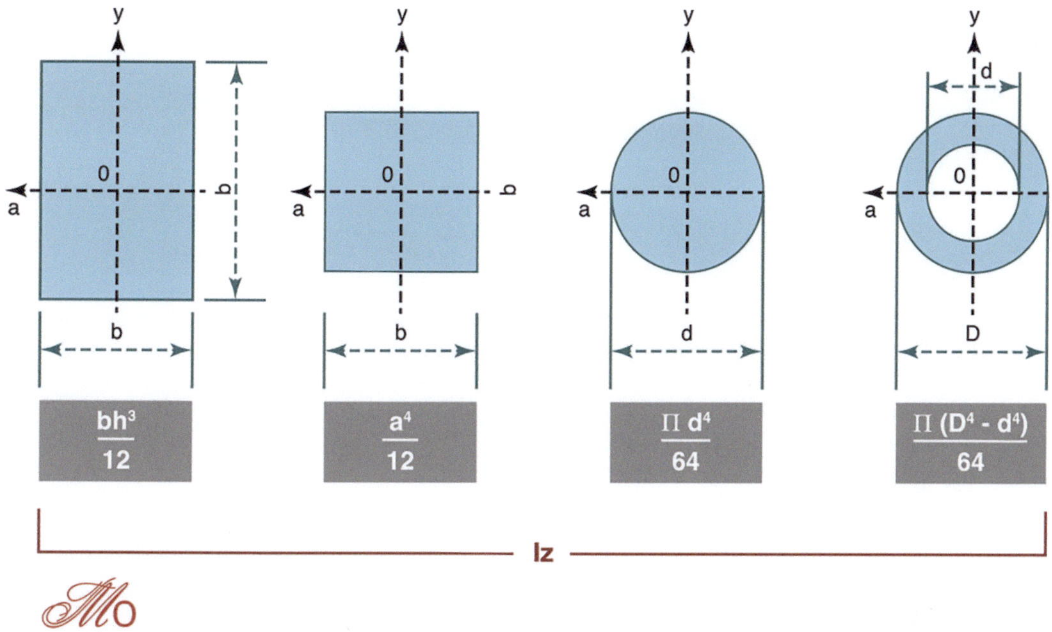

Fig. 6.5 Calculation of the second moment of area (SMA) for basic shapes, representing the object's resistance to loading based on its geometry. The SMA of the hollow tube on the left is not vastly different than the SMA of the full tube on the right, although it requires significantly less matter.

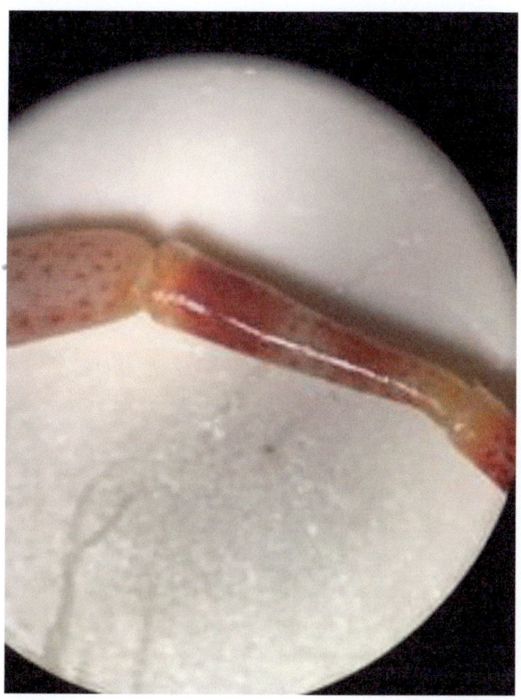

Fig. 6.6 Exoskeleton of an arthropod's leg (here a shrimp). The geometry is like that of Fig. 6.13.

peripheral portion of tubes, composed of cellulose, pectin, lignin, etc. As the tree grows, lignification with cell death makes up the middle wood, while the activity and organization described previously continue in the peripheral portion—the cambium—which is responsible to the trunk's increase in diameter.

6.3.1.3 Calculation of Deflection

What happens with a branch or a bone is subject to a moment? A moment is the force multiplied by the distance to its application point, in $M \times m$. The material bends, over a distance called deflection (Fig. 6.7). The amplitude of this deflection, no matter whether the beam is a bone or plant, is calculated using the SMA and Young's modulus.

$$\text{Deflection} = \frac{F \times L}{C \times E \times I_Z}$$

F force placed on the beam (weight)L length of beam$C$ constant (dimensionless),E Young's modulus,I_z SMA in Z axis.

The magnitude of a beam's deflection is proportional to the force applied, such as weight or

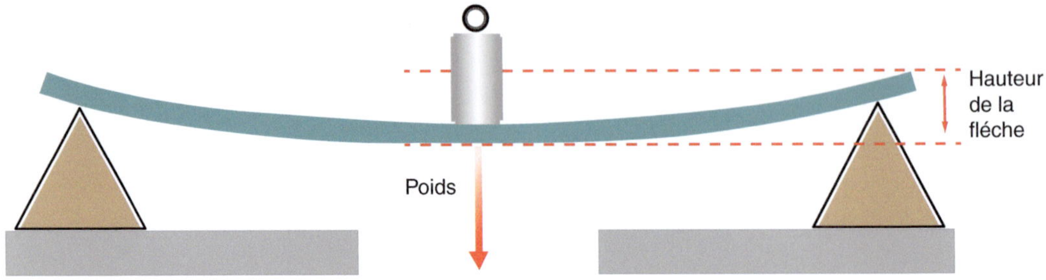

Fig. 6.7 Deflection of a beam due to the effect of weight. It depends on the type of material (Young's modulus) and the object's geometry (SMA).

foliage stuck in the wind. There is less deflection when the resistance to deformation is high (*E*) and/or the geometry of the cross-section of the beam withstands it—bone or branch—(SMA).

The living organism (animal or plant) is able to produce matter to withstand the forces that it is subjected to by modifying the quality and orientation of its materials to optimize the Young's modulus and of its geometry to increase the SMA.

6.3.2 Elements Modifying Young's Modulus

6.3.2.1 Hydroxyapatite and Animal Collagen

Mechanical loading provokes an increase in bone remodeling, although excessive loading can cause overload injuries [8, 9]. Conversely, the absence of stresses leads to rapid loss of bone mass like in astronauts or bedridden patients. One of the evolutionary responses in the animal kingdom was to make the skeleton more rigid by mineralizing it, with mechanical loading being a powerful stimulus. Unstretchable collagen fibers mainly withstand tensile forces, while hydroxyapatite withstands the compressive ones. Thus, it is logical to see that mineralization occurs where the mechanical loads are the highest (Fig. 6.8), so as to locally modify Young's modulus [8].

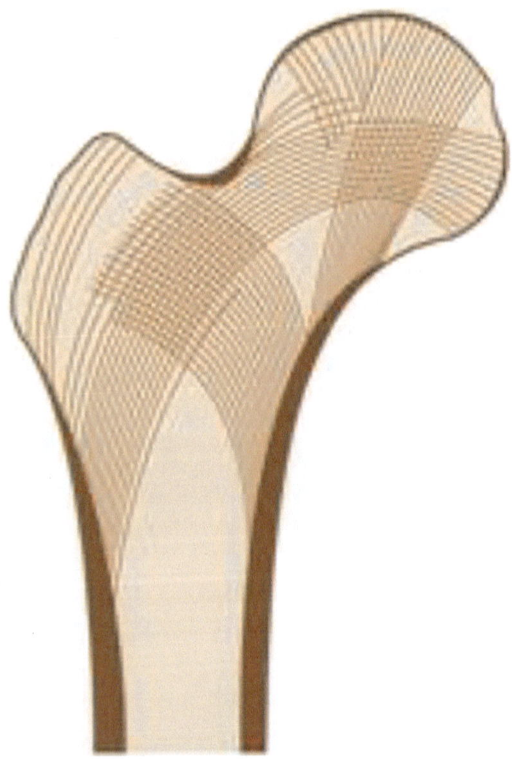

Fig. 6.8 Layout of cancellous bone trabeculae in the femoral neck based on the type and direction of stresses.

6.3.2.2 How Plants Make a Composite Material

A plant's cell walls consist of cellulose and lignin, in combination with xyloglucans (hemicellulose) and pectin, forming an extremely robust composite material. This structure is anisotropic, meaning that its mechanical properties vary by direction, which is how plants adapt to these stresses. The process of reactional lignification (reaction wood) increases its resistance. Moreover, the new wood on the periphery is highly adherent to old wood. Given its larger size, it generates a reserve of mechanical energy in the form of internal forces. Cellulose is better at resisting tensile forces, like collagen. Lignin resists compressive forces, like hydroxyapatite, providing a support function thanks to its mechanical properties and conduction function due to the hydrophobic nature of lignin. Histologically [1] there are modifications in the orientation of cellulose fibers, anatomy, and number of vessels (tracheids) along with lignin deposits.

Depending on the location of the mechanical stress, the tree can produce wood with an appropriate cellulose/lignin distribution. It is logical to observe that lignification always occurs where the mechanical loading is the highest, like for bone mineralization.

6.3.2.3 Change in Orientation of Trabecular Bone

Changes in curvature are detected inside the cancellous bone. The bone is composed of an external cortex that can withstand flexion and torsion that is minimally elastic and that turns over more slowly than trabecular bone. The latter consists of cancellous bone, which makes up 80% of its area, but only 20% of its mass. It turns over very quickly, is not extraordinarily strong but is highly elastic.

In 1892, Julius Wolf [11–13] described the orientation of the trabeculations of cancellous bone (trabecular bone) and observed how they changed their orientation based on the mechanical stresses, in an era where X-rays had not yet been discovered. He proposed that bones change their external shape and internal architecture in response to these stresses, based on the works of the anatomist George Hermann von Meyer and the engineer Karl Culmann. The direction of the trabeculations in the cancellous bone of the proximal femur are aligned with the direction of the maximum stresses (Fig. 6.9), like for the spine, tibia, and calcaneus, describing its anisotropy. This made the cancellous bone stronger.

This can be explained mechanically: when the bone bears a load that is not uniformly distributed, and/or it is already asymmetric (with a concavity and convexity), it will be subjected to excessive compression on the concave side and traction on the opposite side. The muscles mainly oppose traction forces, with the bone being responsible for withstanding compressive loads. In a simplified way, when a load is placed on a console or a cantilevered beam (Fig. 6.10), it causes vertical compression forces where it is applied, and horizontal tensile forces where it is attached (wall, trunk, hip), making it the weak point.

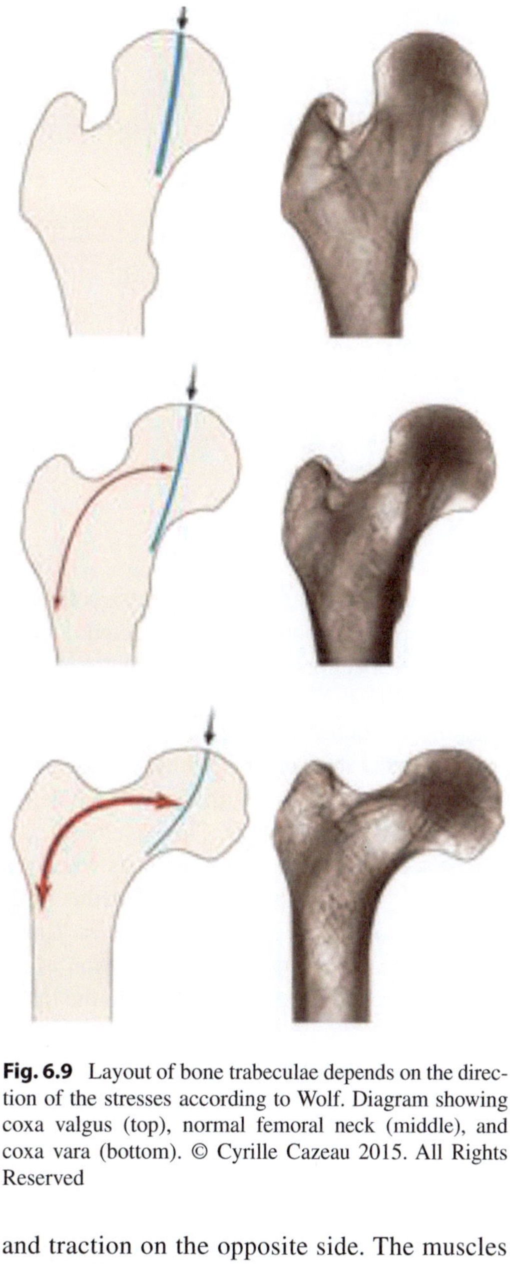

Fig. 6.9 Layout of bone trabeculae depends on the direction of the stresses according to Wolf. Diagram showing coxa valgus (top), normal femoral neck (middle), and coxa vara (bottom).

The appearance of a curvature with verticalization helps to suppress most of the tensile

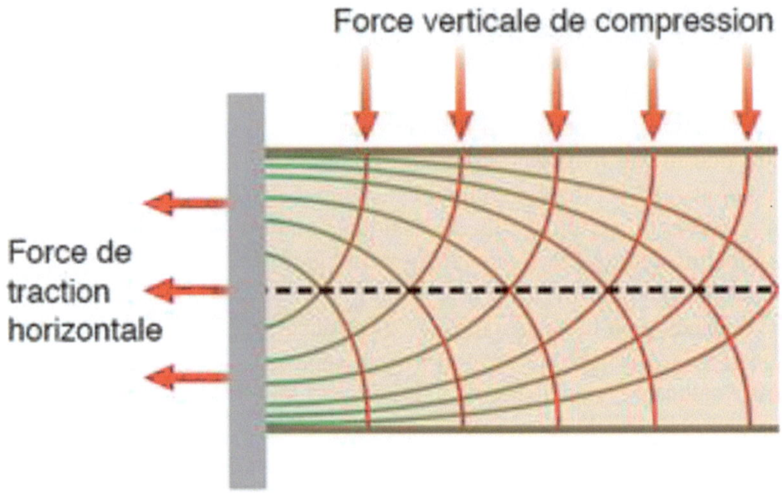

Fig. 6.10 Distribution of vertical compression forces and horizontal traction forces on a cantilever bending system such as a large branch.

forces and to maintain the compressive forces. Qualitatively, the bone areas subjected to the most tensile loading have more collagen fibers in the axis of loading, since collagen is better at resisting traction. In compressive areas, the hydroxyapatite deposits that withstand compression are more numerous, with the collagen being arranged perpendicular to it. These elements can also be seen experimentally in animals when we alter the type of stress, evidence that this phenomenon is not solely dependent on genes. These two examples of anisotropic configuration illustrate how strength increases to adapt to the loading direction without increasing the mass cost.

The works of Julius Wolf were confirmed by recent archaeometry studies on bone ultrastructure [91]. Collagen is studied in several ways, from analyzing its fibrillar structure using polarized microscopy to macromolecular analysis using FTIR/Raman spectroscopy. These methods make it possible to differentiate the rapid bone formation mode through remodeling due to small mechanical stresses where fibrils are deposited anarchically (fibrous tissue) from the remodeling scenario where bone formation is slower, strongly directional and influenced by the mechanical loads placed on the bone. In the first case, the bone's response to the stresses is isotropic, while in the second case, it is anisotropic and completely adapted to the direction of the loads being applied. New analysis methods have shown that remodeling induced by loading impacts the entire bone, from its macroscopic shape to the molecular structure of the collagen and atomic structure of hydroxyapatite.

6.3.3 Elements Modifying the Second Moment of Inertia

6.3.3.1 Increase in Diameter

The increase in the bone diameter due to stress occurs in many situations: skeleton of children subjected to hard manual labor like mining, mechanical load transfer to the lateral rays in cases of functional insufficiency of the first ray of the forefoot shown on Fig. 6.11 as hyperostosis of the second metatarsal.

The same goes for a fracture callus. Figure 6.12 shows the surgical correction of hallux valgus with percutaneous elevation osteotomies of the lateral rays that are not fixed. A bone callus appears early on and quickly evolves because of the immediate full weight-bearing.

This phenomenon was described extensively by Robling [9]. Thickening of the walls of long bones by appositional growth increases the SMA, and thereby the ability to withstand flexion and torsion.

The circular geometry helps to better counter the flexion moments in all axes [5]. On the con-

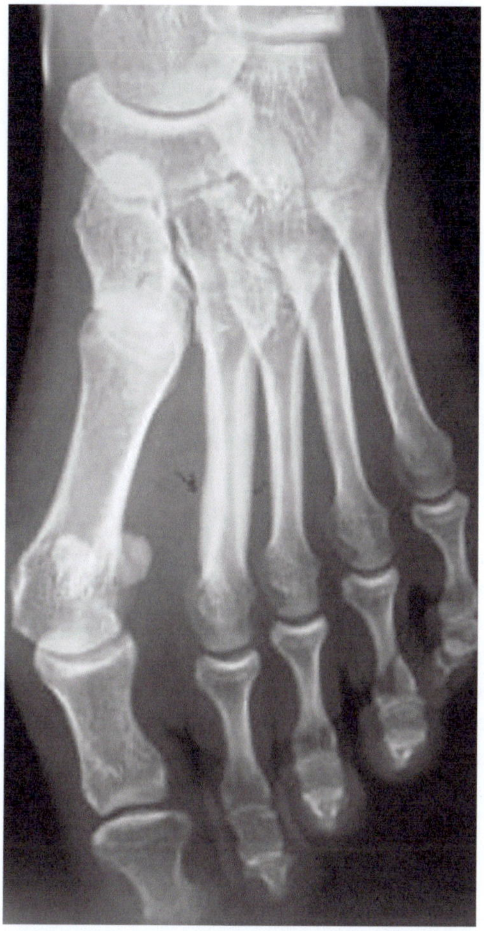

Fig. 6.11 Hyperostosis of cortical surfaces of the second metatarsal is related to excessive stress due to load transfer from metatarsus varus. © Cyrille Cazeau 2015. All Rights Reserved

trary, lack of loading in a growing child leads to long but small-diameter bones with lower-round SMA, like a young tree that was protected from the wind during its growth. Experiments in dogs show bone loss with expansion of the medullary canal, predominately in the distal bones of the legs, the ones that are typically overloaded, close to the ground. Healthy volunteers that were confined to their beds for 17 weeks had significant bone loss, mainly in the calcaneus, lumbar spine, and proximal femur.

The impact of loading is also evident by bone overuse injuries. Their geometry and corticocancellous topography depend on the intensity and direction of the stresses [14–17], with the injuries triggering new repair processes as an attempt to adapt. In botany, during growth, there is an increase in mass and lift to the wind, resulting in an increase in the diameter of the trunk and its branches. This increases the SMA by increasing the outer diameter.

6.3.3.2 Compromise Between a Full and Hollow Tube

Optimization between mass and strength is embodied by the bone being shaped as a hollow tube, which allows for large reduction in mass creation for a lower reduction in SMA. The optimal relationship between the outer and inner diameter is 1:0.9 [18].

In both cases, the hollow tube structure is comparable to the morphology of the exoskele-

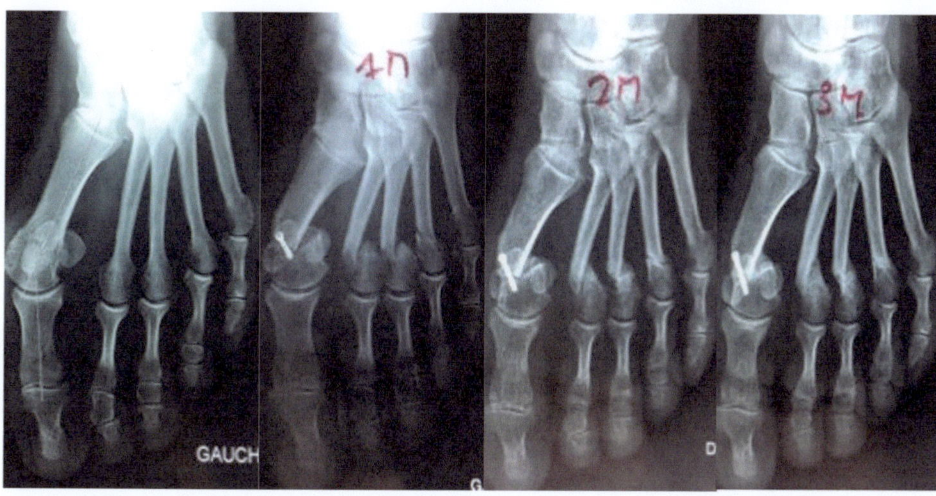

Fig. 6.12 Early appearance and rapid development of bone callus after osteotomy of the first four metatarsals that were loaded immediately. © Cyrille Cazeau 2015. All Rights Reserved

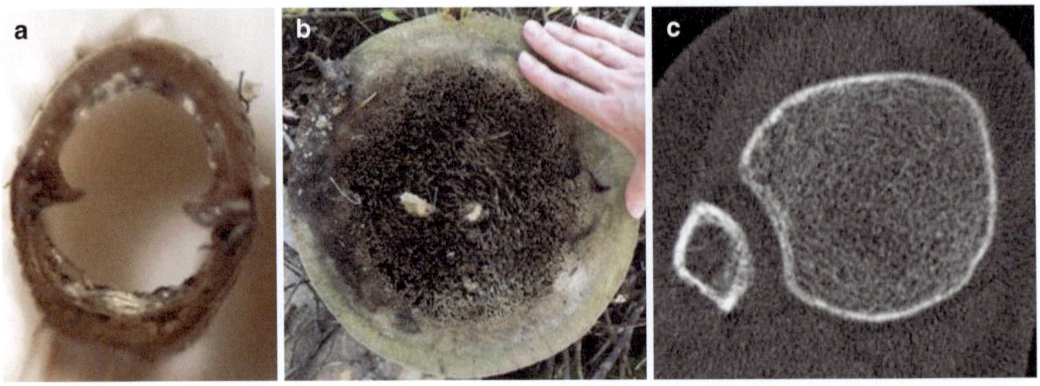

Fig. 6.13 Hollow tube structure shown on transverse slices, (**a**) in an arthropod's leg, (**b**) in bamboo, and (**c**) in a long bone; this optimizes the second moment of area relative to the low cost of creating material.

ton of arthropods, insects, crustaceans, etc., of a slice of bamboo or a long bone (Fig. 6.13a, b, c).

6.3.3.3 Ovalization of the Bone's Cross-Section

The addition of bone or plant material in an area weakened by the repair process makes it possible—due to the asymmetry of the cross-section—to both increase the SMA and to save on material. Experiments in the ulna of adult rats show that new bone formation is higher in the concave areas of the bone where the stresses are the highest (Fig. 6.14a) [9].

The SMA in the experiment increased 70% by changing the bone's geometry, where it needed it the most; conversely, the 7% increase in mineralization shows that Young's modulus was minimally altered. By comparison, on Fig. 6.14b, we can see the oval-shaped growth of a gymnosperm on the left and angiosperm on the right.

6.3.4 Elements Modifying both Parameters

The two parameters are related when calculating the deflection, which represents the bending of a structure subjected to a bending moment. The maximum moment is applied in the middle of the beam at the "point of weakness." In the femur, the biconvex curvature of its cortex in the middle portion of the diaphysis (Fig. 6.15) exists to better withstand these moments. This feature is well known to orthopedic surgeons who carry out non-locked press-fit femoral nailing. This morphology increases both the Young's modulus and the SMA. Ovalization of the cross-section during repair is another example of a mechanism impacting both physical characteristics.

6.3.5 Impact of Frequency of Stress Application

Other experiments have shown how the dynamics of stress application drive bone adaptation. Increased frequency increases osteogenesis considerably [19, 20]. Thus, it would be interesting to study the effect of walking speed (i.e., cyclic loading) in humans and variable winds on treetops. The rate of bone deformations by the intermediary of thousands of repetitive loads seems particularly effective [21]. However, if the duration of loading is too long, the effect on forma-

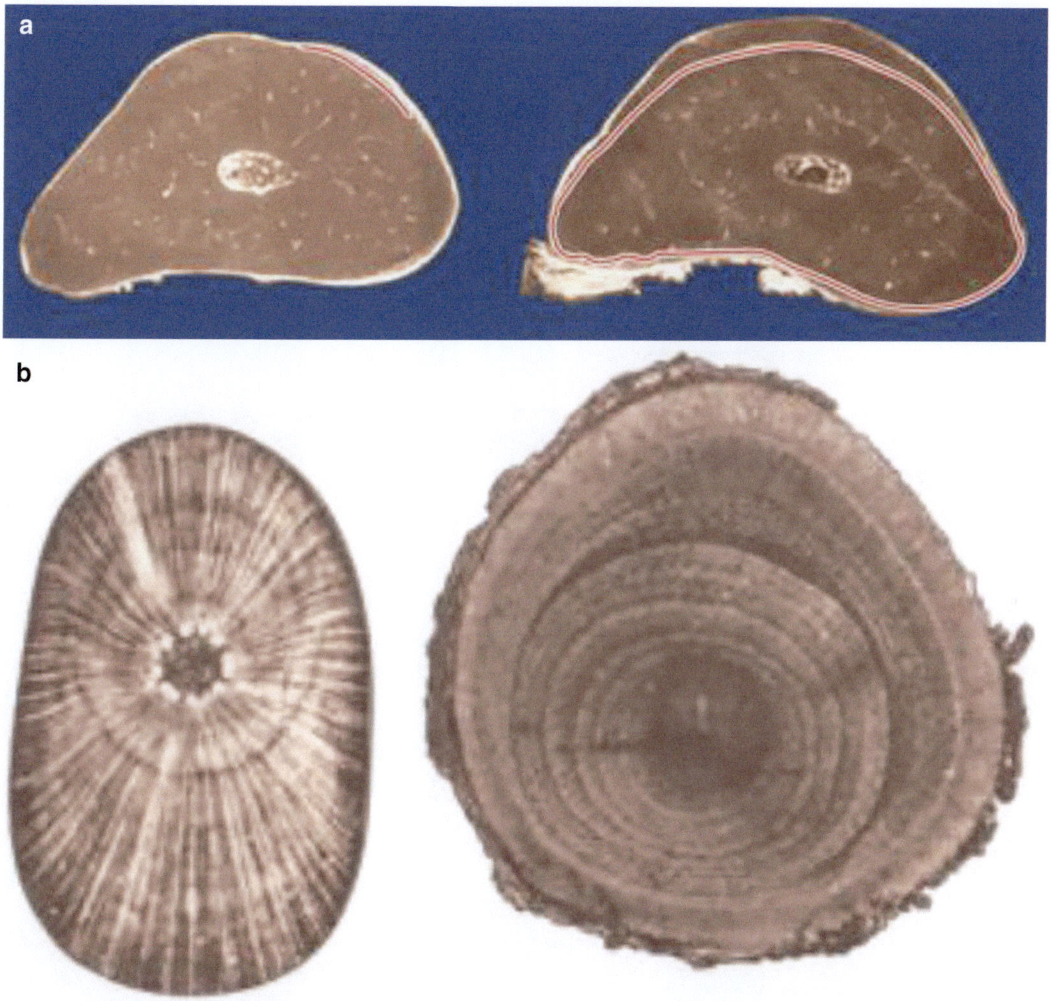

Fig. 6.14 (**a**) Oval-shaped bone growth in response to stresses on the transverse slice of the radius. (**b**) Oval-shaped growth on the inferior face of a branch in a gymnosperm (left) and on the superior face of an angiosperm (right). © Cyrille Cazeau 2015. All Rights Reserved

tion wears out, like if the production chain became desensitized. A rest period is then needed. Given that bone is not highly innervated, the mechanoreceptors do not receive commands from a central unit. This is like plants since they have no innervation.

6.3.6 Summary

There are strong analogies between plants and animals in terms of the dynamic capacity and ability to modify the structure of materials and the external shape of the "individual."

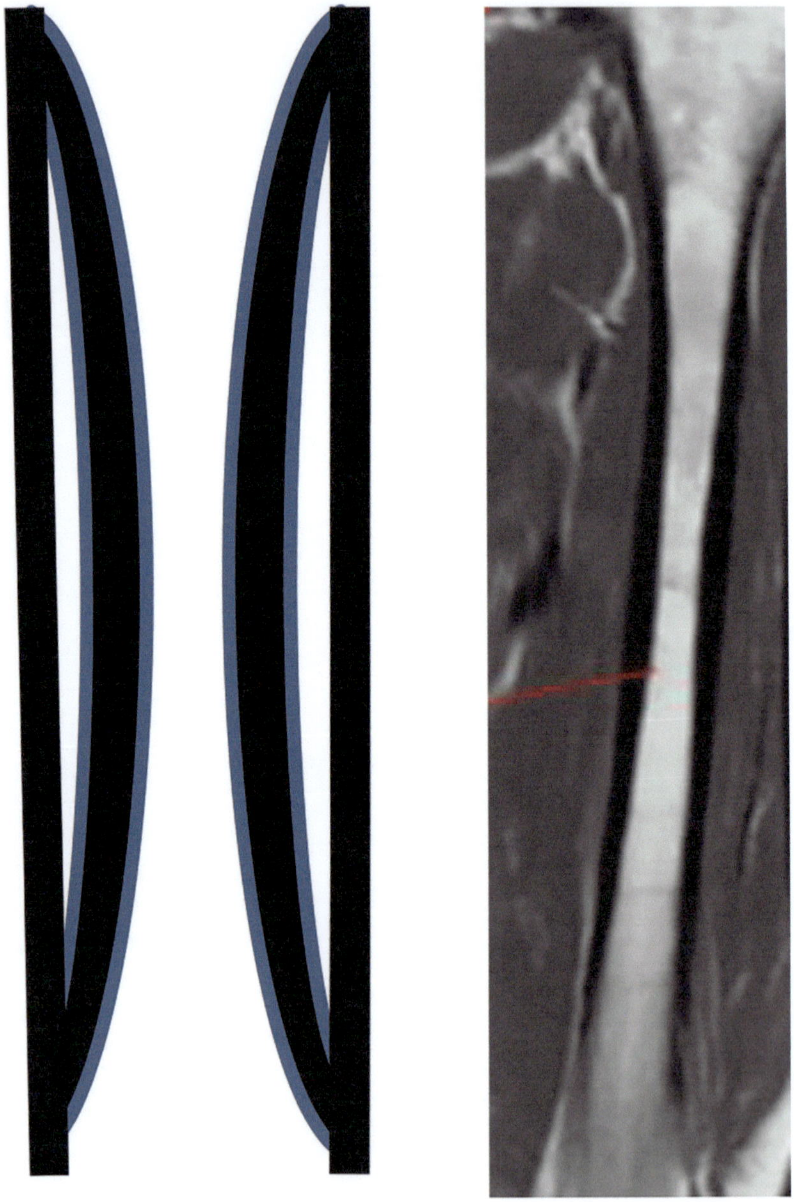

Fig. 6.15 On the anterior side of the femur, the largest amount of material is added where the bone is weakest.

6.4 Conclusion

The remodeling of human tissues varies like in the bone or wood because of mechanical loads, especially those related to gravity. The mechanoreceptive control of growth is remarkably similar between the plant and animal kingdoms. While the exact mechanisms are not known, the sequencing of these phenomena is the same in plants and animals, which at least allows us to draw powerful analogies. The term "analogy" is used here to signify a study of similarities of functions and structures determined by mechanical stresses.

A mechanoreceptor is activated, transmitting the forces in the extracellular matrix to the inside of the cell to the cytoskeleton, resulting in a biochemical cascade. This translates into the production of material to repair damage, withstand stress, and guide the growth necessary for survival. Since gravity is related to the telluric nature of the Earth, they were present before any life appeared. Under these conditions, it is not surprising that they are present in the function of every living being.

7 Exostectomy

Cyrille Cazeau

7.1 Introduction

The term *exostosis* must be used carefully as it designates a benign bone tumor that is unrelated to hallux valgus. The bump observed on the medial side of the big toe corresponds to asymmetric bone growth on the medial side of the head and to varus positioning of the first metatarsal. Surgeons and podiatrists know this, but the continued use of this term causes confusion in some nonspecialists and misleads patients.

In theory, this chapter is completely out of place here since exostectomy is not a treatment for hallux valgus. Nevertheless, it is relevant because it summarizes the general procedures employed during percutaneous surgery: beaver blade use, working space creation, careful burring movement, and meticulous removal of bone debris.

7.2 Technique

The skin entry point is located on the inferomedial side of the first metatarsal head, behind and against the medial sesamoid (Fig. 7.1). The incision is made with a beaver blade, angled 20–40° upward, outward, and forward. The blade penetrates directly into the capsule until it makes con-

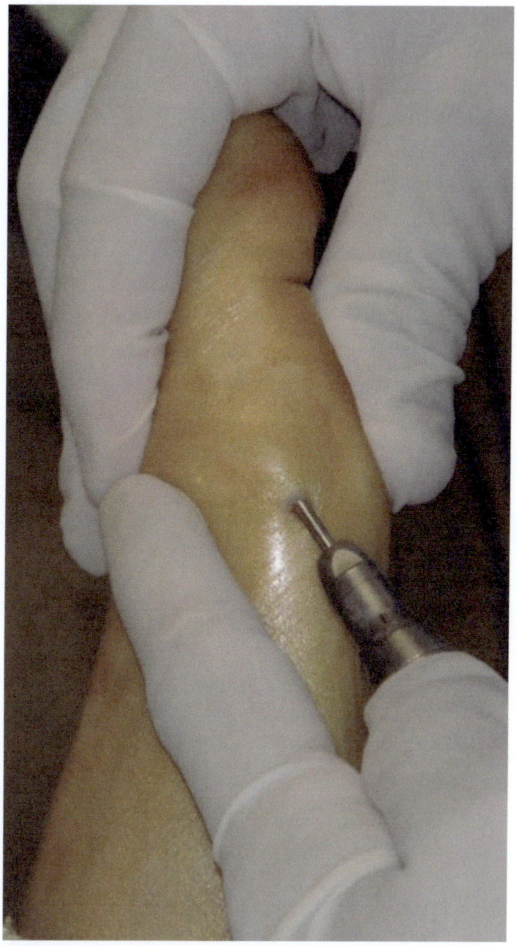

Fig. 7.1 Entry point for exostectomy. © Cyrille Cazeau 2015. All Rights Reserved

C. Cazeau (✉)
Clinique Victor Hugo, Paris, France

C. Cazeau, Y. Stiglitz (eds.), *Percutaneous and Minimally Invasive Foot Surgery*,
https://doi.org/10.1007/978-3-030-98791-6_7

tact with the medial side of the first metatarsal head. The capsule is carefully detached from the bone surface using repetitive motions, in the subperiosteal plane, with a beaver blade then a raspatory or elevator (see Chap.3). We want to emphasize that percutaneous surgery consists of doing manipulations in spaces that we need to create anatomically, unlike arthroscopy where the space already exists. The removal starts with a conical burr, such as a 3.1-mm or 4.1-mm wedge burr (Fig. 7.2). The work of the opposite hand is very important, like in any percutaneous procedure. For a left-handed surgeon operating on a left foot (Fig. 7.1), the right thumb and index finger pinch the metatarsal in front of the entry point. The left hand holds the powered instrument like a pencil, and the left index finger occasionally makes contact with the upper side of the first metatarsal head, such that the working hand can rest on the foot.

This prevents slipping and uncontrolled maneuvers during the procedure and provides useful proprioceptive feedback for locating landmarks. It is also a general rule for percutaneous surgery. Bone resection is done gradually by moving the burr like a windshield wiper against the medial side of the first metatarsal head. It is important to avoid placing traction or excessive tension on the skin entry point, which must remain stationary. The burr must always be buried under the skin. This can be accomplished by having the entry point located at a distance greater than the length of the burr. The bone is resected from the diaphyseal-metaphyseal junction to the articular surface while creating a flat, regular surface.

The more the medial metatarsal bone protrudes out, the lower the entry point. Bone resection is most effective when slower motor speeds are used (hence the importance of using a high torque, powered surgical tool) and the procedure is done without pressure: by applying less force, the motor turns more slowly, making the procedure safer and more effective. Progress should be checked regularly by palpating the bone through the skin and then with fluoroscopy (Fig. 7.3). Percutaneous bone resection is the procedure that generates the most bone debris. This debris must be removed meticulously. Manual pressure is used to directly

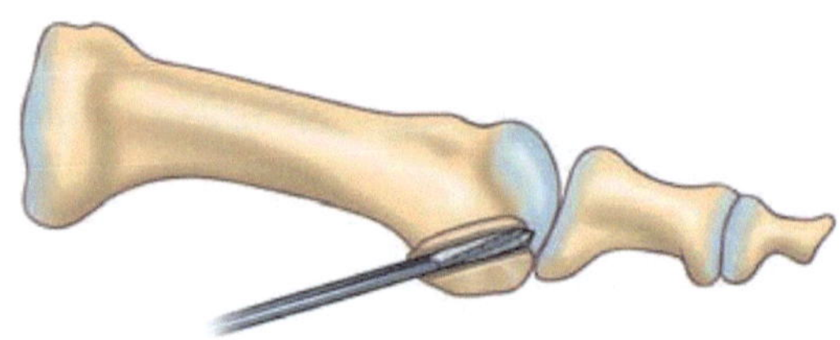

Fig. 7.2 Wedge burr used to remove bone on medial side of first metatarsal head.

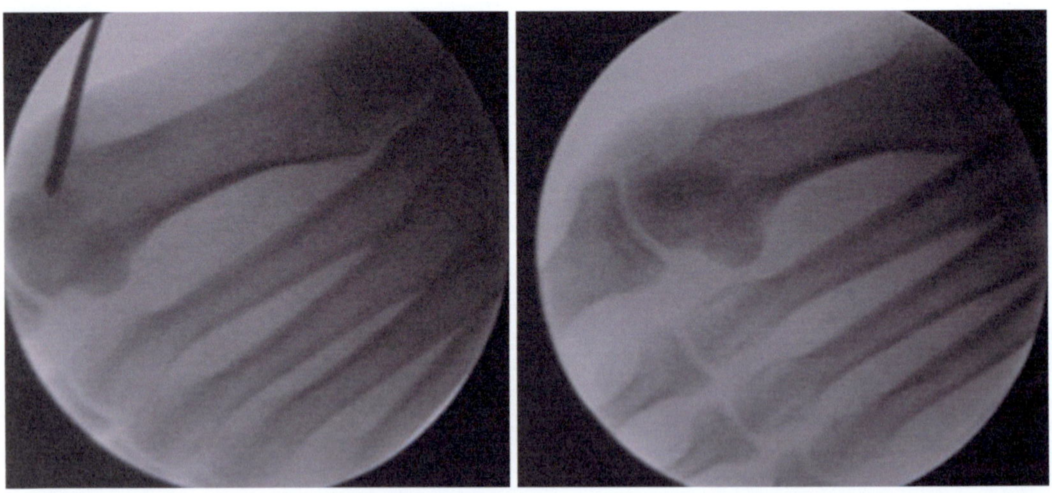

Fig. 7.3 Progress of exostectomy checked with fluoroscopy.

extract the bone paste, and a rasp can be used to scoop out bone by pointing it towards the capsule. This can be finished off by injecting saline into the working space with a pressurized syringe, then manually expelling the residual debris; if needed, a second entry point on the skin can be added to created back-and-forth pathway. A final check is done with fluoroscopy to confirm that all debris has been removed. The patient must be informed that debris could continue to be ejected for several days after the procedure.

7.3 Indications

There is a strong consensus about the fact that hallux valgus has nothing to do with exostosis, as bone did not grow in this location. Of course, exostectomy is not the means to solve the hallux deformity problem (Fig. 7.4). Nevertheless,

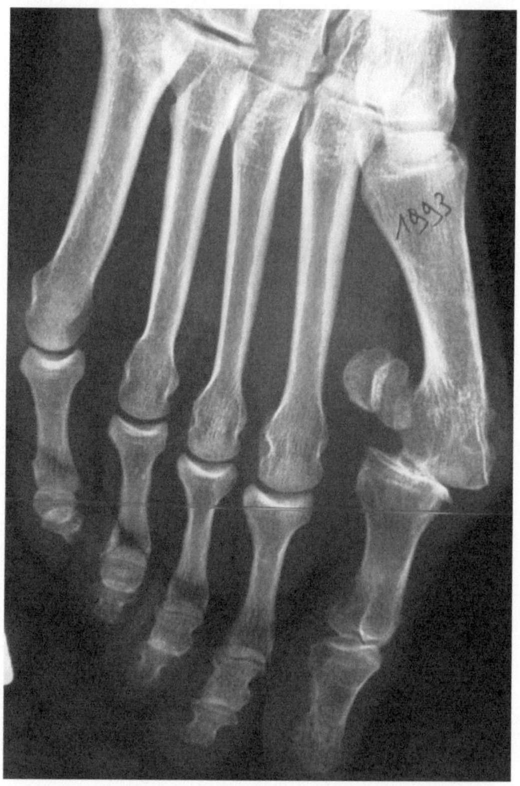

Fig. 7.4 Outcome of a hallux valgus case treated by extensive exostectomy only. © Cyrille Cazeau 2015. All Rights Reserved

decortication of the medial face may help to reduce the size of the bump and make the bone surface flatter for a future M1 osteotomy. Resecting the excess bone on the first metatarsal head eliminates the dorsal and medial rubbing that patients experience when wearing shoes.

This resection can also be done in the context of hallux rigidus where the osteophytes generate pain due to rubbing (see Arthritis chapter 20). The extent of the bone resection must be evaluated and adapted intraoperatively based on the shape of the first metatarsal head, the palpation findings, and the procedure being performed (percutaneous chevron, Reverdin-Isham osteotomy, or proximal osteotomy).

7.4 Dangers

The primary danger is hallux varus due to excessive resection (Fig. 7.5), although the risk is very low with percutaneous forefoot surgical techniques. In a surgeon's early cases, we recommend doing the burring in successive passes that are monitored by fluoroscopy. One has to be especially careful in older, osteoporotic women.

There is a risk of inflammation or necrosis at the incision related to the percutaneous surgery learning curve. Likewise, insufficient or incomplete resection (especially at the diaphysis-metaphysis junction where the capsule is firmly attached) is a typical pitfall when a surgeon is starting out. It goes without saying that it is important to perform the bone procedures only after having created a large working space, which allows the surgeon to resect bone without constraints and to verify the result with fluoroscopy as one goes along. Lastly, removing the bone debris is vital to preventing chronic inflammation and having to re-operate to clear out the remaining debris with the risk of infection and joint stiffening. We also have to point out that performing a procedure against a joint affected by osteoarthritis can trigger sudden worsening on this condition.

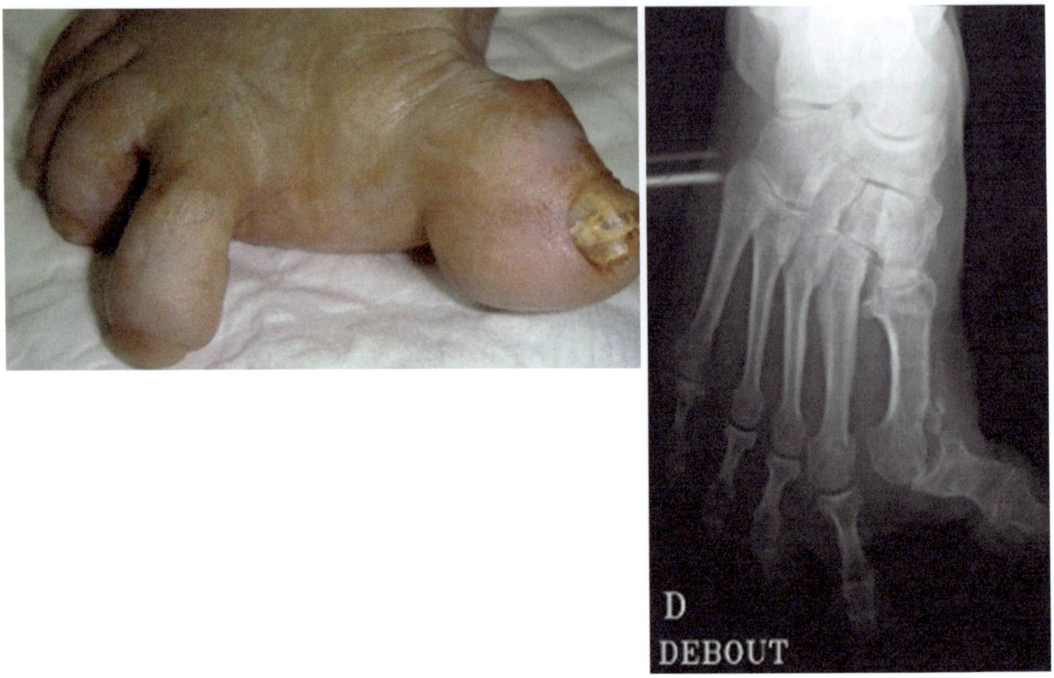

Fig. 7.5 Hallux varus due to excessive resection and excessive lateral release.

Sensing Without Seeing

- Palpate the medial side of M1 before and after the procedure to gain insight on what the patient will see and feel.
- Directly view the whitish bone paste during expulsion maneuvers.
- Feel the slackness in the soft tissues after removing the bone debris.

Editors' Point of View

This technique is included because it is part of the history of percutaneous foot surgery; it is relevant because it summarizes the steps employed during percutaneous surgery. Obviously, it is an intellectual step backward if used solely to treat hallux valgus.

8 Arthrolysis of the First Metatarsophalangeal Joint

Cyrille Cazeau

8.1 Introduction

Arthrolysis of the first metatarsophalangeal (MP1) joint consists in releasing the lateral metatarsophalangeal-sesamoid complex (Fig. 8.1) [1]. This allows the retracted elements on the concave side of the deformity to lengthen, which restores soft tissue balance and helps to correct the hallux valgus.

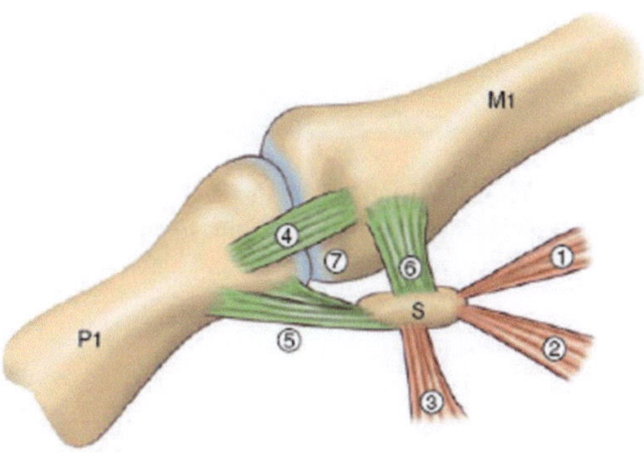

Fig. 8.1 Lateral structures at first metatarsophalangeal joint. (1) Flexor hallucis brevis, (2) Adductor hallucis (oblique head), (3) Adductor hallucis (transverse head), (4) Lateral collateral ligament, (5) Sesamoid phalangeal ligament, (6) Sesamoid metatarsal ligament, (S) Lateral sesamoid, (M1) First metatarsal, (P1) Proximal phalanx. © Cyrille Cazeau 2015. All Rights Reserved

8.2 Surgical Technique

An incision is made on the dorsal side of the MP1 joint on the lateral side of the extensor hallucis longus between 0 and 3 mm using a beaver blade. The skin is incised with the blade parallel to the tendon, to avoid damaging the tendon fibers or nerve structures. The blade penetrates into the lower half of the joint (Fig. 8.2), below the lateral collateral ligament. The correct position is achieved when it feels like the blade is stuck between the head of the first metatarsal (M1) and the base of the proximal phalanx (P1) of the hallux, and synovial fluid leaks out of the incision

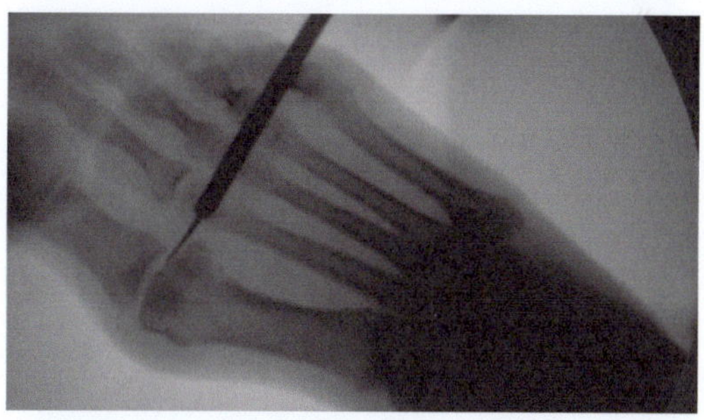

Fig. 8.2 Beaver blade entering lower half of first metatarsophalangeal joint. © Cyrille Cazeau 2015. All Rights Reserved

C. Cazeau (✉)
Clinique Victor Hugo, Paris, France

C. Cazeau, Y. Stiglitz (eds.), *Percutaneous and Minimally Invasive Foot Surgery*,
https://doi.org/10.1007/978-3-030-98791-6_8

(Figs. 8.3 and 8.4). Blade penetration can be facilitated by distracting the MP1 joint by using the opposite hand to apply axial traction on the hallux. It is recommended to angle the blade at 45° (Fig. 8.5) to approach the capsule from below and from the inside, in order to cut it under the lateral collateral ligament (Fig. 8.6). It is vital to preserve this ligament to prevent the development of hallux varus. Fluoroscopy can be used to verify the blade's position during the learning curve.

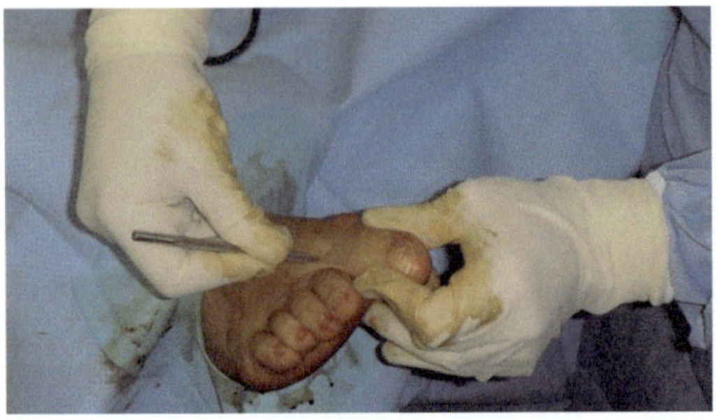

Fig. 8.3 Intraoperative view of correct incision placement.

The blade is then turned to 90°, so it parallels the metatarsophalangeal joint line and is aimed externally at the inferolateral corner of the P1 base (Fig. 8.7), where the adductor hallucis or phalangeal insertional band is inserted. The latter, which is also called the fibular sesamoid phalangeal ligament, is one of the structures that holds the lateral sesamoid to the base of the phalanx. Forcing the hallux into varus places tension on these lateral stays, making them easier to tran-

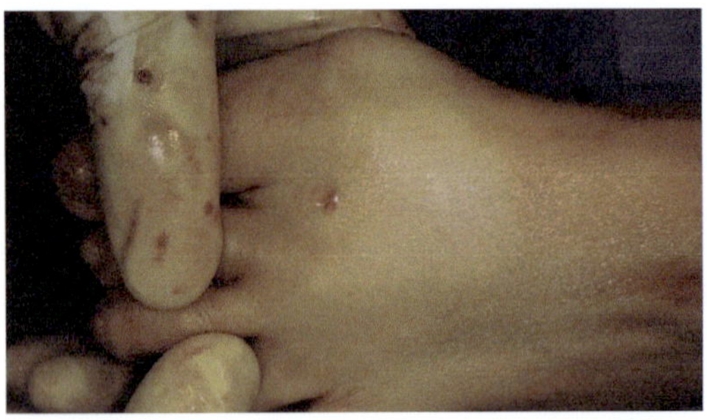

Fig. 8.4 Synovial fluid leaking out of an incision.

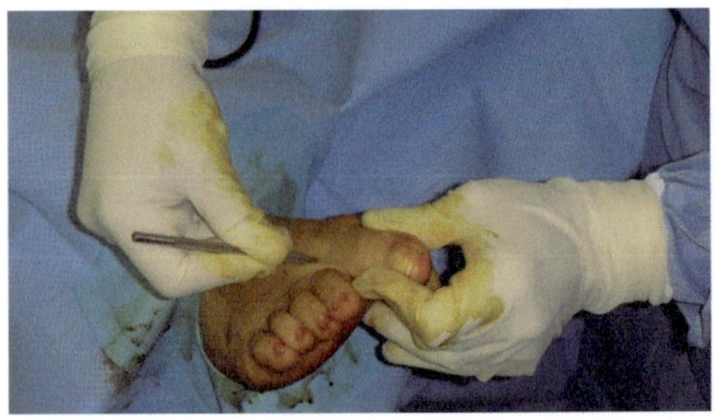

Fig. 8.5 Beaver blade angled at 45° to approach the capsule.

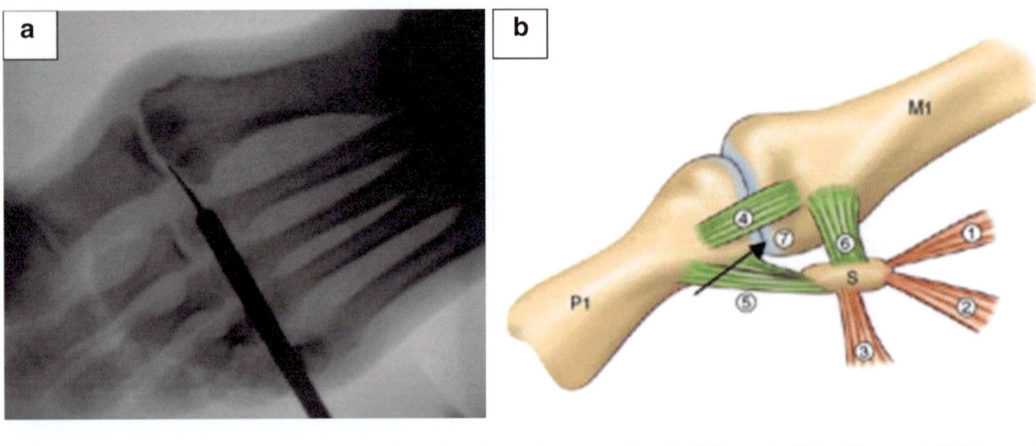

Fig. 8.6 Beaver blade positioned to cut under lateral collateral ligament. Fluoroscopy image (**a**) and drawing with target defined by black arrow (**b**). (1) Flexor hallucis brevis, (2) Adductor hallucis (oblique head), (3) Adductor hallucis (transverse head), (4) Lateral collateral ligament, (5) Sesamoid phalangeal ligament, (6) Sesamoid metatarsal ligament, (S) Lateral sesamoid, (M1) First metatarsal, (P1) Proximal phalanx.

sect with the beaver blade. Separating the lateral sesamoid from the P1 base helps to reposition it below the M1 head without increasing the intra-articular pressure. This transection is performed in the sagittal plane, from back to front, against the lateral side of the P1 base. Starting from the same capsular entry point, but this time going backward, against the lateral side of the M1 head, the sesamoid metatarsal ligament is transected as needed (Fig. 8.8). Cutting it will make it easier to reposition the M1 head above the lateral sesamoid after the osteotomy and prevent it from shifting laterally.

This arthrolysis is the same as the one described theoretically by M. de Prado and S. Isham in the Isham-Reverdin technique for the first ray. It can be very different during a more classical chevron-type osteotomy (minimally invasive or percutaneous), in which the adductor hallucis may not need to be detached from the phalanx base and in which the lateral head of the flexor hallucis brevis must be preserved: once in the joint, the blade is turned 90° toward the back to cut the suspensory ligament above the lateral sesamoid. When doing a minimally invasive procedure, this action can be done through a

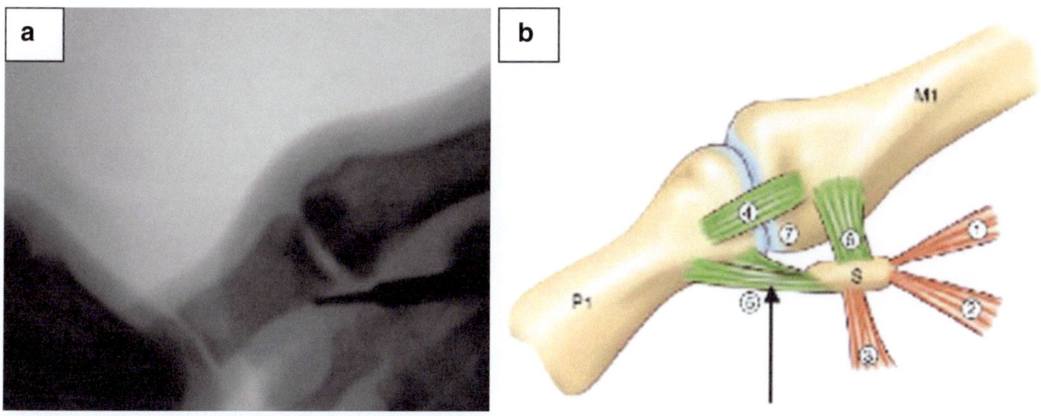

Fig. 8.7 Beaver blade aimed at inferolateral corner of the proximal phalanx base. Fluoroscopy image (**a**) and drawing with arrowing pointing at the target sesamoid phalangeal ligament (**b**).

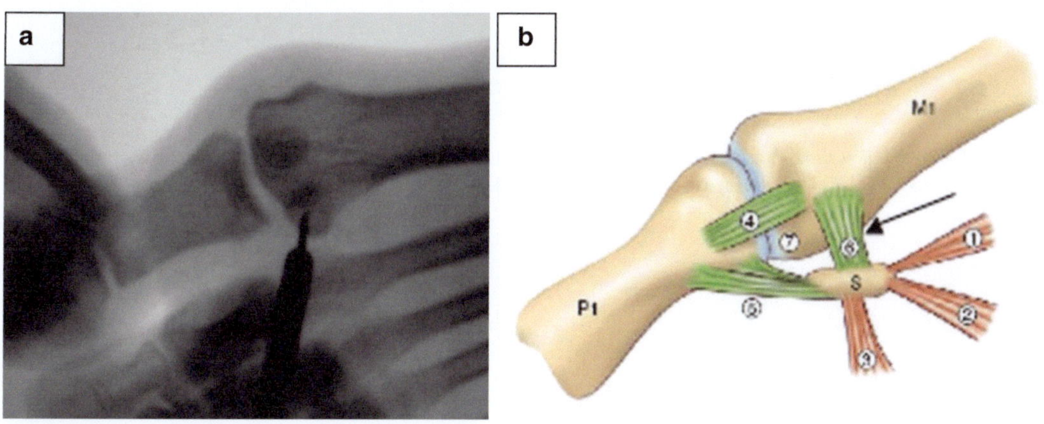

Fig. 8.8 Beaver blade positioned on lateral side of the M1 head. Fluoroscopy image (**a**) and drawing with arrowing pointing at the target sesamoid metatarsal ligament (**b**). (1) Flexor hallucis brevis, (2) Adductor hallucis (oblique head), (3) Adductor hallucis (transverse head), (4) Lateral collateral ligament, (5) Sesamoid phalangeal ligament, (6) Sesamoid metatarsal ligament, (S) Lateral sesamoid, (M1) First metatarsal, (P1) Proximal phalanx.

medial approach through the metatarsal osteotomy, by the submetatarsal approach, or even trans-articular, using Mayo scissors. There is no audible snapping, contrary to transection of the sesamoid phalangeal ligament; thus it may be safer to do it through a minimally invasive chevron approach (Fig. 8.9).

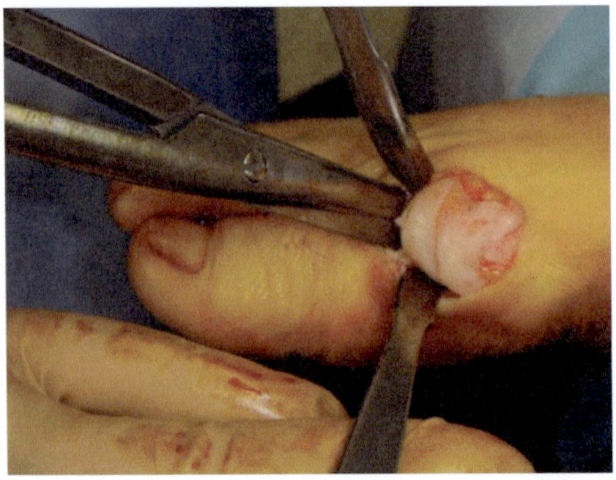

Fig. 8.9 Minimally invasive chevron approach for the arthrolysis.

8.3 Success Criteria

The criteria for success are the perception of a snap and of the joint shifting into varus during these maneuvers. Using fluoroscopy, success is defined as the absence of lateral sesamoid movement when the hallux is placed in varus (Fig. 8.10).

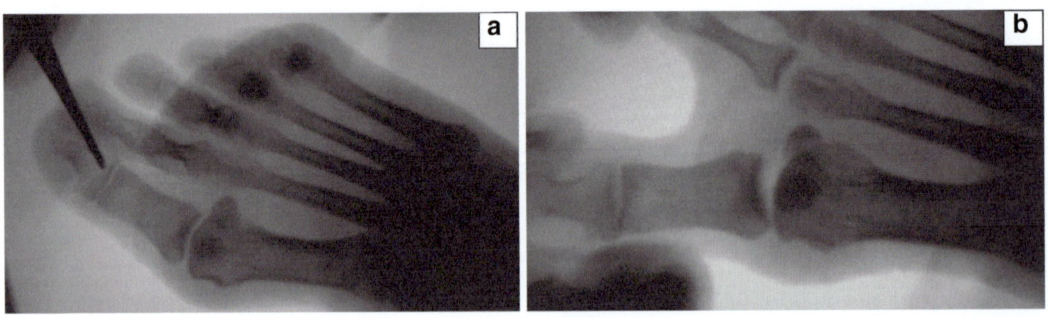

Fig. 8.10 No lateral sesamoid movement when hallux is placed in varus equals success. Original position (**a**) and forced hallux varus (**b**).

8.4 Risks

Excessive lateral release can destabilize the metatarsophalangeal joint. The biggest problem is development of hallux varus (Fig. 8.11), which is disastrous from both the patient's and the surgeon's point of view. The lateral collateral ligament must be preserved in all cases.

With insufficient release, there is a risk of the lateral sesamoid shifting laterally during M1 head translation and a risk of under-correction, with rapid recurrence of the deformity.

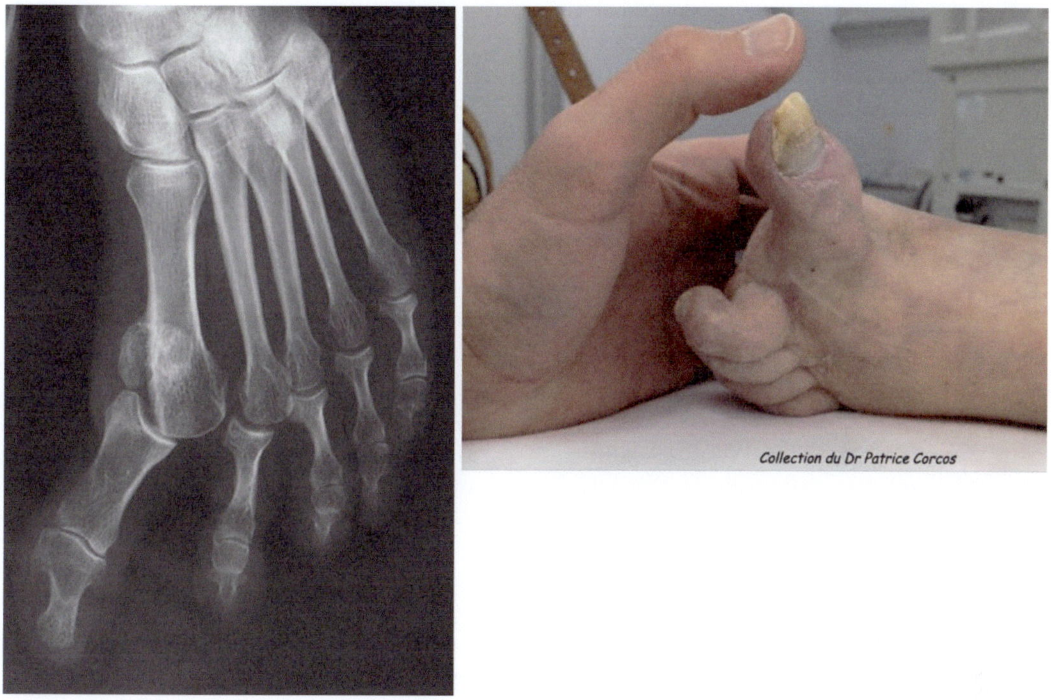

Fig. 8.11 Excessive lateral release resulting in the development of hallux varus. © Cyrille Cazeau 2015. All Rights Reserved

8.5 Indications

This lateral release procedure is a standard feature of hallux valgus correction. When the entire procedure is being done percutaneously, the release is performed before the M1 osteotomy and the hallux osteotomy, in order to work with a solid prop.

However, the strategy is more nuanced now. A partial or complete release can be done gradually, by testing the joint stability after each step while forcing the hallux into varus. Lateral release is performed in the majority of cases, but the extent of the release varies.

Sensing Without Seeing

- Feeling of beaver blade being stuck as evidence of being inside the joint.
- Leak of synovial fluid as evidence of being inside the joint.
- Feeling the contours of the phalanx when moving the bade to the proximal portion of the lateral side of the phalanx.
- Audible snap during forced hallux varus movement.
- Feeling of partial separation between M1 and P1 during varus testing after the tenotomy.

Editors' Point of View

While this procedure is universal, the exact method varies greatly between surgeons depending on which anatomical structure is targeted. This technique is valuable as every procedure can be done in a gradual manner.

Reference

1. Barouk LS, Barouk P. Reconstruction de l'avant-pied. Paris: Springer; 2006.

9 Reverdin-Isham Osteotomy

Christophe de Lavigne and Thomas Bauer

9.1 Principles

The Reverdin-Isham osteotomy is a distal osteotomy of the first metatarsal (M1) that minimally shortens it and also corrects the distal metatarsal articular angle (DMAA) (Figs. 9.1 and 9.2).

This osteotomy, which is derived from the one described by Reverdin in 1881 [1], was modified by Stephen Isham and then popularized by Mariano De Prado, which resulted in it being used to correct hallux valgus percutaneously.

The major modification that Isham made to the Reverdin osteotomy was to perform a 45° osteotomy cut from distal dorsal to proximal plantar relative to the M1 axis and finishing behind the sesamoids. Because of this orientation, the Reverdin-Isham osteotomy is more stable than the Reverdin osteotomy while achieving the same DMAA correction.

Also, intra-articular retraction and stiffness are minimized since it is located behind the sesamoids. The principle of this osteotomy consists in removing the nonfunctional cartilage (dorsomedial portion of metatarsal head) and then reloading the functional cartilage after reorientation due to varus shift and plantar flexion of the M1 head. No bone fixation is required because the oblique osteotomy cut and the lateral cortical hinge are self-stabilizing.

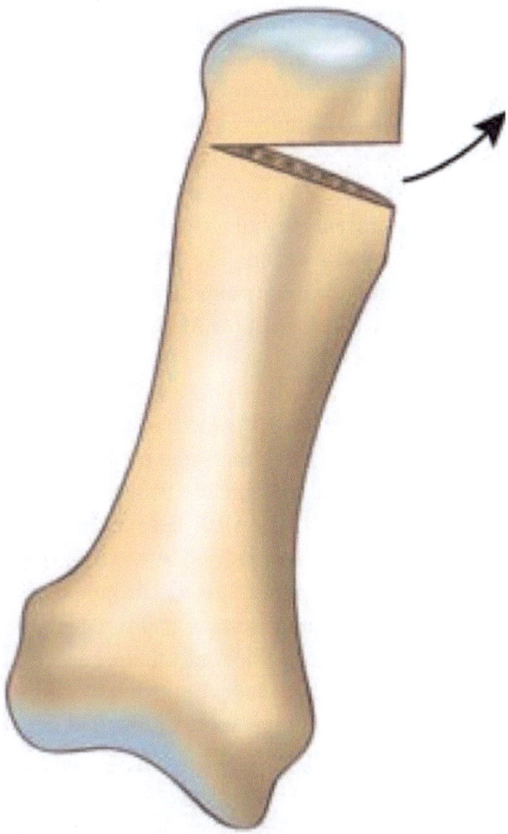

Fig. 9.1 Reverdin-Isham osteotomy of the first metatarsal. © Christophe de Lavigne 2015. All Rights Reserved

C. de Lavigne (✉)
Clinique du Sport, Merignac, France
e-mail: secdrdelavigne@gmail.com

T. Bauer
Orthopedic Department, Ambroise Paré University Hospital, Boulogne-Billancourt, France
e-mail: thomas.bauer@aphp.fr

C. Cazeau, Y. Stiglitz (eds.), *Percutaneous and Minimally Invasive Foot Surgery*,
https://doi.org/10.1007/978-3-030-98791-6_9

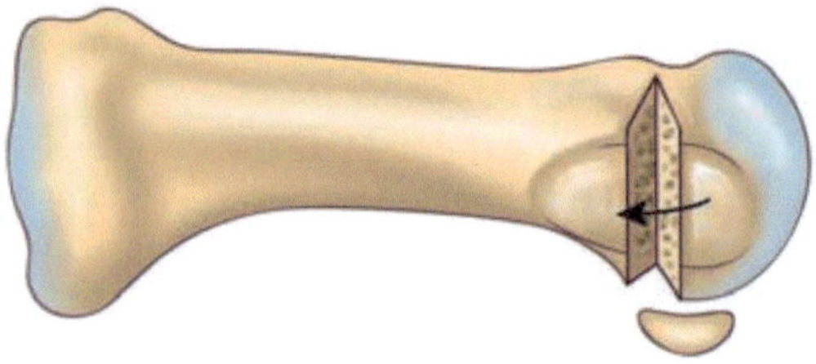

Fig. 9.2 Reverdin-Isham osteotomy of the first metatarsal.

9.2 Surgical Technique

The patient is positioned supine with his foot hanging off the table to facilitate the surgical procedures and fluoroscopy checks. After making a 3–5 mm incision on the medial and plantar side of the M1 head, immediately behind the medial sesamoid, the metatarsophalangeal joint's capsule is detached, and a working space is created around the M1 head using a beaver blade and elevators (see Chap. 3 on instruments). The Reverdin-Isham osteotomy is performed after bone is removed from the medial M1 head. Since this is a closing wedge osteotomy, more bone is resected from the M1 head than in other M1 osteotomies to prevent the reappearance of a medial bump after head rotation. The bone resection is checked with fluoroscopy and then extended into the functional cartilage of the M1 head, inside the medial groove.

After the bone debris is removed, the Reverdin-Isham osteotomy is performed with a straight burr introduced through the same approach. The burr's tip is placed immediately behind the superior articular surface of the M1 head and its position verified with fluoroscopy. The osteotomy cut (Fig. 9.3) is made parallel to the metatarsophalangeal joint's articular surface and directed distal dorsal (immediately behind superior articular surface) to proximal plantar (immediately behind sesamoids) at an average angle of 45° relative to the M1 axis. The metatarsal's lateral cortex must be preserved. The surgeon holds the hallux between his thumb and index finger and then forcefully places it in varus and plantar flexion (Figs. 9.4 and 9.5). This closes the medial wedge, compresses the osteotomy site, and corrects the DMAA (Fig. 9.6). Fluoroscopy is used to check the closure of the osteotomy with the foot placed in 45° dorsiflexion relative to the X-rays, which provides the best view of the osteotomy site. If the DMAA correction is not satisfactory, it means that either the lateral cortical hinge is too thick and the osteotomy cannot close (most common scenario) or the closure and medial compression are not sufficient (this occurs in cases with very large DMAA).

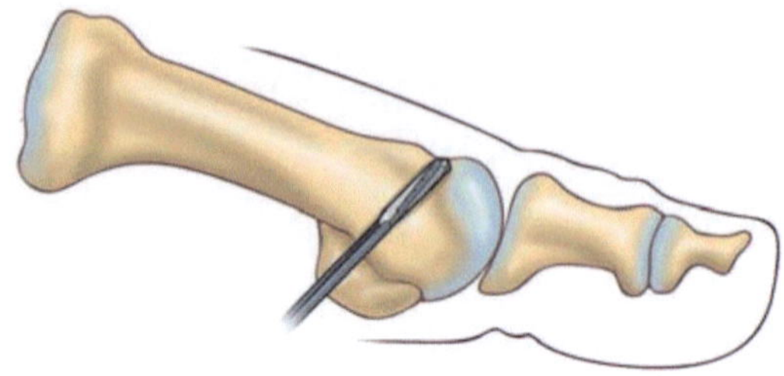

Fig. 9.3 Orientation of the burr to perform the osteotomy.

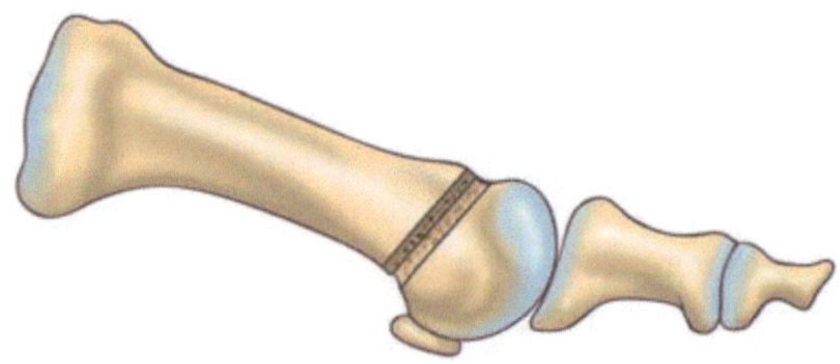

Fig. 9.4 Medial closing wedge and lateral cortical hinge resulting from the osteotomy cut.

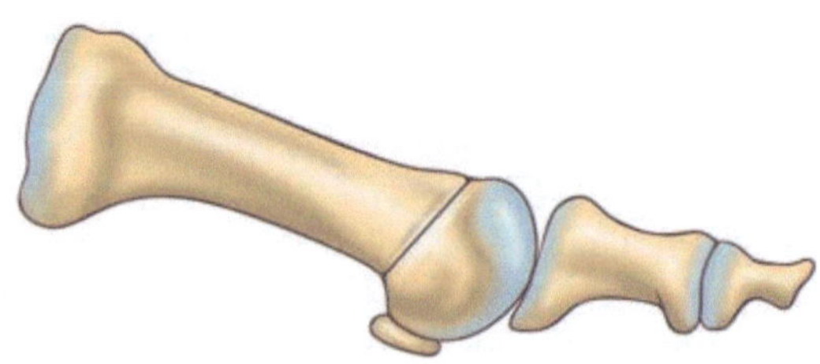

Fig. 9.5 Result after the osteotomy is closed by forcing the hallux into varus.

When the hinge is too thick, it must be thinned out more by introducing the straight burr in the same position but pushing it more laterally to weaken the lateral cortex. Often, the hinge is the

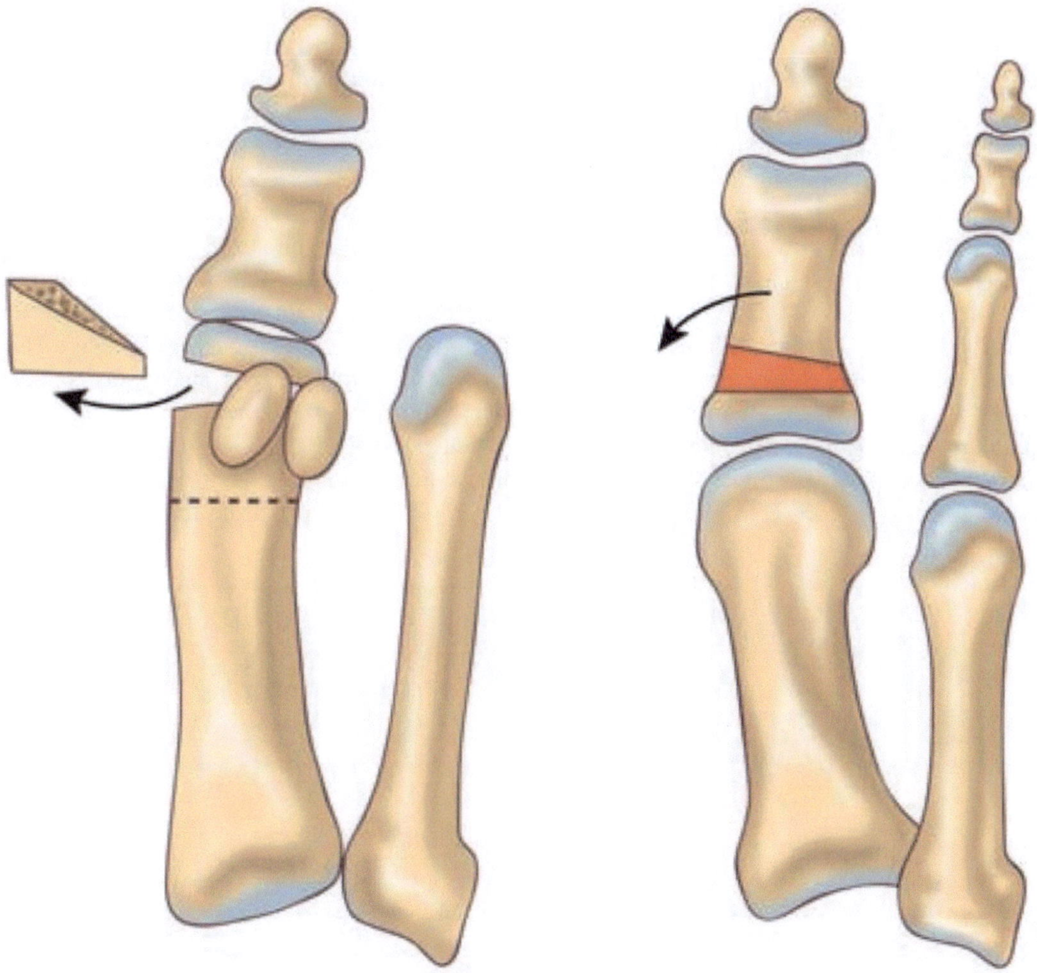

Fig. 9.6 Closing wedge osteotomies: M1 (left) and proximal phalanx (right).

thickest and strongest on the lateral and plantar side of the metatarsal. If the preoperative DMAA is very large, a conical burr may be needed to resect a larger medial wedge, which will subsequently allow for greater correction. Lateral release is performed only after the DMAA has been corrected and after confirming the correction is sufficient and the osteotomy is self-stabilizing. In fact, once the lateral release has been performed, it is impossible to correct the DMAA through varus movements induced on the hallux.

9.3 Indications and Results

The ideal indication for hallux valgus correction using the Reverdin-Isham osteotomy is a foot with moderate deformity (hallux valgus <30° and metatarsus adductus <16°) and a large DMAA (>10°). This procedure has been reported to reduce the hallux valgus angle by 50% (28°–14°), reduce the DMAA by 50% (15°–8°), and alter the metatarsus varus slightly (13°–10°).

9.4 Risks and Complications

The main complication is rupture of the lateral cortical hinge of the osteotomy which can occur intraoperatively or postoperatively. This has been reported in 3% of cases but did not require fixation since the oblique osteotomy cut is intrinsically stable.

The risk of stiffness in the metatarsophalangeal joint of the first ray (MTP1) after Reverdin-Isham osteotomy is related to its very distal position near the joint. Stiffness has been reported in 17% of patients at 1 year of follow-up (90° overall range of motion preoperatively and 75° at 1 year postoperative). The biggest risk is that this will slow down the recovery of range of motion (3–6 months) in patients with preoperative stiffness or pre-existing metatarsophalangeal osteoarthritis; this justifies a rehabilitation prescription after 1 month.

Overcorrection of the DMAA happens because of an incorrect indication (normal or minimally increased preoperative DMAA), a technical error (rupture of lateral cortical hinge, excessive medial resection, overcorrection due to the dressing or toe orthotic use), or poor bone quality (osteoporosis, rheumatoid arthritis). This may cause postoperative incongruity of the MTP1 joint.

The postoperative dressing is critical because no bone fixation is used (Fig. 9.7). This is described in detail in a dedicated chapter.

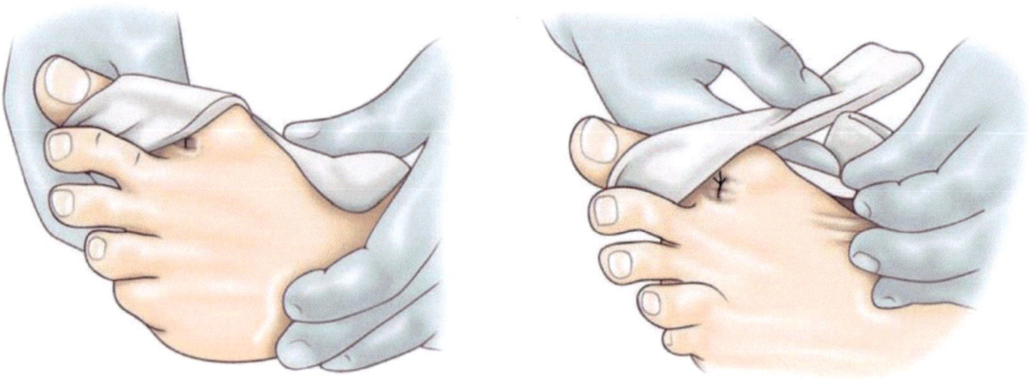

Fig. 9.7 Postoperative dressing. © Christophe de Lavigne 2015. All Rights Reserved

Editors' Point of View

Like exostectomy, this technique is part of the history of percutaneous foot surgery and is a great example of the sequence of essential steps that needs to be performed in the newer techniques. Mathematically, it can only correct the DMMA, not any other deformities, especially metatarsus varus, which is the most important deformity. The way this osteotomy was taught was misleading and inadequate, as it incorporated percutaneous into this very incomplete technique, by combining it with exostectomy. This added fuel to the fire for those who oppose percutaneous surgery, who hold on to their old practices and who ridicule new ones.

Reference

1. Reverdin J. De la déviation en dehors du gros orteil (hallux valgus, vulg. "oignon", "bunions", "Ballen") et de son traitement chirurgical. Trans Internat Med Congress. 1881;2:508–12.

Further Reading

de Prado M, Ripoll PL, Vaquero J, Golanó P. Tratamiento quirúrgico pecutáneo del hallux valgus mediante osteotomías múltiples. Rev Ortoped Traumatol. 2003;47:406–16.

de Prado M, Ripoll PL, Golanó P. Cirugía percutánea del pie: técnicas quirúrgicas, indicaciones, bases anatómicas. Barcelona: Masson; 2003.

Canovas F, Poirée G, Bonnel F, Vergnes N, Nicolau F, el Hammami R. Radiographic analysis of the orientation of the distal articular surface of the first metatarsal in the horizontal plane [article in French]. Rev Chir Orthop Reparatrice Appar Mot. 1998;84:546–9.

Coughlin MJ. Hallux valgus in men: effect of the distal metatarsal articular angle on hallux valgus correction. Foot Ankle. 1997;18:463–70.

Isham SA. The Reverdin-Isham procedure for the correction of hallux abducto valgus. A distal metatarsal osteotomy procedure. Clin Podiatr Med Surg. 1991;8:81–94.

Andreasi A, Coppo M. L'intervento di Reverdin-Gren modificato nel truittamento quirurgico dell'alluce abdono-valgo. In: Gaggi A, editor. Progresi in Medicina e Chirurgia del Piede. L'alluce valgo. Bologna: Aulo Gaggi; 1997. p. 105–14.

Laffenêtre O, Cermolacce C, Coillard JY, et al. Chirurgie mini-invasive de l'hallux valgus. In: Valtin B, Leemrijse T, editors. Cahiers d'enseignement de la SOFCOT: chirurgie de l'avant-pied. Paris: Elsevier SAS; 2005. p. 96–104.

Bauer T, de Lavigne C, Biau D, De Prado M, Isham S, Laffenétre O. Percutaneous hallux valgus surgery: a prospective multicenter study of 189 cases. Orthop Clin North Am. 2009;40:505–14.

Minimally Invasive Chevron Osteotomy

10

Patrice Determe and Stéphane Guillo

10.1 Introduction

Several procedures have been described for correcting hallux valgus. Conventional open techniques are effective and reliable, although they are associated with a certain morbidity given the inevitable soft tissue damage. At the other end of the spectrum, percutaneous techniques are said to be less damaging but have their own set of problems. Command over the bone correction is less effective since; by definition, it is not done under direct visual control. The absence of standard fixation may cause secondary displacements that negatively impact the outcome. Also, the burrs used in percutaneous surgery can cause lesions and burns in the periosseous soft tissues, which can trigger inflammatory flare-ups that can compromise the final outcome and stiffen the joint. Any bone debris left in and around the joint will also contribute to this stiffness and periarticular inflammation.

Our technique combines the advantages of conventional and percutaneous techniques. The qualifier *minimally invasive* is justified here. This technique is one of the GREMIP's trademarks since it is derived directly from the group's integration and evaluation of percutaneous surgery. The underlying principle consists of performing a chevron osteotomy with fixation through a minimally invasive approach. A percutaneous Akin osteotomy can be added if needed.

This is an example of a successful marriage between conventional and percutaneous surgery. We believe our technique combines the best of both.

10.2 Patient Positioning

Nowadays, this surgery is mainly performed in an outpatient setting. As with every forefoot surgery, hallux valgus correction by distal chevron osteotomy is performed with regional anesthesia, which is started in the pre-anesthesia room.

For this procedure, the sciatic nerve or its terminal branches innervating the surgical incision area, and all the foot bones must be anesthetized. Ultrasound is used to identify the nerves in question, which improves the reliability of this nerve block and induces very distal anesthesia that preserves the foot's motor control. Long-lasting local anesthesia (naropeine or levobupivacaine) contributes to postoperative analgesia. Dexamethasone, which is used as an adjuvant for local anesthetics (intravenous or perineural), helps to extend their action beyond the first 24 h. Consequently, the postoperative pain can be controlled fully by the paracematol–NSAID combination.

P. Determe (✉)
Clinique Médipôle Garonne, Toulouse, France

S. Guillo
Clinique du Sport, Merignac, France

C. Cazeau, Y. Stiglitz (eds.), *Percutaneous and Minimally Invasive Foot Surgery*,
https://doi.org/10.1007/978-3-030-98791-6_10

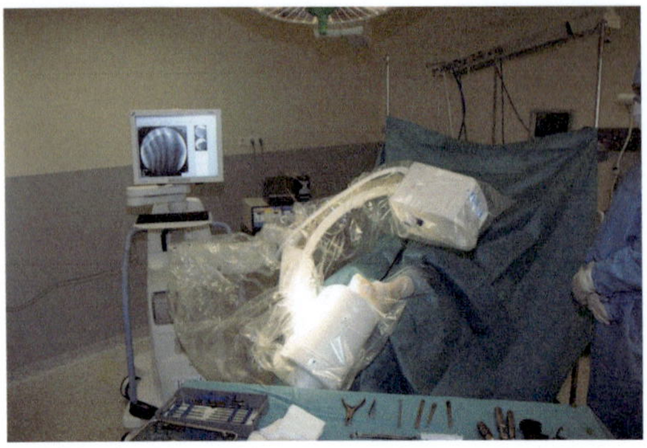

Fig. 10.1 Fluoroscopy used intraoperatively.

The procedure is done with a tourniquet and the patient supine on the operating table. The foot is prepared as usual. For practical reason, one should make sure the contralateral foot is not in the way; the knee of the non-operated leg can be flexed, or this foot lowered if the surgical table allows it.

Fluoroscopy is used throughout the procedure to verify the bone cuts and the positioning of the fixation devices (Fig. 10.1).

10.3 Surgical Technique

10.3.1 Skin Incision

A 2–3 cm incision is made on the medial side of the hallux metatarsophalangeal joint at the junction between the plantar and dorsal skin. A small wedge of skin can be removed to improve the exposure. The capsule is opened while making sure to avoid the sensory subcutaneous branch typically found on the medial side of the capsule. Another quarter wedge can be removed from the capsule to optimize the view of the surgical site (Fig. 10.2).

10.3.2 Arthrolysis

Arthrolysis is not performed automatically in every case. It is important to remember that its role is to allow the bone structures to be repositioned correctly. If overly flexible, it can be useless or even dangerous. Excessive lateral release, even when performed percutaneously, increases the risk of overcorrection.

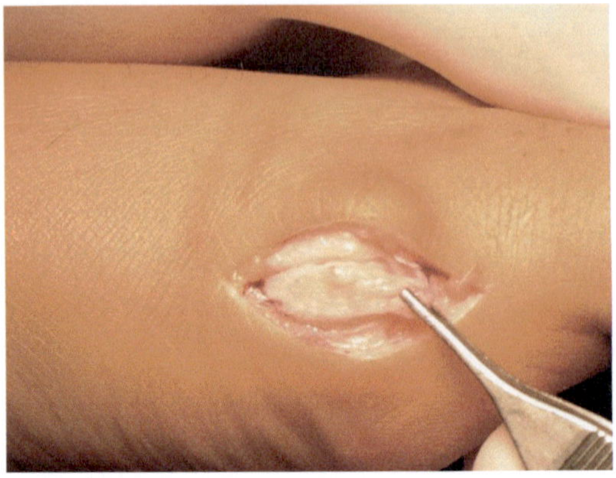

Fig. 10.2 Skin incision and removal of capsule wedge.

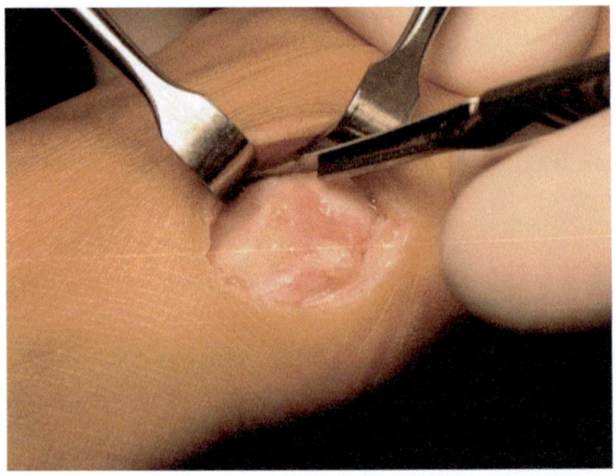

Fig. 10.3 Metatarsophalangeal arthrolysis.

The first step of the correction consists of meticulous metatarsophalangeal arthrolysis. For us, this arthrolysis consists mainly in transecting the metatarsosesamoid ligament or lateral sesamoid phalangeal ligament to allow mobilization of the sesamoid band and allow the head to be repositioned correctly on the sesamoids after the osteotomy (Fig. 10.3).

In many cases, a medial meniscus-like structure will be present. It must be removed. This is one reason why the minimally invasive approach is best here, since percutaneous first metatarsal

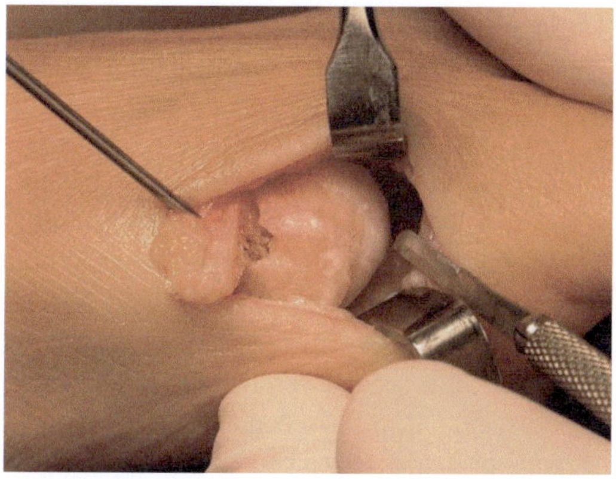

Fig. 10.4 Trans-articular lateral capsulotomy.

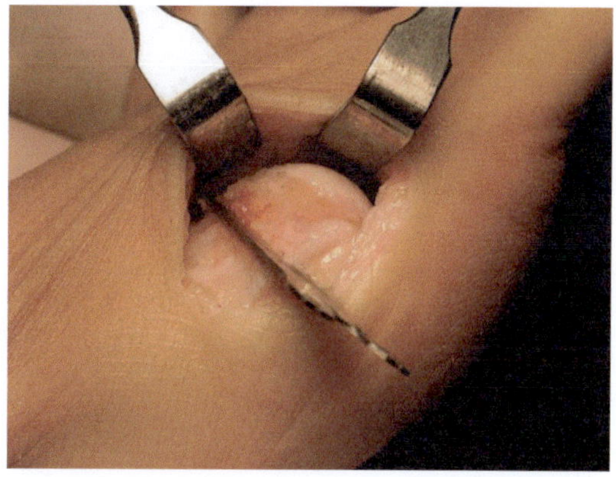

Fig. 10.5 Metatarsal osteotomy: the first cut is dorsal, 5 mm proximal to the articular surface.

surgery does not allow for intra-articular exploration. The degeneration of this meniscus may explain why certain cases of moderate hallux valgus are very painful, especially congenital ones.

In cases where the chevron osteotomy has been performed but the head does not translate easily, lateral capsulotomy (Fig. 10.4) with or without tendon detachment (adductor hallucis, lateral band of flexor hallucis brevis) may be necessary. Obviously, this release is performed only in cases of excessive contracture.

The metatarsal head and phalanx base are released from their capsular attachments, while preserving the feeder vessels, especially in the area of the metatarsal head.

10.3.3 Metatarsal Osteotomy

The metatarsal osteotomy requires a combination of two or three bone cuts:

- The first cut is roughly vertical and parallel to the metatarsophalangeal joint. It is located about 5 mm behind the articular surface and is 5 mm deep (Fig. 10.5). This is the opportunity to shorten the metatarsal (Fig. 10.6) or redo a second cut behind it (Fig. 10.7).
- The second cut is more horizontal (Fig. 10.8). Its distal origin is the deep portion of the first (verti-

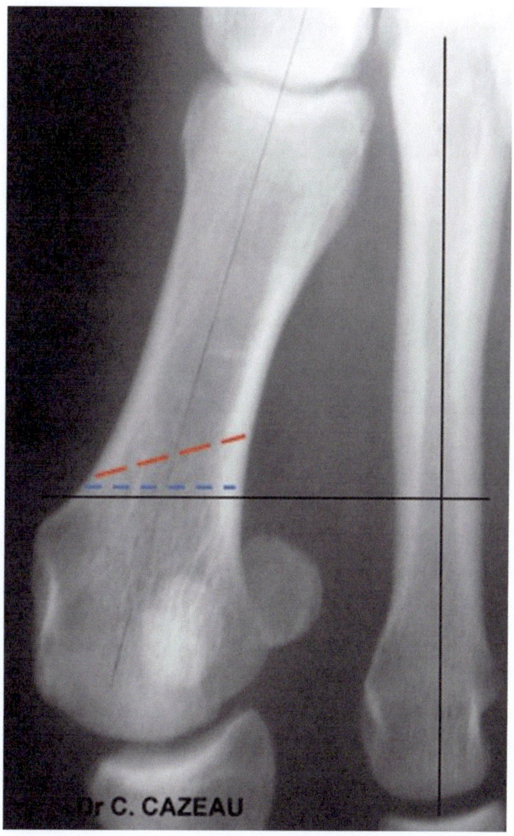

Fig. 10.6 The metatarsal can be shortened making a superior oblique cut directed backwards and laterally (red dotted line). A cut perpendicular to the second metatarsal axis (blue dotted line) will maintain the metatarsal's current length.

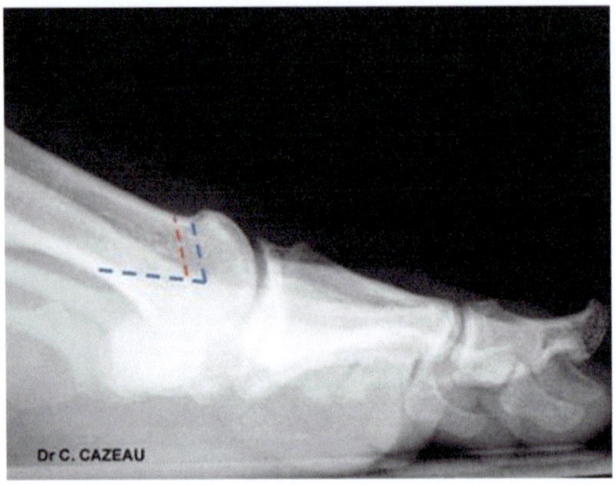

Fig. 10.7 Shortening of metatarsal after making the second cut (red dotted line) behind the first vertical cut (blue dotted line).

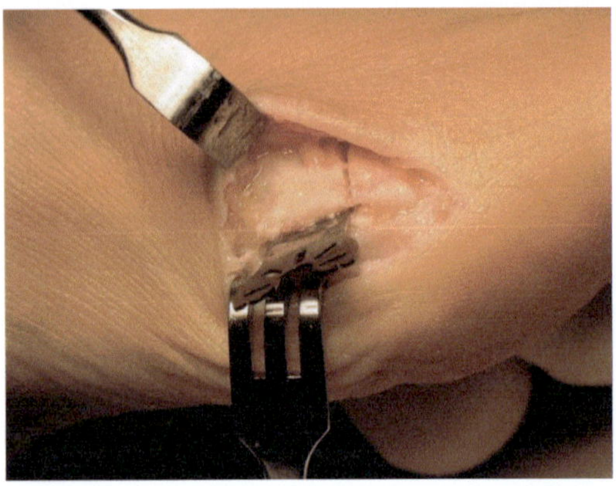

Fig. 10.8 Second osteotomy cut is closer to horizontal.

cal) cut. It is angled downward and backward, ending behind the feeder vessels at the head. The saw will be roughly oriented toward the fifth metatarsal, although it can be aligned more dorsal or plantar as needed. This cut is the opportunity to perform lowering (Fig. 10.9). Some surgeons inverse the order of these two cuts.

- If the metatarsal head angle (DMAA) also needs to be corrected or the metatarsal bone shortened, a second vertical cut can be done perpendicular to the second metatarsal axis to remove a parallelepiped of cortical bone (Fig. 10.10). This brings the articular surface of the first metatarsal perpendicular to this axis, thereby bringing the DM2A angle to zero [1], which increases the probability the correction will be maintained over the long term.

At this stage, it is important to release the soft tissues around the osteotomy cuts to facilitate M1 head translation. This can be done using an osteotome, which is placed medially and laterally against the bone cuts (Fig. 10.11). This releases the periosteum and all the attachments, especially any remnants of the lateral sesamoid phalangeal ligament.

Generally, the head translation occurs without any problems. The head can be pushed manually; small forceps can be used to stabilize the proximal portion of the metatarsal at the same time (push-pull maneuver).

Fig. 10.9 Lowering can be achieved with this osteotomy by orienting the second cut downward.

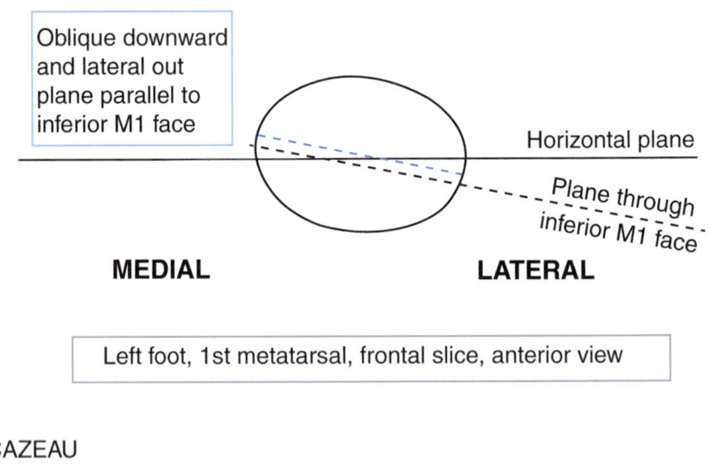

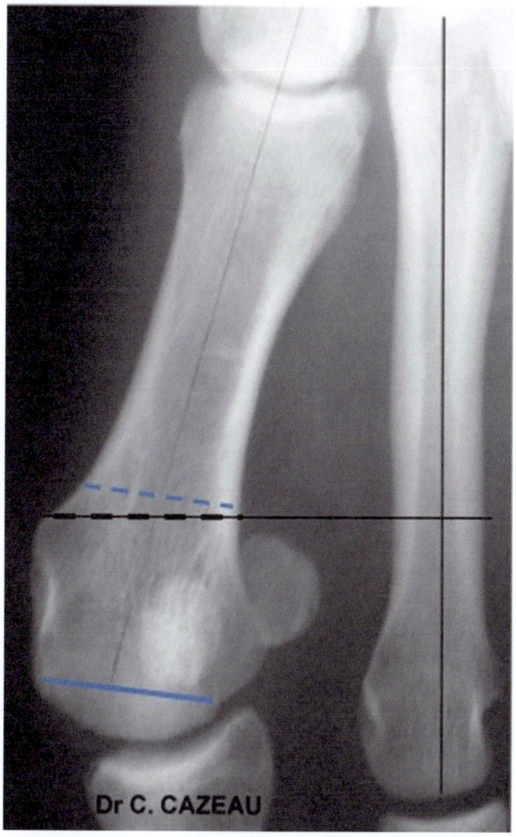

Fig. 10.10 The first cut (black dotted line) is made perpendicular to M2, and the second cut (blue dotted line) is parallel to the M1 articular surface (solid blue line) to correct the DMAA.

However, the head may unintentionally rotate during this translation. Most of the time, this rotation happens because of excess tension in the skeleton, which may require additional metatarsal shortening or supplemental arthrolysis as described previously.

Once the head is in the correct position, it is stabilized temporarily with a K-wire (Fig. 10.12), which acts as a clamp and allows the resulting correction to be checked with fluoroscopy. A load simulation is also done at this point.

10.3.4 Correction Checks

Since this is a bone correction, it is important for the foot to be aligned and stable before the capsule is closed. Several parameters must be verified to ensure good correction. These checks are done with simulated loading:

- Confirm good congruency of the P1 base by making sure it is aligned correctly with the head (no medial overhang, no lateral subluxation).
- Uniform mobility and no impingement with fixation devices.
- Good balance of the metatarsal loading points.

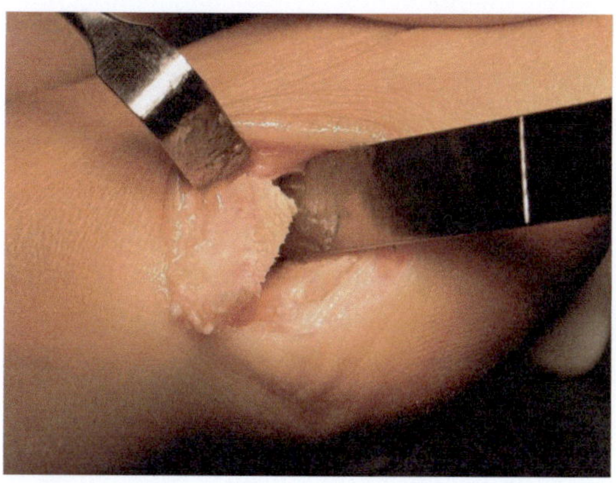

Fig. 10.11 Osteotome used to release soft tissues around osteotomy site.

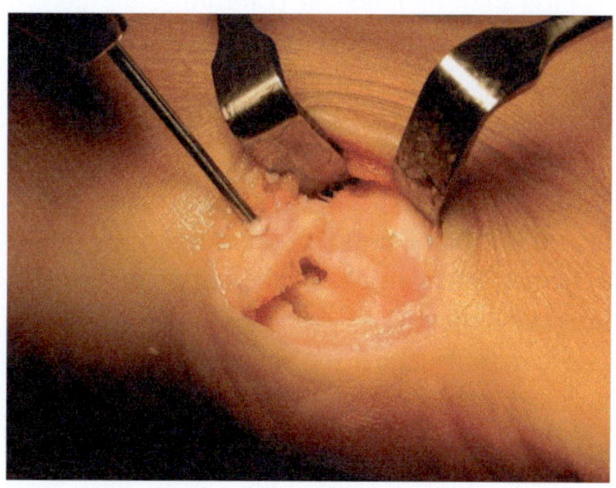

Fig. 10.12 K-wire inserted to stabilize osteotomy site temporarily.

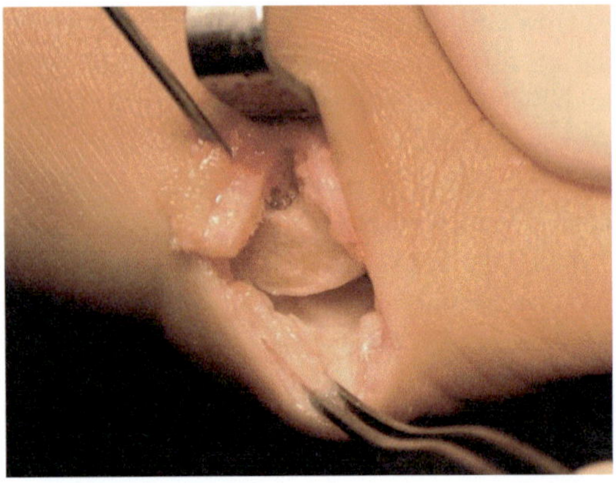

Fig. 10.13 Medial sesamoid position is verified to ensure it is recentered correctly under the M1 head.

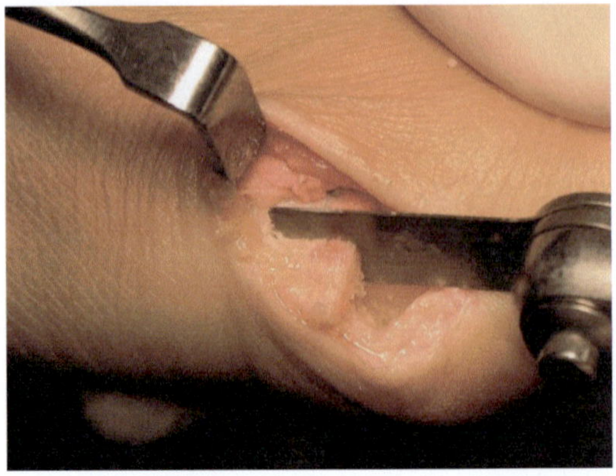

Fig. 10.14 Oscillating saw used to recut the extra-articular bone overhang.

- Classically, the sesamoids must be recentered under the M1 head; this is verified at the medial base of the sesamoids (Fig. 10.13).
- Of course, a fluoroscopy check is desirable here.

10.3.5 Fixation

The correction is fixed using the surgeon's preferred method. One or even two screws are preferable to other fixation methods, especially K-wires that provides less good hold. Double fixation may be better at controlling the head's rotation. This variation is especially relevant when more than 50% offset is present. These screws must be stable to prevent displacement upon weight-bearing.

When using double-screw fixation, the first is inserted from the dorsal cortex toward the center of the metatarsal head, and the second is typically inserted vertically.

We remove the temporary K-wire after the first screw has been inserted and then use an oscillating saw to recut the extra-articular bone overhang present after the head has been translated (Fig. 10.14). The final position of the head will be set after the second screw has been inserted.

10.3.6 Additional Procedures

10.3.6.1 Akin Osteotomy

In cases of lateral toe deviation, required shortening or derotation, an Akin osteotomy is performed as described in the dedicated chapter.

10.3.6.2 Lengthening of Extensor Mechanism

Stable correction requires that dislocating forces be eliminated. The extensor hallucis longus can destabilize the joint; thus, one of the roles of the Akin osteotomy is to recenter this tendon's moment arm. Tendon lengthening may be required to achieve this balance. This can be done in two ways, depending on the clinical findings:

- In the case of distal IP hyperextension, lengthening can be performed percutaneously over the dorsal face of the IP joint. Dorsal capsulotomy is performed at the same time using a beaver blade. The blade is inserted under the skin, and the capsule opened from superficial to deep.
- If the tendon bows dorsally, lengthening is achieved with a Z-plasty. Two-tiered transverse semi-cuts are made near the metatarsophalangeal joint, one distal lateral and the

other proximal medial. Plantar hyperflexion is then applied to the metatarsophalangeal joint to allow the two half-tendons to slide relative to each other.

10.4 Closure and Dressing

Closure is initiated once the correction has been achieved, fixed, and confirmed. The standard procedure is to lavage the operated area with saline to remove any remaining bone debris generated by the bone cuts. The capsule is closed without tension using absorbable suture. By initially performing exostectomy, the resulting bone decortication greatly contributes to repairing the medial ligament and capsule layer. No drain is used. The superficial and cutaneous layers are closed as usual.

The foot is bandaged using saline-soaked gauze, which acts as a soft cast that helps to maintain the correction. It is redone after 15 days during the follow-up visit with the surgeon. The postoperative dressing is fashioned depending on whether additional surgical procedures were done on the lateral rays. It is left in place for 10–15 days.

10.5 Postoperative Course

Immediate full weight-bearing is allowed with an appropriate rigid postoperative shoe. The rockered sole protects the forefoot while preserving the mechanics of walking and balance as much as possible.

Special care is taken to combat edema, with the patient instructed to keep the foot elevated and given a prescription for NSAIDs and for lymphatic drainage. If the patient has no risk factors, it is not necessary to prescribe anticoagulants.

The dressing is redone after 15 days and the patient allowed to resume activities gradually.

The ideal indication for hallux valgus correction by minimally invasive chevron osteotomy is a foot with minor to moderate deformity (hallux valgus <40° and metatarsus adductus <20°). This procedure has been reported to correct the hallux valgus angle by 70% (30°–8.5°), reduce the DMAA by 42% (13°–7.5°), and reduce the metatarsus adductus angle by 40% (13°–7.6°) [2].

This strategy expands the indications for an Isham-Reverdin-like percutaneous technique, while copying the management from a percutaneous-only surgery.

Editors' Point of View

The chevron stems from early distal M1 osteotomies that were introduced in the late 19th century. Between the initial technique described by Reverdin (1881) and the one adopted by Richardson (1999), modifications were made by Green, Laird, Todd, Mitchel, Wilson, and Lindgren. The V-cut described by Austin was a true innovation and was repeated by Johnson and Cofield; it was popularized in France by Patrice Diebold. The chevron was reduced as much as possible in the context of MIS. It provides surgeons with an opportunity to correct deformities in all three planes and confers mechanical stability that allows immediate full weight bearing. The instantaneous lateral displacement of the M1 head after separating the final bone bridge shows the difference in the elastic potential energy between the lateral and medial elements of the MTP1 joint. The spontaneous displacement, which can be "encouraged" by a pull-and-push action, stops when the static equilibrium (force and moment) occurs. This is highly likely correlated with a reduction in pain.

References

1. Coillard JY, Determe P, Diebold P, Roussignol X. Poster 86: the use of a new angle (DM2AA) for the surgical planification of hallux valgus. In: 2nd Joint Meeting of International Federation of Foot and Ankle Societies (IFFAS). 2005, Groupe Talus Naples.
2. Lahrach H. Chirurgie de l'hallux valgus par chevron mini-invasif: suivi prospectif de 172 pieds. Mémoire pour le DIU de Chirurgie du Pied et de la Cheville, Université Victor Segalen Bordeaux 2. 2008.

Hallux Valgus Correction via Distal Metaphyseal Osteotomy

11

Mark A. Hardy, Troy J. Boffeli, and Jennifer L. Prezioso

11.1 Introduction

Research has made significant strides toward the subject of hallux abductovalgus (HAV) correction. The deformity plagues millions across the world and is considered one of the most common deformities affecting the foot and ankle. Twenty-three percent of adults age 18–65 suffer from this condition, and the prevalence continues to increase with age [1].

HAV is characterized by abduction of the hallux with accompanying medial deviation of the first metatarsal resulting in a prominence of the first metatarsal head. An accompanying valgus rotation of the hallux may also be seen. Over time, this deformity may lead to significant patient morbidity with pain limiting shoe gear, activities of daily living, ability to exercise, and one's quality of life.

11.2 Etiology

It is the authors' opinion that HAV tends to be an acquired, progressive deformity caused by abnormal pronatory biomechanics. Subtalar joint pronation—often observed in a pes planus foot—or instability along the medical column may contribute to a structurally unstable first ray, increasing the incidence of a concomitant HAV deformity.

HAV can develop in the setting of abnormal first metatarsal phalangeal joint (MTP) mechanics and usually progresses in severity as the hallux continues to sublux laterally. As this happens, ground reaction forces and dynamic muscular forces begin to overpower the normal alignment of the first MTP. As the hallux deviates laterally, the long axis of the first metatarsal is placed more medially, and the center of rotation of the first MTP is shifted laterally. The long extensors and flexors now have a lateral mechanical advantage further exacerbating the deformity. Combined with medially applied ground reaction forces, these forces contribute to lateral sesamoid displacement, plastic deformation, and adaptation of soft and osseous tissue of the first MTP over time. There are progressive stages of HAV described in the literature which correspond to the degree and severity of the deformity [2].

11.3 Evaluation

Selection of the proper procedure begins with a thorough clinical and radiographic evaluation of the patient. The patient's concerns, objectives, and expectations must be elicited to ensure the goals of both the patient and surgeon are met.

M. A. Hardy (✉) · T. J. Boffeli · J. L. Prezioso
Balance Foot & Ankle Wellness Center, Lakewood, OH, USA
e-mail: hardy@balanceCLE.com

C. Cazeau, Y. Stiglitz (eds.), *Percutaneous and Minimally Invasive Foot Surgery*, https://doi.org/10.1007/978-3-030-98791-6_11

11.3.1 Clinical Evaluation

A thorough interview of the patient with regard to symptomatology and complaints should be undertaken. Specifically, the surgeon should differentiate pain from pressure over the first metatarsal head versus pain during ambulation within the first MTP joint. The latter suggests a more severe deformity in which arthritic degeneration has occurred with destruction of cartilage within the joint. Physical examination will reveal varying degrees of hallux abduction with or without valgus angulation of the digit.

Examination of the first MTP should include the range of motion testing with attention directed to any limitation, tracking, or crepitation. The presence of these signs may be indicative of degenerative changes within the joint. Deficits within the cartilage may be recognized by performance of a grind test—an axial load applied to the hallux, while at the same time, circumducting against the first metatarsal head. The test is deemed positive if pain is elicited.

First ray range of motion and any concomitant hypermobility should be noted. Hypermobility is often subjective but is defined by total excursion of the first ray greater than 15 mm or 8 mm of dorsal excursion (Fig. 11.1) [2–4]. Deviations at the interphalangeal joint should also be noted although this is often better appreciated radiographically. Weight-bearing examination should always be performed as this deformity is commonly accentuated when fully weight-bearing. Concomitant pathology during this stage of evaluation should also be investigated—pes planus, metatarsus adductus, and equinus, to name a few.

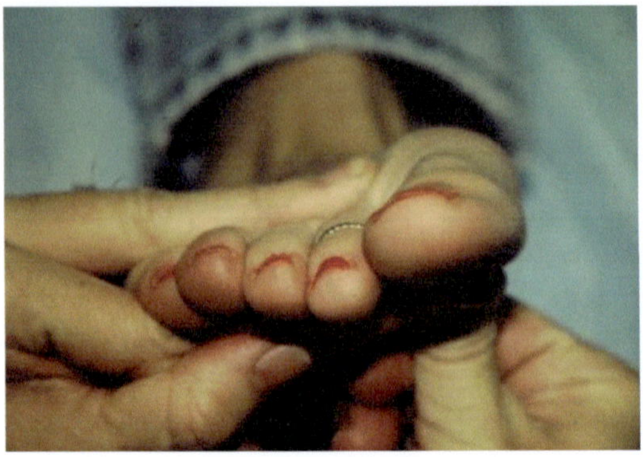

Fig. 11.1 Clinical evaluation of hypermobility with increased dorsiflexion of the first ray evident.

Table 11.1 Normal values

IM 1–2	0–9°
HAA	0–15°
HAI	0–10°
PASA	0–7.5°
DASA	0–7.5°
TSP	<4
Met protrusion	+2 to -2 mm
Med adductus	0–15°
Seiberg index	(−)value-plantarflexion; (+)value-elevatus

11.3.2 Radiographic Evaluation

Radiographic evaluation plays a role in procedure selection for correction of HAV deformities. Weight-bearing films including anteroposterior, oblique, lateral, and sesamoid axial views may be utilized in the evaluation of HAV. Common measurements used in the assessment include intermetatarsal 1–2 angle (IM 1–2), hallux abductus angle (HAA), hallux interphalangeal angle (HIA), proximal articular set angle (PASA), distal articular set angle (DASA), tibial sesamoid position (TSP), metatarsal protrusion, metatarsus adductus, and Seiberg index (Table 11.1).

IM 1–2 is the most common parameter used for the determination of procedure [5]. This is in part due to the implication of the angular measurement on the level of correction. Classically, IM 1–2 angles less than 16° have been addressed with distal metaphyseal osteotomies, whereas angles 16° or greater have necessitated proximal or midshaft procedures [6, 7]. Recent literature has supported the use of distal metaphyseal osteotomies for moderate to severe HAV deformities, citing similar outcomes in comparison to more proximal procedures [6–8].

Radiographs should be used as a guide for potential operative correction (Fig. 11.2a, b). Final decisions regarding positioning should be made intraoperatively once the goal of re-establishing congruity of the first MTP joint has been achieved.

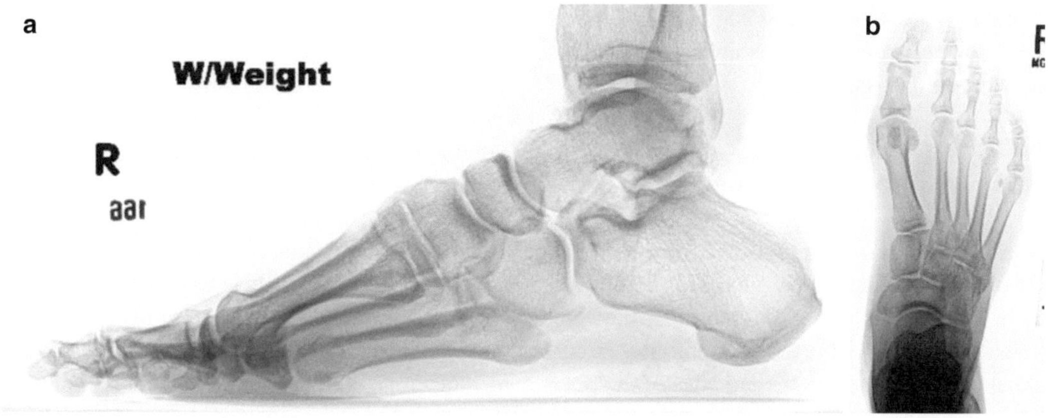

Fig. 11.2 Preoperative (**a**) lateral and (**b**) AP radiographs on the right foot demonstrating hallux valgus deformity.

11.4 Surgical Correction

There are a multitude of procedures available for surgical correction of HAV deformity. Soft tissue procedures as well as those involving osseous work are commonly utilized, yet the goals remain consistent. Surgical correction is aimed at decreasing pain and improving function by restoring congruity to the first MTP joint. Improved cosmesis is a result but it is not the primary goal.

11.5 Dorsal Locking Plate Fixation in Distal Metatarsal Osteotomy

While screw fixation remains the most popular fixation construct for distal metatarsal osteotomy, there are patients where traditional fixation may be insufficient. This may be related to the desire for maximum transposition, need for frontal plane correction, bone quality issues, revision surgery, or intra-operative fixation challenges. Plate fixation allows the surgeon to span the osteotomy and anchor the fixation to the stable proximal shaft. Plates need to be properly sized, and the authors have found that an L-shaped plate best fits the post-transposition shape of the metatarsal head.

Screw fixation works well for conservative transposition in patients with adequate bone quality. It's the authors' opinion that stability of screw fixation becomes compromised as the surgeon pushes the limits of transposition beyond 30% of the metatarsal width. The distal transverse locking screws from the dorsally applied plate are able to provide proper stability in this scenario and help to prevent the metatarsal head from displacing dorsally, plantarly, or laterally into the inter-metatarsal space. A variety of osteotomy configurations are amenable to dorsal plate fixation including the traditional Chevron, which is most stable, the long plantar arm osteotomy, which allows a central screw to cross the osteotomy, and a transverse flat cut that allows frontal plane correction.

Another circumstance where dorsal plate fixation is useful involves failed screw fixation. This can occur intraoperatively with repeated stripping of screws due to poor bone quality. Screws can also fail in the early postoperative period requiring revision. Distal metatarsal osteotomies do not have many fallback fixation options, and the surgeon should be ready to apply a plate when the need arises. Patients with osteoporosis either identified preoperatively or intraoperatively should also be considered for this advanced fixation technique. Large cysts within the metatarsal head are also commonly found in patients with long standing hallux valgus and may compromise stability of standard screw fixation constructs.

11.6 Authors' Technique

A traditional dorsal medial incision is used for the distal metatarsalosteotomy. This is followed by a lateral joint release including the deep transverse intermetatarsal ligament and release along the fibular sesamoid and base of the proximal phalanx. The lateral collateral ligament was left undisturbed to minimize the chance of hallux varus. A vertical medial capsulotomy is performed about 1.5 cm proximal to the metatarsal phalangeal joint to create a ligamentous flap to allow medial collateral ligament reconstruction after the osteotomy. Joint exposure is otherwise routine.

As taught by the senior author (TJB), the osteotomy involves a long plantar arm distal metatarsal osteotomy. Our preferred osteotomy technique involves a short vertical dorsal osteotomy that is conducive to screw fixation. This is similar to a Waterman-type osteotomy although there is no double-dorsal cut which is commonly used for joint decompression in hallux limitus. An osteotomy guide pin is placed above the midline of the metatarsal to allow a more substantial plantar arm. Lateral transposition of the metatarsal head can easily be pushed to 50% overlap when using the L-shaped locking plate fixation technique. A temporary 0.045″ K-wire is used for temporary fixation. This is placed from proximal medial to distal lateral as shown in Fig. 11.3.

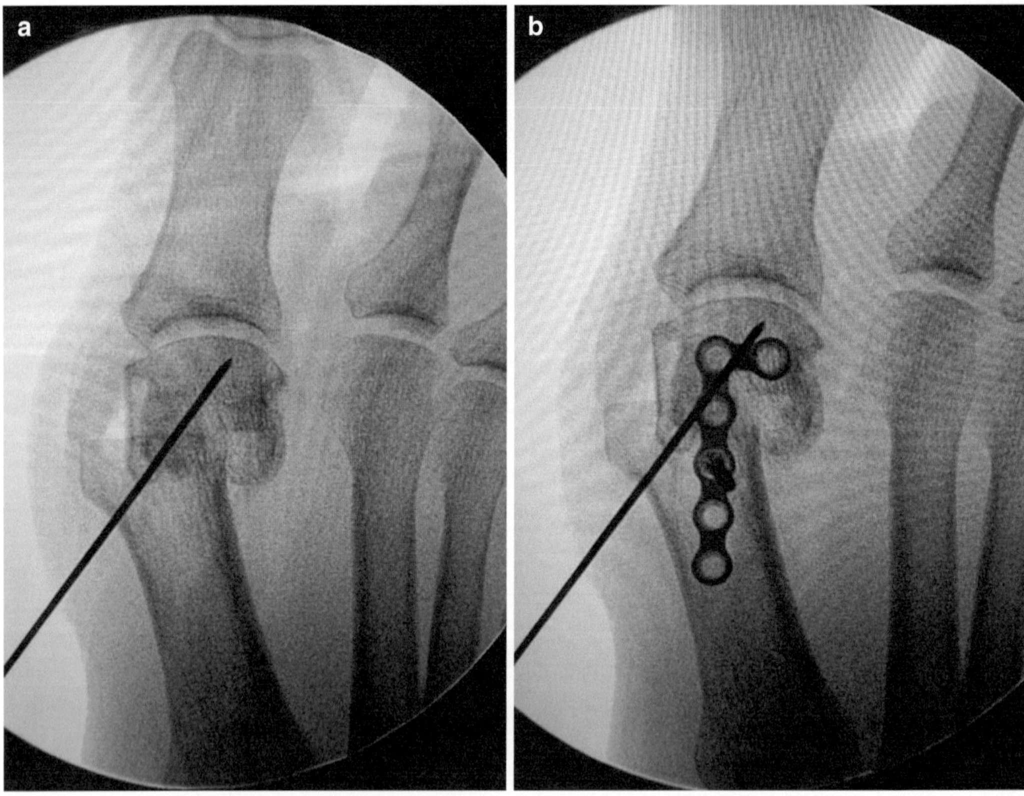

Fig. 11.3 Long plantar arm Waterman-type osteotomy was performed with lateral transposition of the metatarsal head. (**a**) Temporary pin fixation was performed using a 0.045″ K-wire inserted from proximal medial. This pin position allows application of the dorsal plate without interference. (**b**) An L-shaped locking plate was applied dorsally. Note how the distal L shape of the plate matches the offset of the metatarsal after transposition. Ideal plate length allows multiple proximal screws for stability yet does not extend excessively along the metatarsal.

The procedure up to this point is a routine approach although the dorsal osteotomy is intentionally placed slightly more proximal to allow a larger metatarsal head surface area for plate fixation. This allows the plate to be positioned just proximal to the joint surface to avoid dorsal impingement on MTP dorsiflexion. A saw is used to flatten the metatarsal head distal to the osteotomy which reduces dorsal prominence and allows the plate to lay flat and in line with the metatarsal shaft. An L-shaped locking plate works well to allow two distal screws and three proximal screws. We typically use a locking plate from one of our industry partner's hand system. A hand plate is lower profile and allows fixation with 2.4-mm screws which have a very low profile head. Most systems have these smaller plates, but it is worthwhile to look at hand fixation devices which we use commonly in the lesser metatarsals and first proximal phalanx. The distal screws are "unicortical" although the dorsal cortex has been cut to expose cancellous bone. The proximal screws are bicortical for better strength (Fig. 11.4). The medial eminence is then removed, and the medial collateral ligament is reconstructed (Fig. 11.5). The medial collateral ligament reconstruction procedure is performed using a 2–0 braided polyester for upper and lower mattress sutures within the ligamentous flap (Figs. 11.6 and 11.7). These are passed from medial to lateral through drill holes in the metatarsal head and tied dorsal laterally under ana-

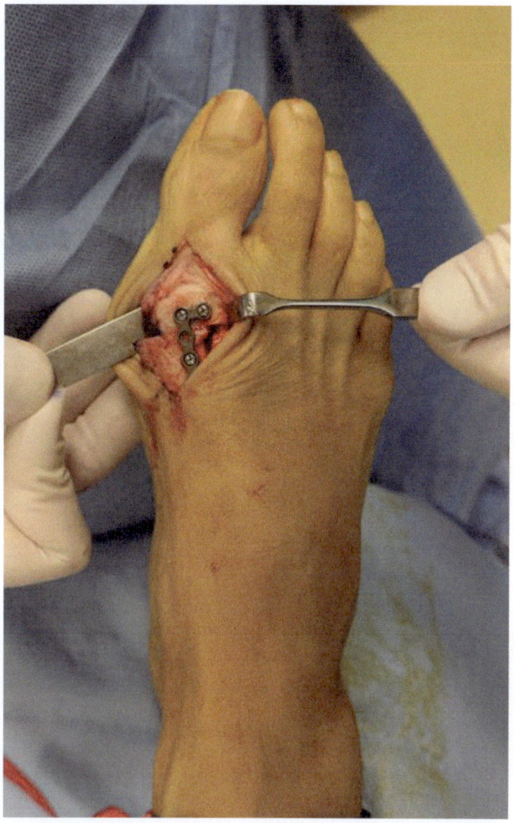

Fig. 11.4 2.4-mm locking screws were used in all but the center hole that crossed the dorsal vertical osteotomy. The plate is held compressed against the bone manually rather than using non-locking screws to seat the plate. We prefer locking screws to avoid the potential for hardware loosening and later removal. Hand plates are intentionally low profile to avoid dorsal prominence.

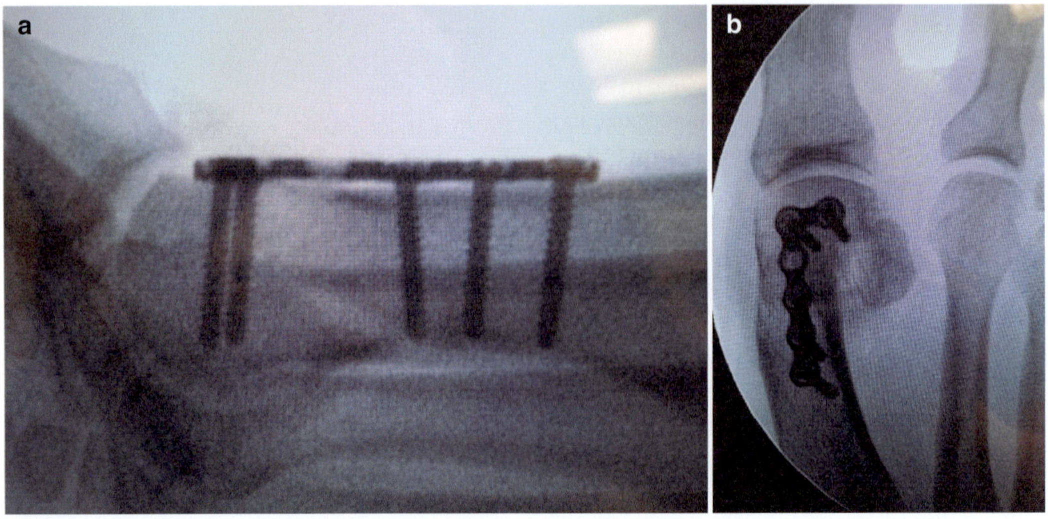

Fig. 11.5 Intraoperative imaging (**a**) lateral and (**b**) AP after fixation and resection of the medial overhang. Note the flat dorsal metatarsal head, lack of hardware prominence, unicortical nature of the distal screws, and bicortical nature of the proximal screws. The plate is centered on the metatarsal head and proximal shaft. The oblique plantar osteotomy is slightly visible on the lateral view. Note how the plate is intentionally positioned just proximal to the joint surface to avoid dorsal impingement which is possible at extreme range of motion.

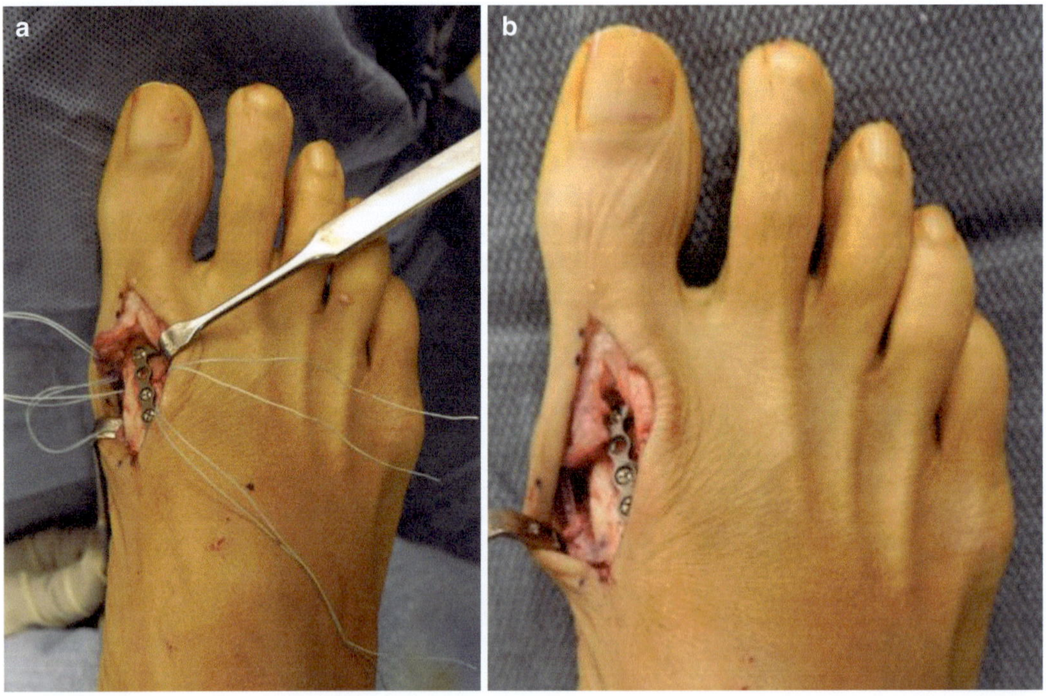

Fig. 11.6 Intraoperative repair of the medial collateral ligament during (**a**) and after (**b**).

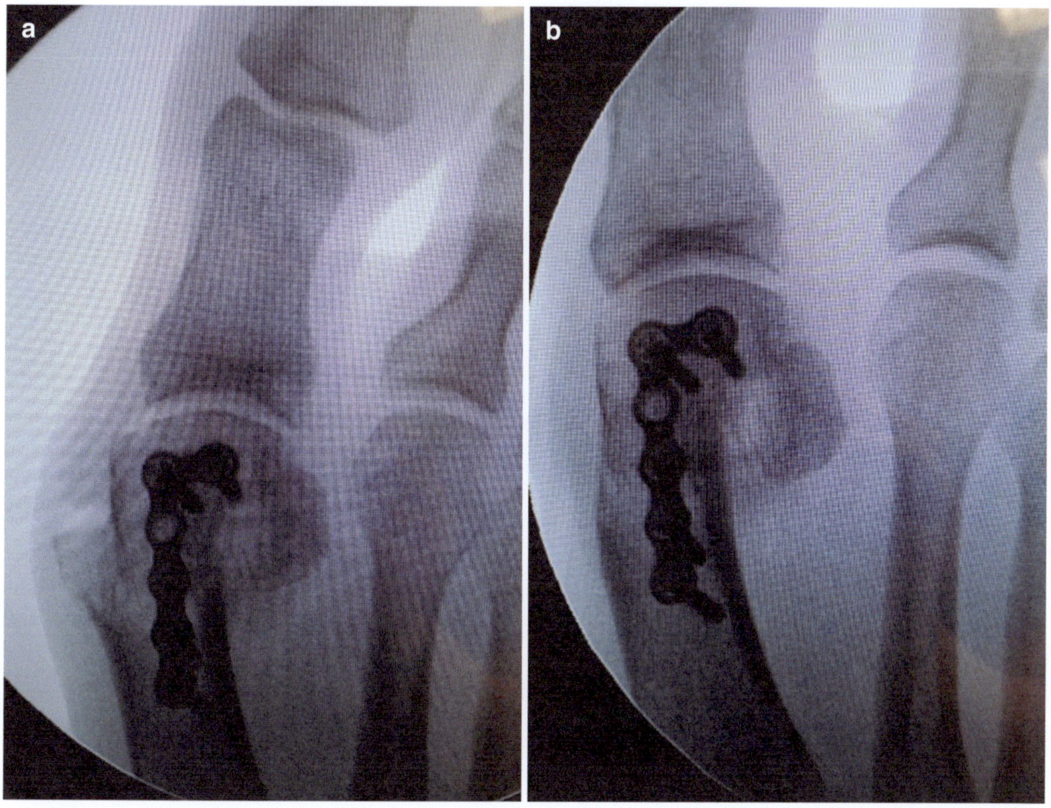

Fig. 11.7 Image intensification of the first MTP before (a) and after (b) medial collateral ligament repair. © Mark A. Hardy 2015. All Rights Reserved

tomic tension, while the hallux is held in a rectus position. Drill holes are intentionally proximal to the joint to maintain range of motion without excessive adhesions. The skin is then closed after dorsal periosteal closure over the dorsal plate.

11.7 Postoperative Care

Protected weight-bearing in a surgical shoe is sufficient with locking plate fixation although we typically use a below knee pneumatic walking boot for 6 weeks in distal metatarsal osteotomy cases. Sutures are removed at 2 weeks (Fig. 11.8). An example of a 6-week postoperative result is shown in Fig. 11.9 which demonstrates improved intermetatarsal angle and desirable joint alignment.

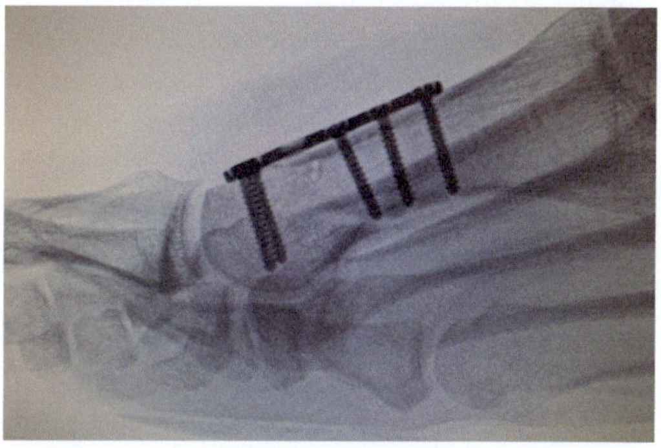

Fig. 11.8 Weight-bearing lateral view 2 weeks postoperative allows confidence with early range of motion and weight-bearing. © Mark A. Hardy 2015. All Rights Reserved

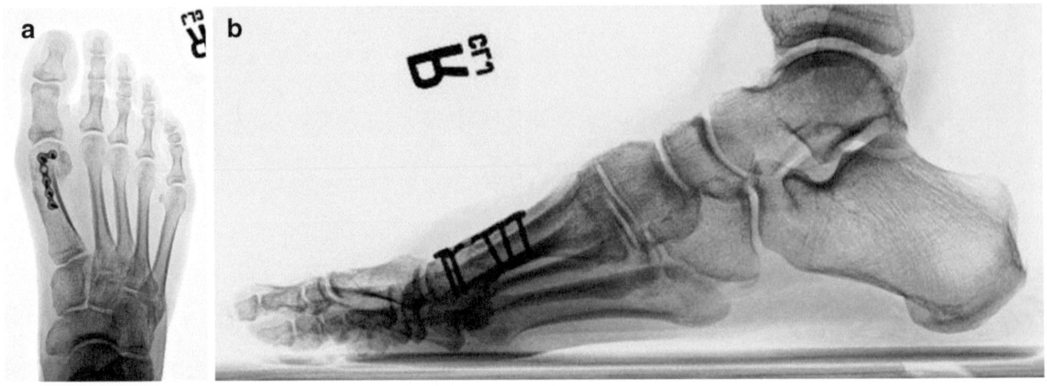

Fig. 11.9 (**a**, **b**) Six-week postoperative radiographs with progressive healing of the osteotomy. © Mark A. Hardy 2015. All Rights Reserved

11.8 Discussion

Screw and pin fixation are traditionally used for distal metatarsal osteotomy. This remains our mainstay fixation construct although there are patients where traditional fixation may be insufficient. One situation involves failed screw fixation. This can occur intraoperatively with repeated stripping of screws during the index procedure. A distal metatarsal osteotomy does not have many options for fallback fixation although conversion to pin fixation is possible. Patients with osteoporosis either identified preoperatively or intraoperatively should be considered for this advanced fixation technique. An L-shaped plate also matches the postoperative metatarsal shape and provides substantial stability against displacement of the osteotomy.

Revision of cases involving postoperative failure of fixation is another indication. The capital fragment has a tendency to shift plantarly which results in shortening of the metatarsal or tips into the interspace, both of which can predispose to hallux varus and undesirable results. We also run into patients who insist on being more active or less protected during the healing process. This might be a physician or a lawyer who expects to be back in the clinic or courtroom in 2 weeks or someone who has an undue DVT risk with prolonged immobilization.

Plate fixation in general has been shown to have less incidence of capital fragment displacement compared to screw fixation [9]. Plate fixation has also been shown to be a stronger construct compared to screw fixation [10]. The L plate fixation allows for greater lateral translocation of the capital fragment as well as provides a stable construct. Yearian et al. used an L-shaped locking plate and retrospectively found only one postoperative complication of screw loosening that was visible on radiographs, and no patients required hardware removal [11].

The main downside of locking plate fixation is cost. It also takes slightly longer to apply the plate compared to pins or a compression screw. This technique should be reserved for special cases, but we have not identified other negative factors. While the plate does not provide direct compression across the osteotomy, the proximal metatarsal shaft is sandwiched between the plantar arm of the distal fragment and the dorsal plate. This sandwich compression technique plus inherent stability provided by spreading fixation along the length of metatarsal from midshaft to metatarsal head imparts far more stability than one or two compression screws.

Medial collateral ligament reconstruction is more commonly used in Lapidus fusion where there is no distal hardware. However, we employ a similar technique for distal metatarsal osteotomy although the medial to lateral drill holes need to bypass fixation. For this reason, we commonly skip the middle hole of the plate which is at the level of the dorsal vertical osteotomy which provides a window where the drill holes can pass from medial to lateral.

References

1. Nix S, Smith M, Vincenzio B. Prevalence of hallux valgus in the general population: a systematic review and meta-analysis. J Foot Ankle Res. 2010;3:21.
2. Palladino SJ. Preoperative evaluation of the bunion patient. In: Gerbert J, editor. Textbook of bunion surgery. 3rd ed. WB Saunders; 2001.
3. Faber F, Mulder P, Verhaar J. Role of first ray hypermobility in the outcome of the Hohmann and the Lapidus procedure: a prospective, randomized trial involving one hundred and one feet. J Bone Joint Surg. 2004;86:486–95.
4. Voellmicke K, Deland J. Manual examination technique to assess dorsal instability of the first ray. Foot Ankle Int. 2002;23(11):1040–1.
5. Malik J, Mathieson I. Clinical usage and influence of radiographs in the assessment of hallux valgus. J Foot Ankle Surg. 2013;52(3):291–4.
6. Brosky T, Hall P. Distal metaphyseal osteotomies in hallux abductovalgus surgery. In: Southerland J, Bopberg J, Downey M, Aprajita N, Rabjohn L, editors. McGlamry's comprehensive textbook of foot and ankle surgery. 4th ed. Philadelphia: Lippincott Williams and Wilkins; 2013. p. 279–89.
7. Stienstra J, Lee J, Nakadate D. Large displacement distal chevron osteotomy for the correction of hallux valgus deformity. J Foot Ankle Surg. 2002;41(4):213–20.
8. Park H, Lee K, Chung J, Kim M. Comparison of outcomes between proximal and distal chevron osteotomy, both with supplementary lateral soft-tissue release, for severe hallux valgus deformity. A prospective randomized controlled trial. Bone Joint J. 2013;95(4):510–6.
9. Andrews BJ, Fallat LM, Kish JP. Screw versus plate fixation for Chevron osteotomy: a retrospective study. J Foot Ankle Surg. 2016;55(1):81–4.
10. Windhager R. Biomechanical analysis of two fixation methods for proximal chevron osteotomy of the first metatarsal. Int Orthop. 2014;38(5):983–9.
11. Yearian PR, Brown T, Goldman F. Chevron bunionectomy with microplate and screw fixation: a retrospective follow-up of 26 feet. J Foot Ankle Surg. 1996;35(6):532–6.

Minimally Invasive Scarf Osteotomy

12

Pierre Barouk

12.1 Introduction

The minimally invasive scarf osteotomy was born from a desire to reproduce the good outcomes of the standard scarf osteotomy while reducing its invasiveness, both superficial (skin, soft tissues) and bony.

Over the past 25 years, a consensus has developed around using midshaft osteotomy procedures for hallux valgus correction: scarf and chevron (metaphyseal-diaphyseal or metaphyseal-epiphyseal). While these two techniques were initially in competition, the best of each has been incorporated over time. The major difference between the two is that, in the scarf, a third proximal cut is made.

When performing a minimally invasive scarf osteotomy, it is essential that the technique used preserves this procedure's advantages, namely, its solidness and versatility.

12.2 History

The scarf osteotomy was first used in the 1980s by American podiatrists to treat hallux valgus [1, 2]. Samuel Barouk introduced this technique in France and Europe and helped to popularize it worldwide through his book *Forefoot Reconstruction* [3, 4] and various other articles and presentations. He was the first to use screws with a threaded head for bone fixation. He also described in detail the various displacement possibilities based on the orientation of the cuts [3–9]. Thus, the scarf became virtually the only hallux valgus reconstruction technique used in our daily practice. In response to the shift toward minimally invasive techniques, the scarf osteotomy has been modified to reduce its invasiveness, both at the bone level and the soft tissue level.

12.3 Anatomy

There are two critical anatomical features when performing a scarf osteotomy:

12.3.1 Vascularization of the First Metatarsal Head

The vascularization of the first metatarsal head is mainly ensured by the plantar pedicle. The dorsal pedicle is less important [9, 10]; however, both are preserved by the scarf osteotomy cuts (Fig. 12.1).

P. Barouk (✉)
Centre de Chirurgie Orthopédique et Sportive,
Merignac, France

C. Cazeau, Y. Stiglitz (eds.), *Percutaneous and Minimally Invasive Foot Surgery*,
https://doi.org/10.1007/978-3-030-98791-6_12

12.3.2 Three Faces of the Metatarsal

- The medial face is a landmark for making the longitudinal cut (Fig. 12.2).
- The plantar face is angled downward and outward (Fig. 12.2). The diaphysis of the first metatarsal has a triangular cross-section in the coronal plane (Fig. 12.2).
- Its lateral face, which is also called lateral "wall" or "beam," is vertical. The scarf's solidness is based on this beam being preserved, with the cut reaching the lower portion of this wall (Fig. 12.3).

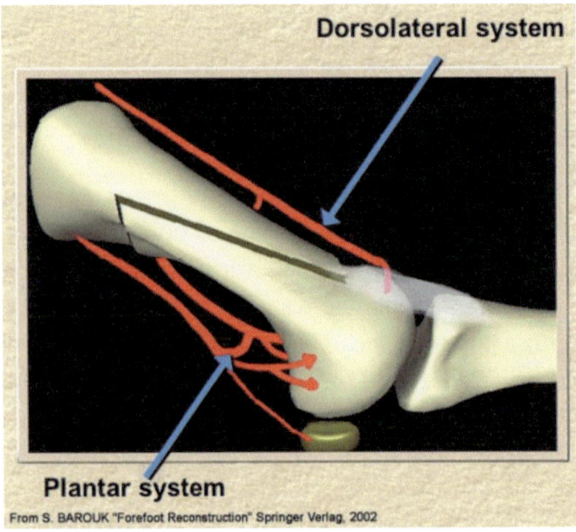

Fig. 12.1 Dorsal and plantar vascularization of first metatarsal head. © Pierre Barouk 2015. All Rights Reserved

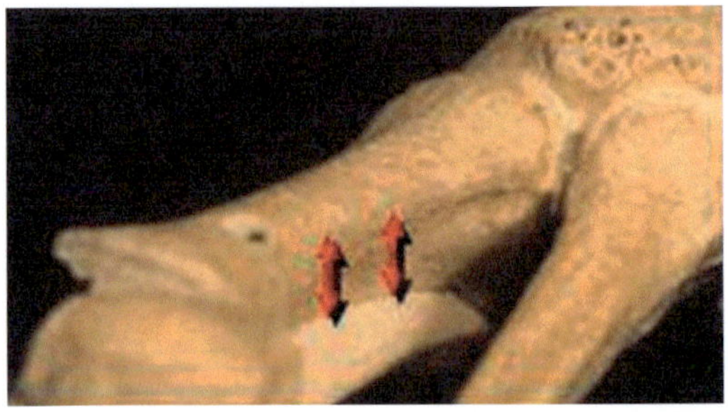

Fig. 12.3 Lateral wall of first metatarsal. © Pierre Barouk 2015. All Rights Reserved

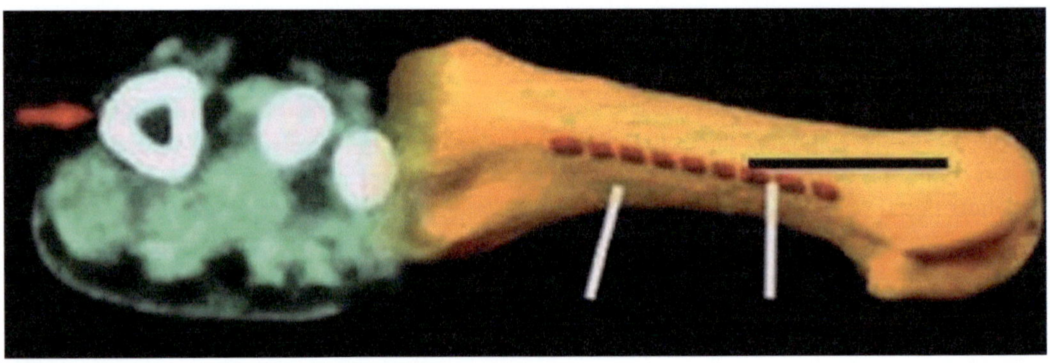

Fig. 12.2 Medial and plantar faces of first metatarsal; the diaphysis has a triangular cross-section in the coronal plane. © Pierre Barouk 2015. All Rights Reserved

12.4 Surgical Technique

12.4.1 Release

Historically, the release has been done through a dorsal approach in the first web space [3, 4]. But in most cases, we now prefer using the trans-articular approach between the head and lateral sesamoid, since only the accessory sesamoid ligament needs to be cut (Fig. 12.4).

12.4.2 Surgical Exposure

The approximately 5-cm-long incision is centered over the medial eminence of the head of the first metatarsal (Fig. 12.5). The capsule is incised along the bone axis and detached from the medial portion of the head. Its dorsal and plantar attachments are preserved. A saw is used to remove the pseudo-exostosis, which is actually a flattened portion of the head. The plantar face of the distal end of the diaphysis is exposed by subperiosteal detachment using a thin bone rasp (Fig. 12.6), while preserving the plantar vascularization of the head immediately in front of it.

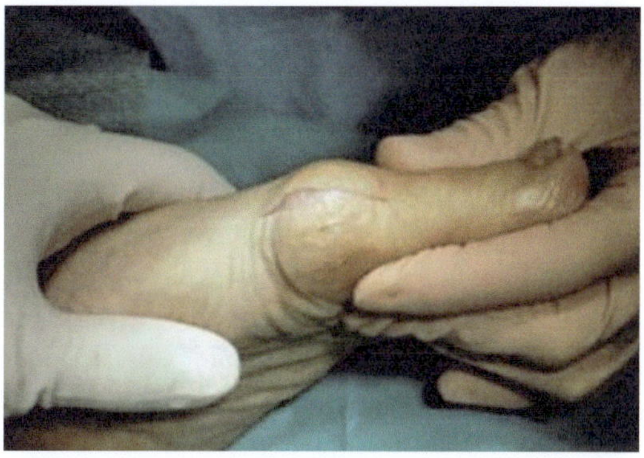

Fig. 12.5 Incision over the first metatarsal head. © Pierre Barouk 2015. All Rights Reserved

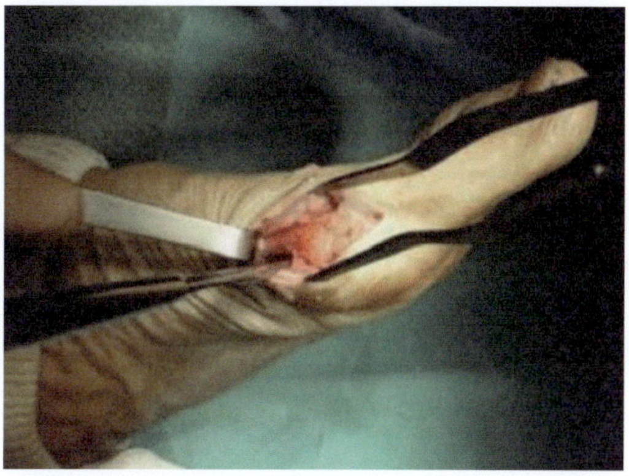

Fig. 12.6 Exposure of the distal end of diaphysis. © Pierre Barouk 2015. All Rights Reserved

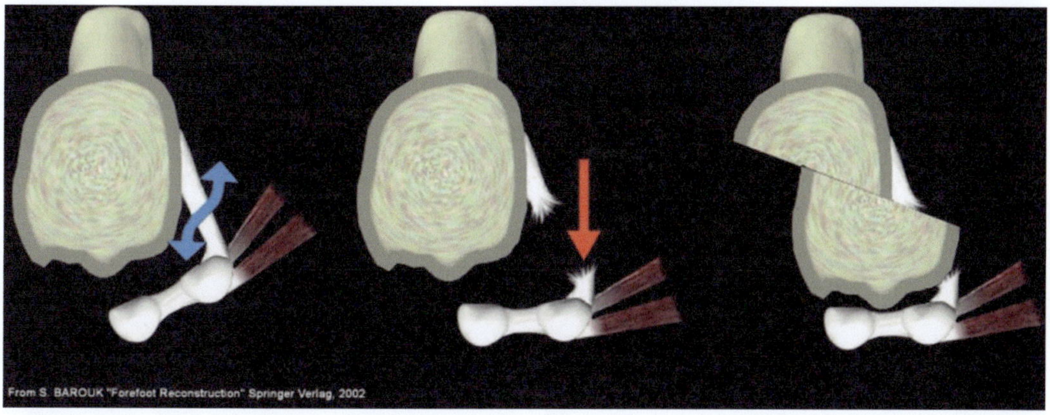

Fig. 12.4 Trans-articular approach between metatarsal head and lateral sesamoid. © Pierre Barouk 2015. All Rights Reserved

12.4.3 Osteotomy Cuts

The first cut is longitudinal. The goal is to reach the lower portion of the lateral face to ensure the construct is solid. Thus its exact orientation will depend on whether the first metatarsal will be lowered or not. To lower the metatarsal, the cut must start fairly high on the head. One must lift the hand to be parallel to the plantar side and then to reach the lower portion of the lateral side (Fig. 12.7). If horizontal translation is the goal instead of lowering (most common scenario), one must start from the center of the head (Fig. 12.8).

The proximal cut is made using a thinner saw to prevent the plantar soft tissues from being damaged (Fig. 12.9). Its direction also depends on whether the first metatarsal will be shortened or not. If the first metatarsal will not be shortened, one must be perpendicular to the second metatarsal; otherwise, the direction must be more proximal (Fig. 12.10). The level at which this diaphyseal cut is made will determine the length of the scarf. Generally, it is made in the middle of the diaphysis. Thus a minimally invasive scarf osteotomy is not necessarily a very short scarf. One advantage of its relative length when compared to a very

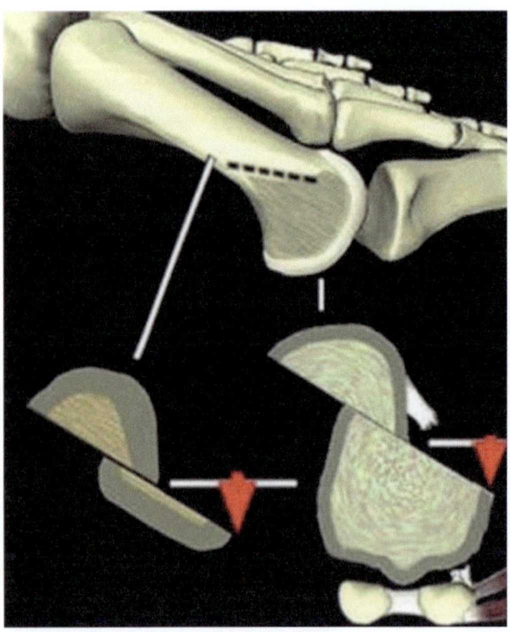

Fig. 12.7 Lowering osteotomy. © Pierre Barouk 2015. All Rights Reserved

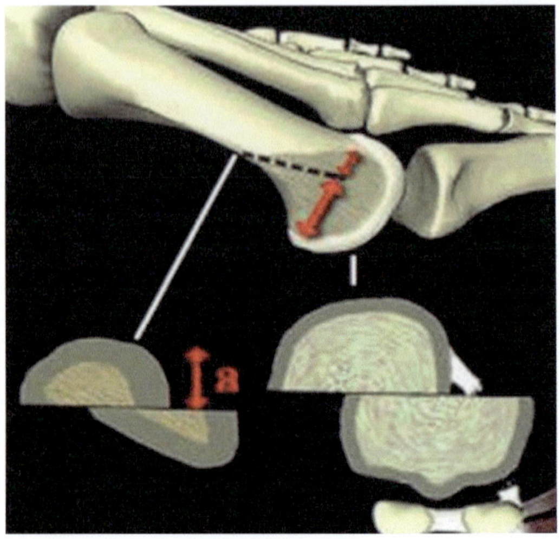

Fig. 12.8 Horizontal translation osteotomy. © Pierre Barouk 2015. All Rights Reserved

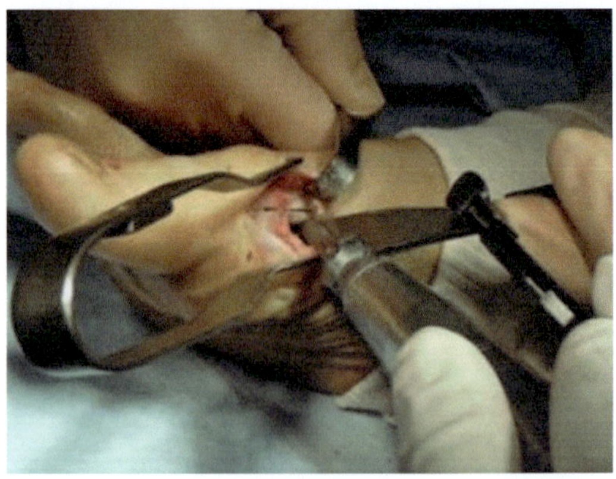

Fig. 12.9 Proximal osteotomy cut. © Pierre Barouk 2015. All Rights Reserved

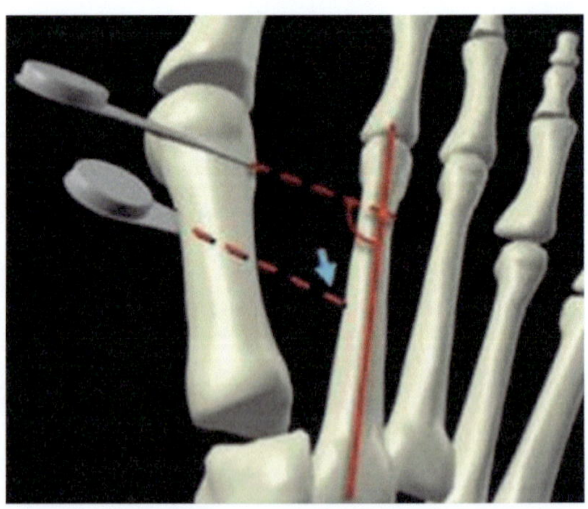

Fig. 12.10 Two options for the proximal osteotomy cut. © Pierre Barouk 2015. All Rights Reserved

short scarf is that it provides a larger contact area and allows near-normal restoration—once union has been achieved—of the first metatarsal's morphology (Figs. 12.11 and 12.12).

The distal cut is made with the largest saw blade proximal to the capsule, thereby preserving the capsule's insertion. This cut must be parallel to the proximal cut or diverge slightly from it in order to achieve good distal impaction. Lack of proximal contact is not detrimental to the solidness of the construct, or at least not as much as lack of distal contact.

12.4.4 Displacement

Lateral translation is carried out using a push-pull technique. The dorsal fragment is pulled on using a surgical clamp, and the plantar fragment is pushed on as much as possible until it makes contact with the head of the second metatarsal (Fig. 12.13).

The surgical assistant holds the reduction by applying compression in the axis of the big toe.

12.4.5 Fixation

Fixation is done using a 2.5-mm-diameter cannulated screw with threaded head. A K-wire is inserted from the lateral side of the dorsal fragment, 1 cm from the cut and aligned in the new metatarsal axis. Ideally, it should exit in the medial half of the head (Fig. 12.14). The screw is then inserted. A pilot hole may need to be drilled

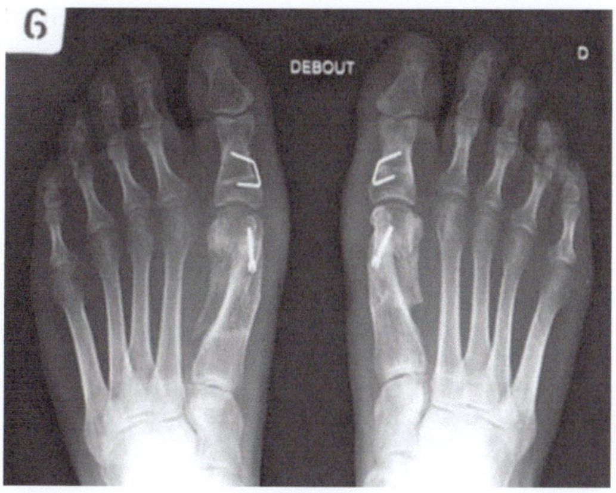

Fig. 12.11 Immediately postoperative. © Pierre Barouk 2015. All Rights Reserved

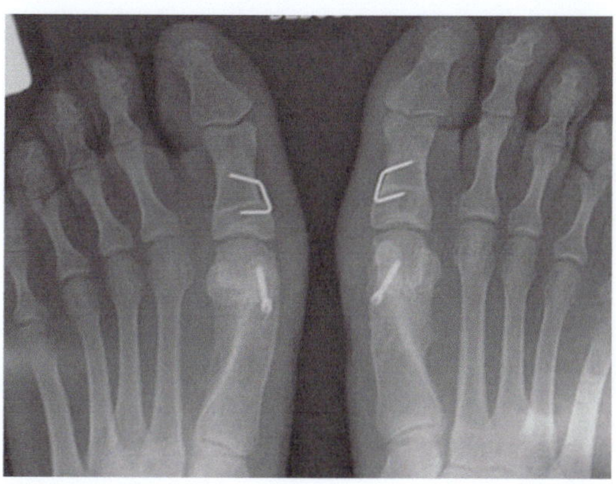

Fig. 12.12 At 1 year postoperative. © Pierre Barouk 2015. All Rights Reserved

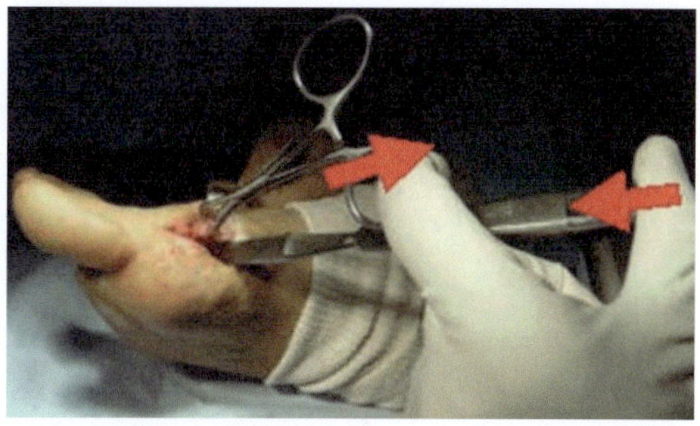

Fig. 12.13 Push-pull technique used to translate metatarsal head laterally. © Pierre Barouk 2015. All Rights Reserved

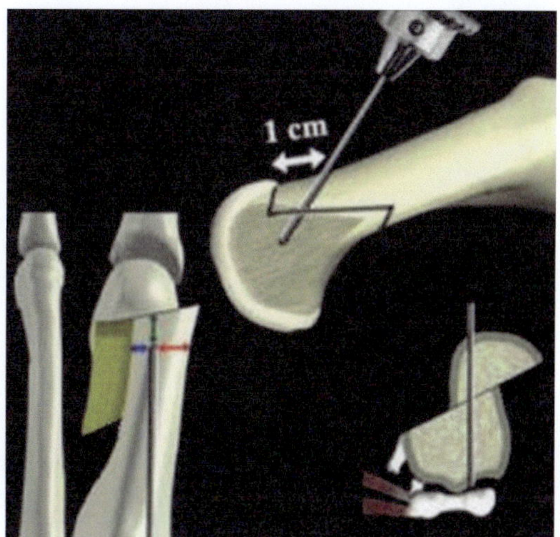

Fig. 12.14 Positioning of the fixation screw. © Pierre Barouk 2015. All Rights Reserved

depending on the manufacturer's instructions. Of course, the screw must not protrude into the joint!

12.4.6 Final Steps

Any excess medial bone is resected, turned over, and impacted in the plantar side of the dorsal fragment to strengthen the construct, fill the diaphysis, and recreate the plantar cortex (Fig. 12.15).

If this fragment is not self-stabilizing, it is best to remove it. A final rounding of any sharp bone edges under the skin is done using a saw; then the capsule is closed with a cross stitch at the center of the head with a solid absorbable suture. This stitch helps to reset the sesamoids under the head; however, in principle, they are already in this position if the displacement was sufficient. If the lateral sesamoid is verticalized in the first web space, the scarf's lateral translation may not be sufficient. If this is the case, retensioning the capsule will help to reset the sesamoid in the proper position.

Osteotomy of the first phalanx can now be carried out, either open or percutaneous, with or without fixation.

Fluoroscopy is then used to verify the construct, preferably with simulated loading. All the criteria for good reduction must be met before closing: good sesamoid reduction, good joint congruency, and 0 to 5° of residual valgus.

12.4.7 Postoperative Care

The patient is discharged on the day of surgery with a rigid-soled postoperative shoe that is slightly elevated in front. It is no longer mandatory to wear a shoe with heel lift except in specific cases: osteoporosis, associated Weil osteotomy of the lateral rays. The first follow-up visit is scheduled for 15 days later. The dressing is removed. The physical therapist who works with the foot surgery unit massages the foot and then applies Hypafix® tape strapping: metatarsal bracelet and support for the big toe and other toes as needed (Fig. 12.16). The patient is now allowed to shower.

This strapping is left in place for 15 days and then replaced if needed with a simple metatarsal bracelet or another strapping configuration suitable to the patient's foot. Radiographs are made during this visit at 1 month postoperative.

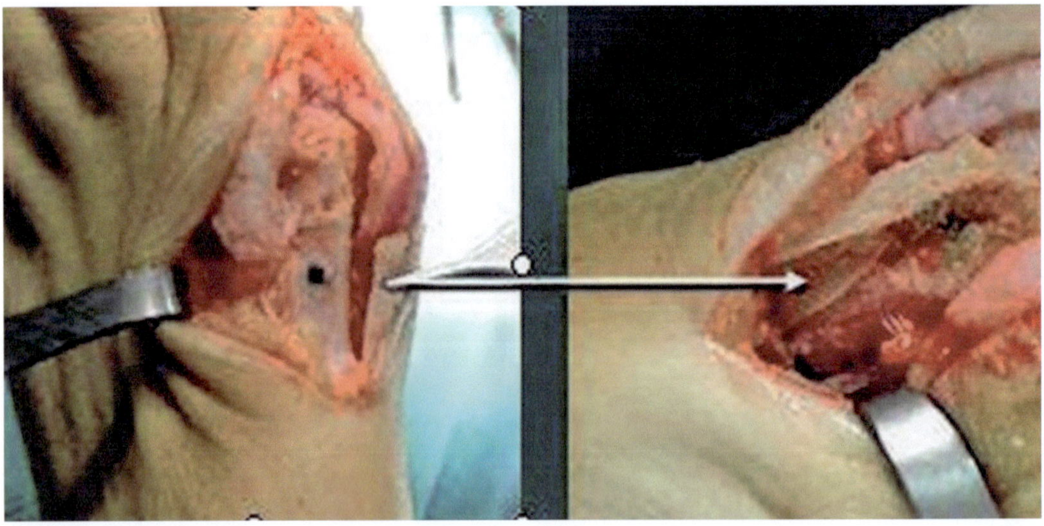

Fig. 12.15 Excess bone used to reconstruct the plantar cortex.

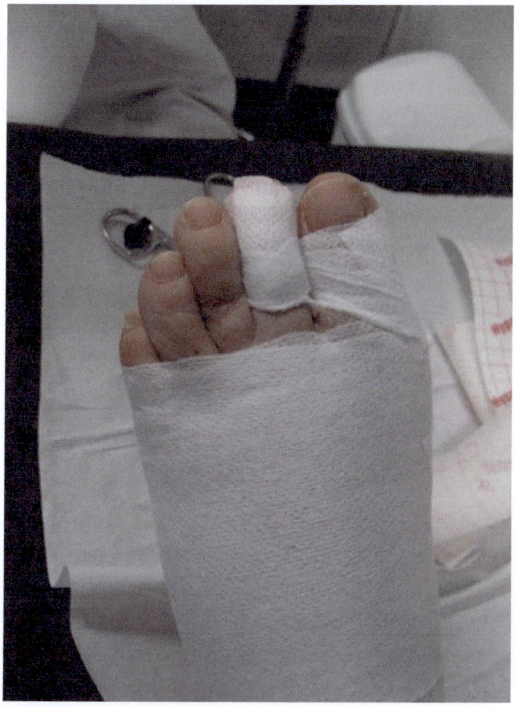

Fig. 12.16 Postoperative strapping at day 15.

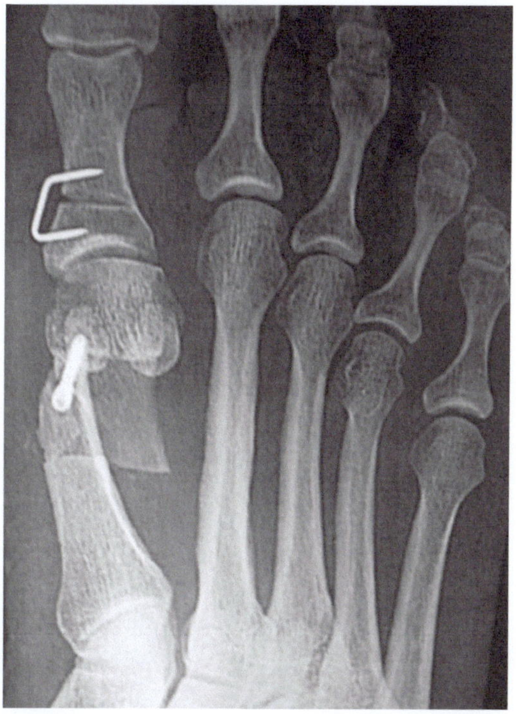

Fig. 12.17 Immediately postoperative.

12.5 Displacement Options

One of the advantages of the scarf osteotomy is its versatility. Surgery for hallux valgus is planned during the in-office consultation with the surgeon. The type of displacement to apply to the first metatarsal is one of the decision points.

12.5.1 Lateral Translation

Lateral translation is accomplished using the push-pull technique. Maximum translation must be applied. Cortex-to-cortex contact is very stable when the osteotomy cuts have been done correctly and the screw implanted properly (Figs. 12.17 and 12.18).

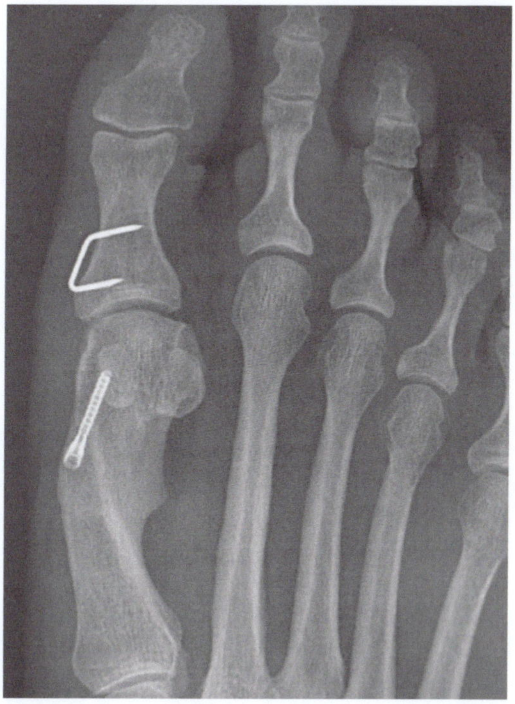

Fig. 12.18 At 1 year postoperative.

12.5.2 Lowering

For lowering, the saw cut must be more vertical; thus, start from a higher point on the head to prevent it from finishing inside the joint and to make sure it always reaches the lower portion of the lateral face (Fig. 12.7). Indications are defective M1 support, flat feet, and transfer metatarsalgia.

12.5.3 Distal Metatarsal Articular Angle Correction

The plantar fragment must be translated more than the proximal portion (medial rotation of head in the horizontal plane) to correct the distal metatarsal articular angle (Fig. 12.19). Indications are juvenile or iatrogenic hallux valgus.

12.5.4 Shortening

There are two ways to induce shortening with a scarf osteotomy:

- More proximal angling of the transverse cuts—in this case, the amount of recoil will depend on the translation. In practice, this is done when only a small amount of shortening is needed.
- The Maestro technique which is more accurate (exact amount of recoil) and more stable (Figs. 12.20 and 12.21). This is best suited for cases when considerable shortening is required, especially with a decompensated forefoot.

12.5.5 Supination

Supination is achieved by removing a medial corner of the plantar portion of the dorsal fragment. While it is easy to carry out, it is more difficult to determine exactly when it is needed. This can be supplemented by derotation of the hallux.

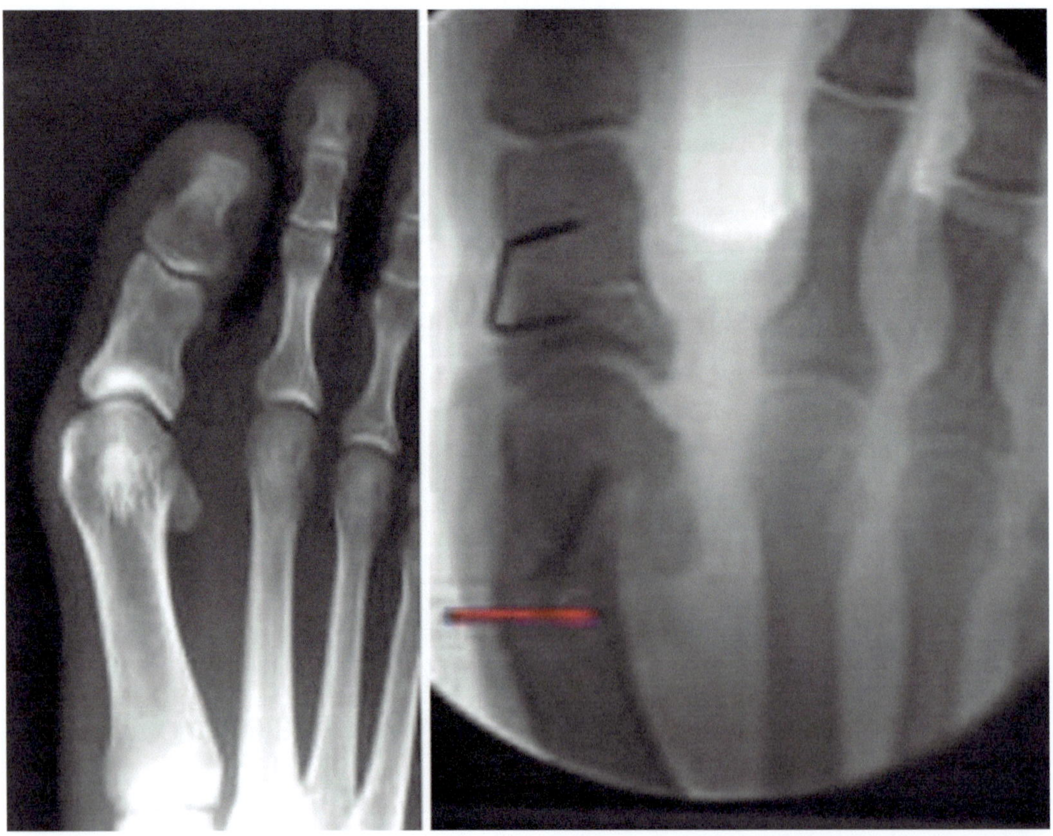

Fig. 12.19 Distal metatarsal articular angle (DMAA) correction.

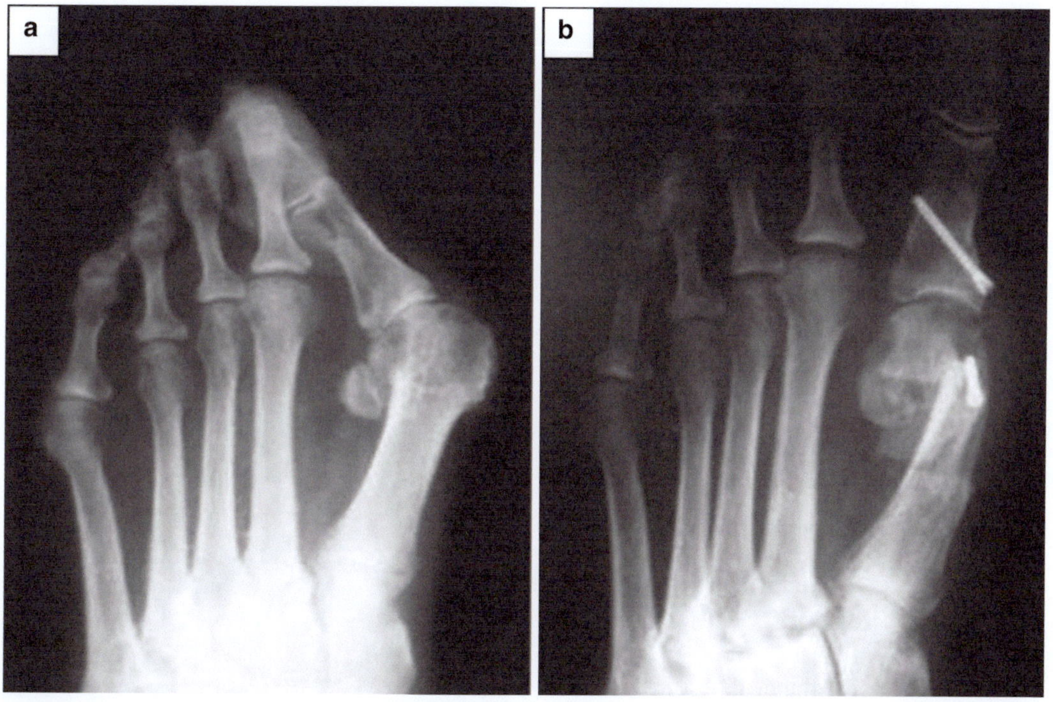

Fig. 12.20 Maestro technique. Preoperative (**a**) and immediately postoperative (**b**). © Pierre Barouk 2015. All Rights Reserved

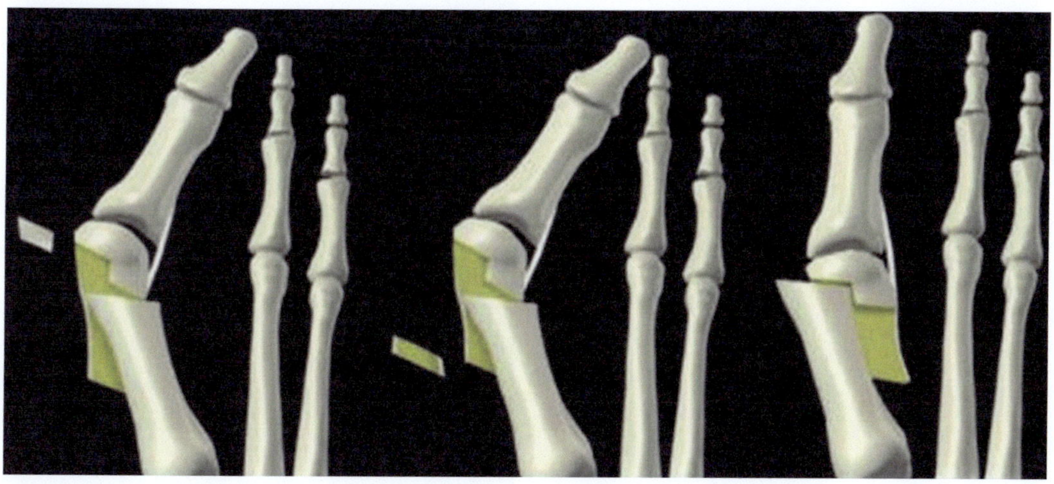

Fig. 12.21 Visual summary of osteotomy cuts and bone shifts during the Maestro technique. © Pierre Barouk 2015. All Rights Reserved

12.5.6 Elevation

Elevation is achieved by removing a plantar fragment from the dorsal fragment. In this scenario, the construct is a bit more fragile because the lateral wall is thinner.

12.5.7 Combinations

One of the advantages of the scarf osteotomy is that these displacements can be combined to shift the first metatarsal exactly into the desired position. The biggest challenge may be analyzing which displacements are needed for a specific patient.

12.6 Complications

The most common complications are proximal fracture and secondary displacement.

Proximal fracture occurs when weight-bearing is done too quickly, the bone is fragile (osteoporosis) or because the lateral beam is weak because the longitudinal cut was made too high. If the metatarsal has not elevated itself too much, unloading the foot is the best strategy.

Secondary displacement generally occurs as medial rotation of the head (Fig. 12.22). It can be avoided by having solid fixation and adding a proximal screw as needed. When detected, it should be treated rapidly before the osteotomy has healed (Fig. 12.23).

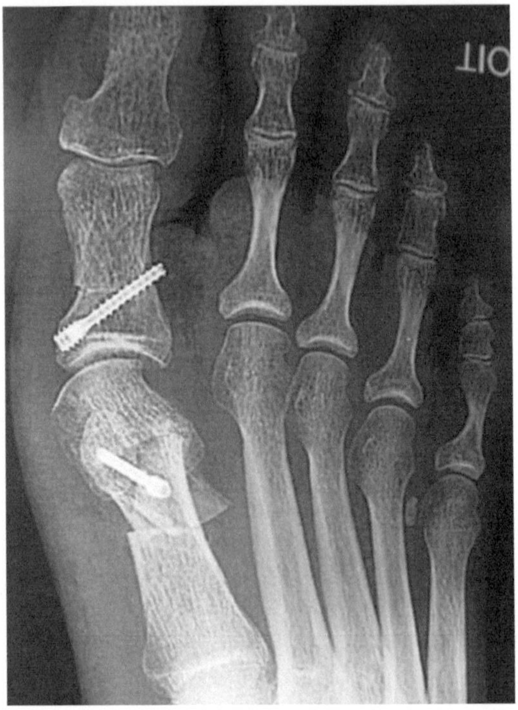

Fig. 12.22 Secondary displacement.

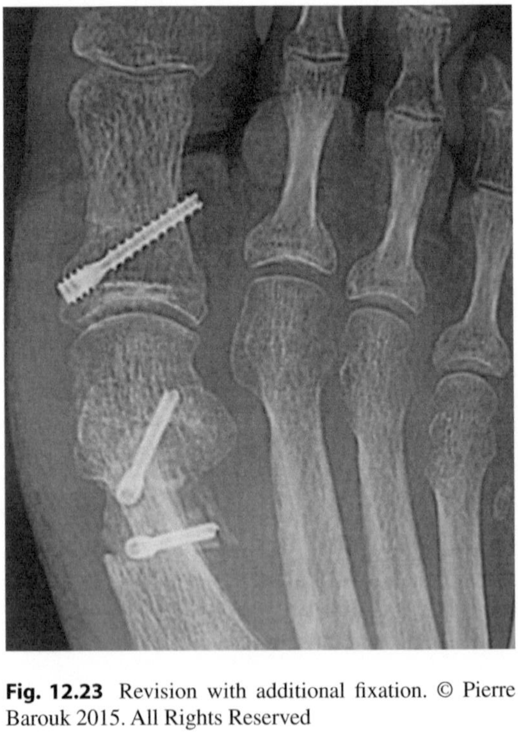

Fig. 12.23 Revision with additional fixation.

12.7 Discussion

The scarf osteotomy is a reliable method for correcting moderate to severe [11–18], congenital [19], recurring [20], or rheumatoid hallux valgus [21, 22]. The minimally invasive scarf osteotomy has evolved from the conventional procedure.

The spirit of the scarf is preserved with its multiple displacement options and solid construct. However, since no published study has compared the conventional to the minimally invasive scarf procedure, it is impossible to claim that this new version is better than the original one. Nevertheless, it seems logical that a smaller incision, less plantar tissue detachment and smaller bone cuts will reduce the postoperative pain and edema. Using a thinner saw blade for the proximal cut is critical to making this a minimally invasive procedure.

For a surgeon who has mastered this technique, the question is not *Which type of osteotomy should be done for this case of hallux valgus?* but *Which type of scarf osteotomy should be done for this case of hallux valgus?*

The evolution of the scarf toward shorter cuts and that of the chevron toward longer cuts means that these two osteotomy techniques are becoming more similar. Should we call it the *scarvron* or *charf*? Studies have found no evidence that one is superior to the other [23, 24]. Nevertheless, the scarf has advantages over the chevron:

- The scarf has an additional stabilization point (proximal chevron). The construct's stability is such that some authors have decided not to insert a screw [25].
- The scarf is better suited to shortening because of the Maestro cut (Fig. 12.21).

The development of percutaneous techniques by De Prado and the GRECMIP (French research group on foot and ankle minimally invasive surgery) has made it possible to perform a shorter scarf percutaneously. This procedure, which is performed by E. Rabat in Spain, may reconcile the advantages of a scarf osteotomy and percutaneous techniques, but requires further evaluation.

12.8 Conclusion

Over the past 30 years, the scarf osteotomy has become one of the preferred treatments for hallux valgus. This technique has evolved over time, first to eliminate the complications during the initial steps and second to increase its versatility—and hence its suitability—for treating the majority of hallux valgus cases. By reducing the size of the incision and cuts, it is feasible to use it with less severe deformities, thus making it a better match for the less-invasive surgery trend. In parallel, the *long* scarf still has its place for treating more severe deformities.

Editors' Point of View

The Scarf osteotomy needs no introduction—it can correct every type of deformity. This has been the gold-standard osteotomy since 1990 when Samuel Barouk introduced it in France. The current version makes use of MIS techniques.

References

1. Zygmunt KH, Gudas CJ, Laros GS. Z-Bunionectomy with internal screw fixation. J Am Podiatr Med Assoc. 1989;79:322–9.
2. Schwartz N, Groves ER. Long term follow up of internal threaded Kirschner wire fixation of the scarf bunionectomy. J Foot Surg. 1987;26:313–6.
3. Barouk LS. Forefoot reconstruction. Paris: Springer; 2003.
4. Barouk LS, Barouk P. Reconstruction de l'avant-pied. Paris: Springer; 2006.
5. Barouk LS. Scarf osteotomy for hallux valgus correction. Local anatomy, surgical technique, and combination with other forefoot procedures. Foot Ankle Clin. 2000;5:525–8.
6. Barouk LS. Scarf osteotomy of the first metatarsal in the treatment of hallux valgus. Foot Dis. 1995;II(1):35–48.
7. Barouk LS. Scarf osteotomy for the hallux valgus correction. Foot Ankle Clin. 2000;5:525–8.
8. Barouk LS. Nouvelles ostéotomies de l'avant-pied et leur rôle thérapeutique. In: Valtin B, editor. Cahiers d'enseignements de la SOFCOT. Paris: Expansion scientifique française; 1996. p. 49–76.

9. Barouk LS. Eléments d'anatomie chirurgicale du premier métatarsien. In: Med Chir pied. Paris: Expansion scientifique française; 1994. p. 76–82.
10. Sarrafian SK. Anatomy of the foot and ankle. Philadelphia: JB Lippincott; 1983.
11. Adam SP, Choung SC, Gu Y, O'Malley MJ. Outcomes after scarf osteotomy for treatment of adult hallux valgus deformity. Clin Orthop Relat Res. 2010;469:854–9.
12. Kristen KH, Berger C, Stelzig S, Thalhammer E, Posch M, Engel A. The SCARF osteotomy for the correction of hallux valgus deformities. Foot Ankle Int. 2002;23:221–9.
13. Larholt J, Kilmartin TE. Rotational scarf and akin osteotomy for correction of hallux valgus associated with metatarsus adductus. Foot Ankle Int. 2010;31:220–8.
14. Robinson AH, Bhatia M, Eaton C, Bishop L. Prospective comparative study of the scarf and Ludloff osteotomies in the treatment of hallux valgus. Foot Ankle Int. 2009;30:955–63.
15. Garrido IM, Rubio ER, Bosch MN, Gonzalez MS, Paz GB, Llabres AJ. Scarf and akin osteotomies for moderate and severe hallux valgus: clinical and radiographic results. Foot Ankle Surg. 2008;14:194–203.
16. Berg RP, Olsthoorn PG, Poll RG. Scarf osteotomy in hallux valgus: a review of 72 cases. Acta Orthop Belg. 2007;73:219–23.
17. Aminian A, Kelikian A, Moen T. Scarf osteotomy for hallux valgus deformity: an intermediate follow-up of clinical and radiographic outcomes. Foot Ankle Int. 2006;27:883–6.
18. Freslon M, Gayet LE, Bouche G, Hamcha H, Nebout J, Pries P. Scarf osteotomy for the treatment of hallux valgus: a review of 123 cases with 4.8 years follow-up. Rev Chir Orthop Reparatrice Appar Mot. 2005;91:257–66.
19. John S, Weil L Jr, Weil LS Sr. Chase K scarf osteotomy for the correction of adolescent hallux valgus. Foot Ankle Spec. 2010;3:10–4.
20. Bock P, Lanz U, Kröner A, Grabmeier G, Engel A. The scarf osteotomy: a salvage procedure for recurrent hallux valgus in selected cases. Clin Orthop Relat Res. 2010;468:2177–87.
21. Roukis TS. Scarf and Weil metatarsal osteotomies of the lateral rays for correction of rheumatoid forefoot deformities: a systematic review. J Foot Ankle Surg. 2010;49:390–4.
22. Barouk LS, Barouk P. Joint-preserving surgery in rheumatoid forefoot: preliminary study with more-than-two-year follow-up. Foot Ankle Clin. 2007;12:435–54.
23. Deenik A, van Mameren H, de Visser E, de Waal MM, Draijer F, de Bie R. Equivalent correction in scarf and chevron osteotomy in moderate and severe hallux valgus: a randomized controlled trial. Foot Ankle Int. 2008;29:1209–15.
24. Deenik AR, Pilot P, Brandt SE, van Mameren H, Geesink RG, Draijer WF. Scarf versus chevron osteotomy in hallux valgus: a randomized controlled trial in 96 patients. Foot Ankle Int. 2007;28:537–41.
25. Besse JL, Maestro M. First metatarsal SCARF osteotomies. Rev Chir Ortop Reparatrice Appar Mot. 2007;93:512–23.

Minimally Invasive Bevel Osteotomy of First Metatarsal without Fixation

13

Michel Benichou

13.1 Introduction

The long plantar arm modified chevron osteotomy was described independently by Elleby in 1992 [1] and Donnelly in 1994 [2]. The plantar cut ends 5–7 mm behind the metatarsal head. A bevel osteotomy of the first metatarsal (M1) is a compromise between a short scarf and a long chevon osteotomy [3]. It has two cuts: the main cut is oblique in the sagittal plane from dorsal distal to plantar proximal, extending in the middle of the metatarsal shaft. The second, shorter cut is dorsal transverse at the metatarsal neck. This bevel osteotomy resembles a distal osteotomy more than a diaphyseal one because its translation and stabilization occur at the distal epiphysis of the metatarsal.

The long plantar arm of the modified chevron osteotomy is more stable than the scarf osteotomy as shown by Vienne in a Sawbones® study [4] and also more stable than the long dorsal arm version based on Ravenell's Sawbones® study on the offset-V osteotomy [5]. The primary stability of the bevel osteotomy, combined with its minimally invasive nature that preserves a large portion of the capsule and periosteal attachments, has reduced the amount of fixation to the point where a screwless osteotomy is now performed in which a bone graft is harvested from the superomedial side of the dorsal fragment obtained after bone translation. This recut fragment is embedded dorsal to plantar through the osteotomy cut and provides the same stability as screw fixation in a large portion of cases.

However, the indication for bevel osteotomy without fixation is limited to minor or moderate deformities in which the bone translation results in sufficient bone contact to allow graft placement. This technique is not recommended in patients with osteoporosis or who are overweight.

13.2 Surgical Technique

13.2.1 Lateral Release

Lateral release is the first step of the surgery and is done percutaneously. It is performed in the first intermetatarsal space with a beaver blade angled lateral to medial to enter the lateral metatarsosesamoid space (Fig. 13.1). The beaver blade is set parallel to the sagittal plane to transect the lateral metatarsal sesamoid ligament. In cases with large deformity, setting the blade parallel to the coronal plane allows the phalangeal attachment of the adductor hallucis brevis to be transected.

M. Benichou (✉)
Centre Medical St Roch, Montpellier, France

C. Cazeau, Y. Stiglitz (eds.), *Percutaneous and Minimally Invasive Foot Surgery*,
https://doi.org/10.1007/978-3-030-98791-6_13

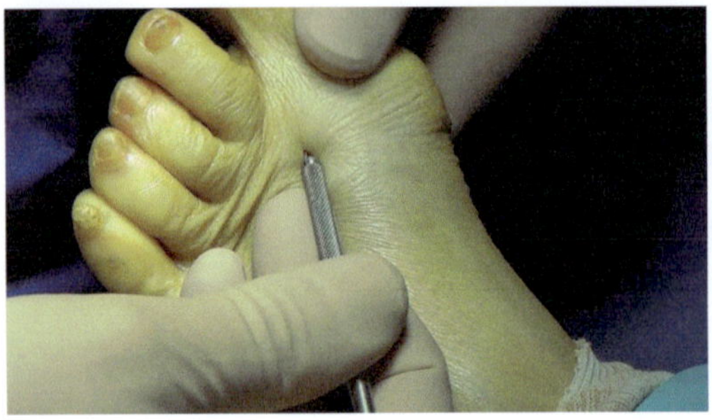

Fig. 13.1 Percutaneous lateral release.

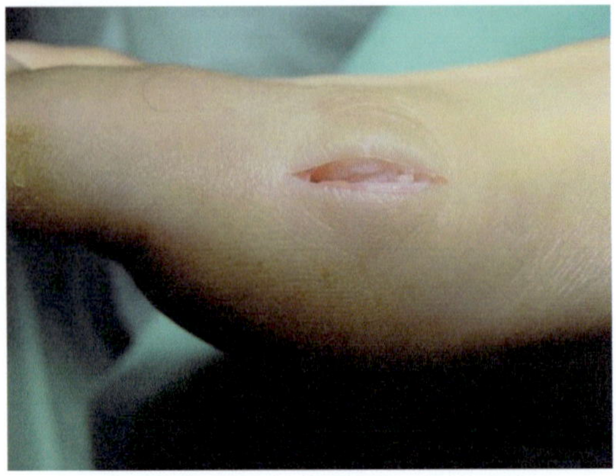

Fig. 13.2 Skin incision.

13.2.2 Incisions

A medial 2–3 cm-long skin incision is centered on the medial side of the metatarsal head, not over the joint line (Fig. 13.2). A medial capsule incision is then made parallel to the skin incision, directly down to the bone; excess capsule tissue is removed to provide a better view of the bone. Minimal decortication of the bone on the medial side of the metatarsal head is performed with a saw.

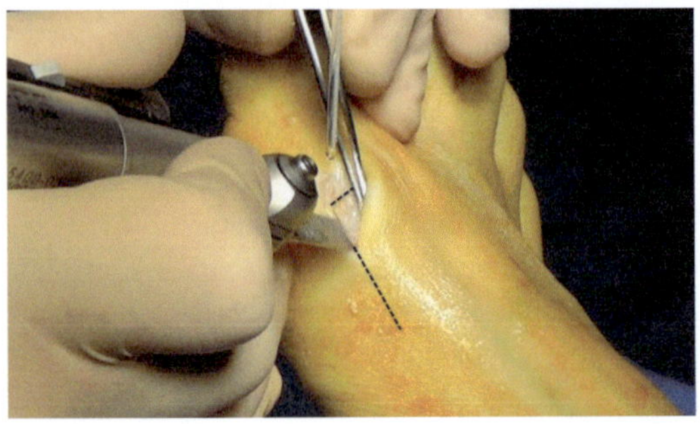

Fig. 13.3 Bevel osteotomy.

13.2.3 Metatarsal Osteotomy

The bevel osteotomy consists of two cuts (Fig. 13.3). The primary cut is oblique in the sagittal plane from distal dorsal to plantar proximal. This cut starts 5 mm behind the articular surface, at the 1/3 dorsal and 2/3 plantar junction of the M1 head. It is angled backward toward the middle of the plantar cortex that it crosses. Because of the small skin incision, the saw blade is angled backward and starts to cut the medial cortex from distal to proximal and then returns proximal to distal through the lateral cortex. At the metatarsal head, the cut is in the coronal plane, either horizontal or lowering. The second distal epiphyseal cut is transverse dorsal, is performed under direct visual control, is perpendicular to the first cut, and is extra-articular, behind the synovial membrane. This second cut is perpendicular to the second metatarsal or angled backward to provide shortening.

A cutting guide can be used to make the cut easier. The cutting guide is placed subcutaneously on the medial face of the metatarsal, with the superior edge of the guide flush with the dorsal cortex of the metatarsal metaphysis. The guide has a slot for the saw blade and a proximal needle that is placed on the inferior face of the diaphysis. Two fingers are used to hold the guide in place on the medial side of the metatarsal (Fig. 13.4).

Once the osteotomy has been completed, an osteotome is inserted through the long plantar arm to distract the two bone fragments and release the periosteal attachments. This maneuver must be performed carefully so as to not break the M1 head. A scalpel is inserted into the dorsal arm to cut the lateral capsular attachments between the two bone fragments.

13.2.3.1 Bone Translation

Bone translation is accomplished by applying traction on the dorsal fragment and pressure on the plantar fragment (Fig. 13.5). Depending on the magnitude of the deformity, it can be done over two-thirds of the epiphyseal's width. Medial derotation is accomplished through proximal, as opposed to distal, translation. The greatest DMAA correction is achieved by excising a bone wedge with medial base through the dorsal cut, from the distal head segment. The osteotomy site is stabilized through pressure on the phalanx in dorsal flexion and forced varus.

13.2.4 Bone Graft

13.2.4.1 Preparing the Bone Graft

The medial overhang of the dorsal fragment is cut with a saw, while staying parallel to the medial side of the metatarsal over a minimum length of 2 cm (Fig. 13.6). This bone fragment is placed inside a cutting guide and then recut to make a triangle-shaped graft that is 20 mm long and has a 5-mm-wide base (Fig. 13.7). Because of its slight thickness, which corresponds to the medial cortex of the metatarsal, it appears flat not conical (Fig. 13.8).

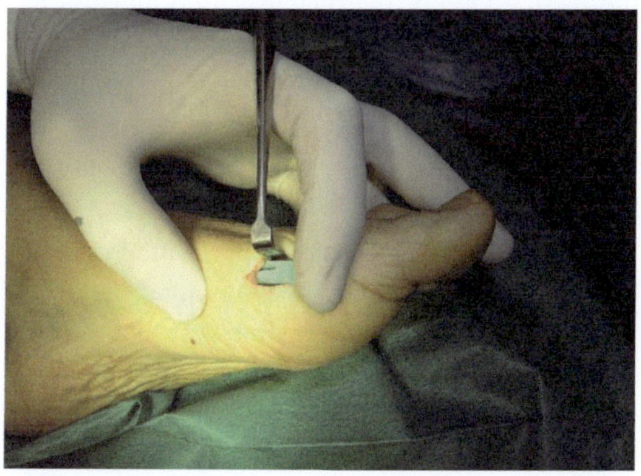

Fig. 13.4 Cutting guide. © Michel Benichou 2015. All Rights Reserved

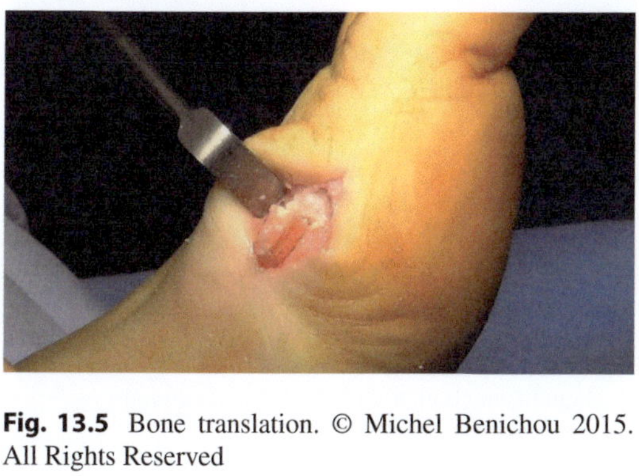

Fig. 13.5 Bone translation. © Michel Benichou 2015. All Rights Reserved

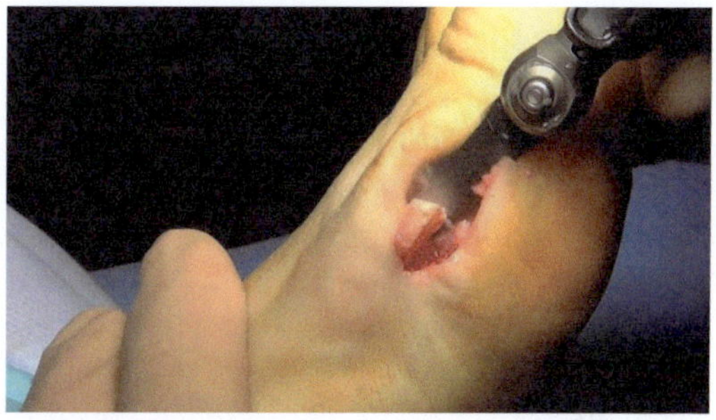

Fig. 13.6 Harvesting the graft. © Michel Benichou 2015. All Rights Reserved

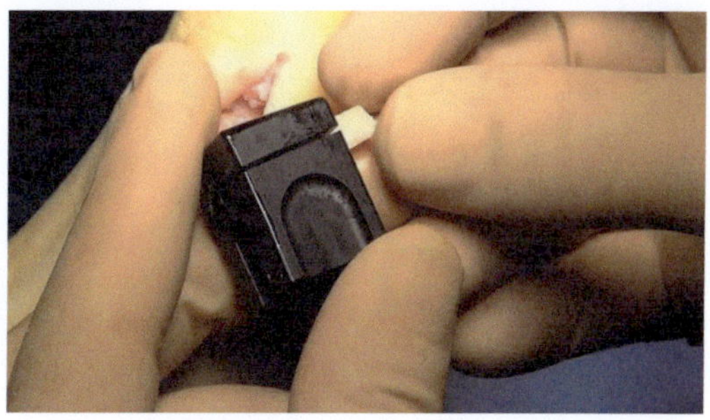

Fig. 13.7 Trimming the graft. © Michel Benichou 2015. All Rights Reserved

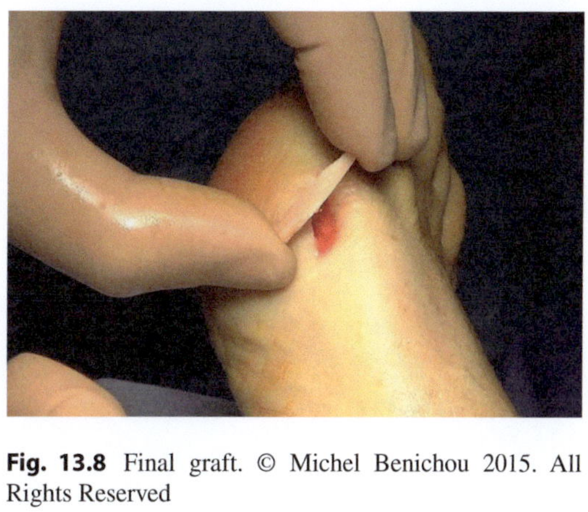

Fig. 13.8 Final graft. © Michel Benichou 2015. All Rights Reserved

13.2.4.2 Preparing the Graft Implantation Site

The dorsal side of the metatarsal neck is exposed. A thin conical burr is used to drill through the metatarsal neck in a plantar and distal direction toward the center of the metatarsal head, thus crossing the distal portion of the osteotomy site (Fig. 13.9). The dorsal hole is widened using a burr of the same length as the graft's width and the same width as the graft's thickness, which results in an elongated slit overall.

13.2.4.3 Inserting the Graft

The graft is embedded in the bone tunnel and impacted carefully using a bone tamp until fully inserted or to minimum depth of 15 mm (Fig. 13.10). If this technique is not feasible, fixation is performed using one or two standard-length screws (17 or 19 mm) inserted dorsal to plantar in the epiphysis through a single cortex.

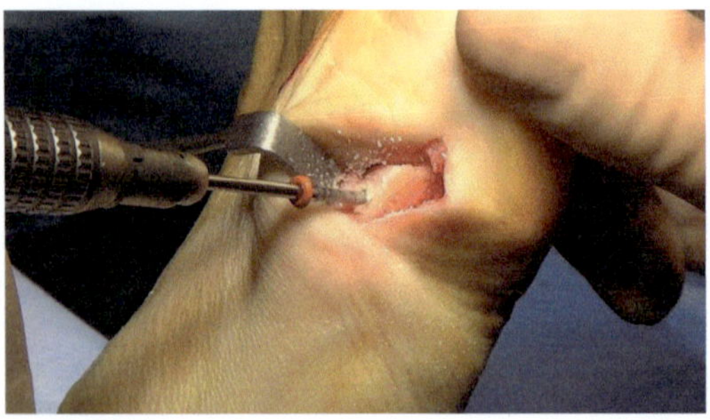

Fig. 13.9 Drilling. © Michel Benichou 2015. All Rights Reserved

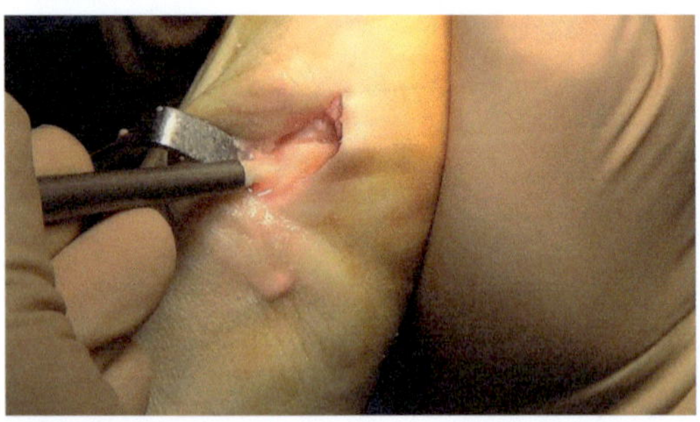

Fig. 13.10 Impacting the graft. © Michel Benichou 2015. All Rights Reserved

13.2.4.4 Phalangeal Osteotomy

A varus-producing phalangeal osteotomy is done percutaneously without screw fixation. It is either proximal or distal for cases of cross-over toe deformity. It can either be transverse with lateral cortical hinge or chevron. A phalangeal chevron osteotomy will provide better stability. The burr crosses the medial cortex midway between the dorsal and plantar sides of the phalanx. The two oblique cuts are proximal to distal through the dorsal cortices and then the plantar ones (Fig. 13.11). The burr is inserted back through the dorsal cut and progressively starts cutting the lateral cortex distal to proximal until one feels the phalanx shift into varus. It is important not to force the burr and crack the lateral cortex. In the distal chevron osteotomy, the dorsal and plantar cuts are reversed, from distal to proximal.

This varus-producing osteotomy is stabilized with an absorbable subcutaneous suture place on the medial side of the phalanx. Two incision are made with the beaver blade: distally just proximal to the medial edge of the interphalangeal joint and proximally just distal to the medial edge of the metatarsophalangeal joint. A No. 1 VICRYL® suture with large needle is passed through the two incisions, first proximal to distal then distal to proximal while staying close to the phalanx and on the dividing line between the dorsal and plantar layers (Fig. 13.12).

Tightening the suture proximally ensures stable closure of the osteotomy by placing tension

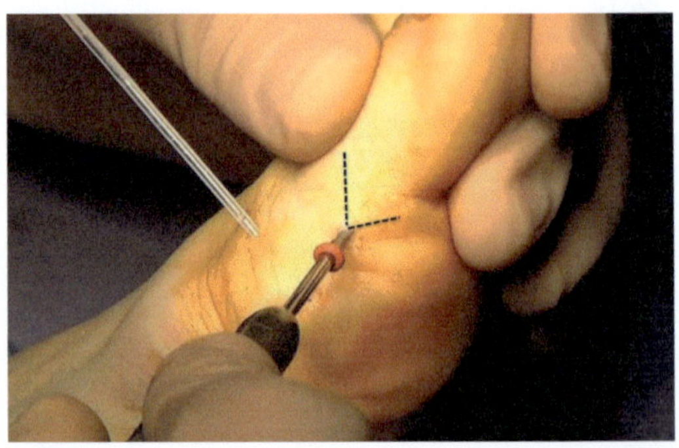

Fig. 13.11 Percutaneous varus-producing osteotomy. © Michel Benichou 2015. All Rights Reserved

on the fibrous and periosteal structures located on the medial edge of the phalanx. The proximal knot is buried.

Tensionless capsular closure is performed with inverted throws, without drainage. Any excess skin is removed, and the skin incision is closed with an absorbable running intradermal suture.

The patient is allowed immediate postoperative weight-bearing while wearing a postoperative shoe.

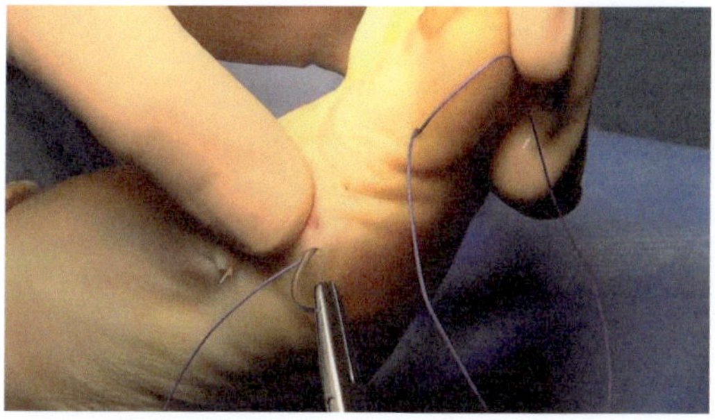

Fig. 13.12 Stabilization with suture. © Michel Benichou 2015. All Rights Reserved

13.3 Conclusion

This minimally invasive bevel osteotomy without screw fixation integrates the principles of minimally invasive surgery, which aims to reduce the morbidity related to the extensive approaches and bone fixation (Fig. 13.13). While its indications are broad, they are limited by the amount of metatarsus varus and by the context. The learning curve requires that conventional M1 osteotomy techniques be mastered followed by minimally invasive ones.

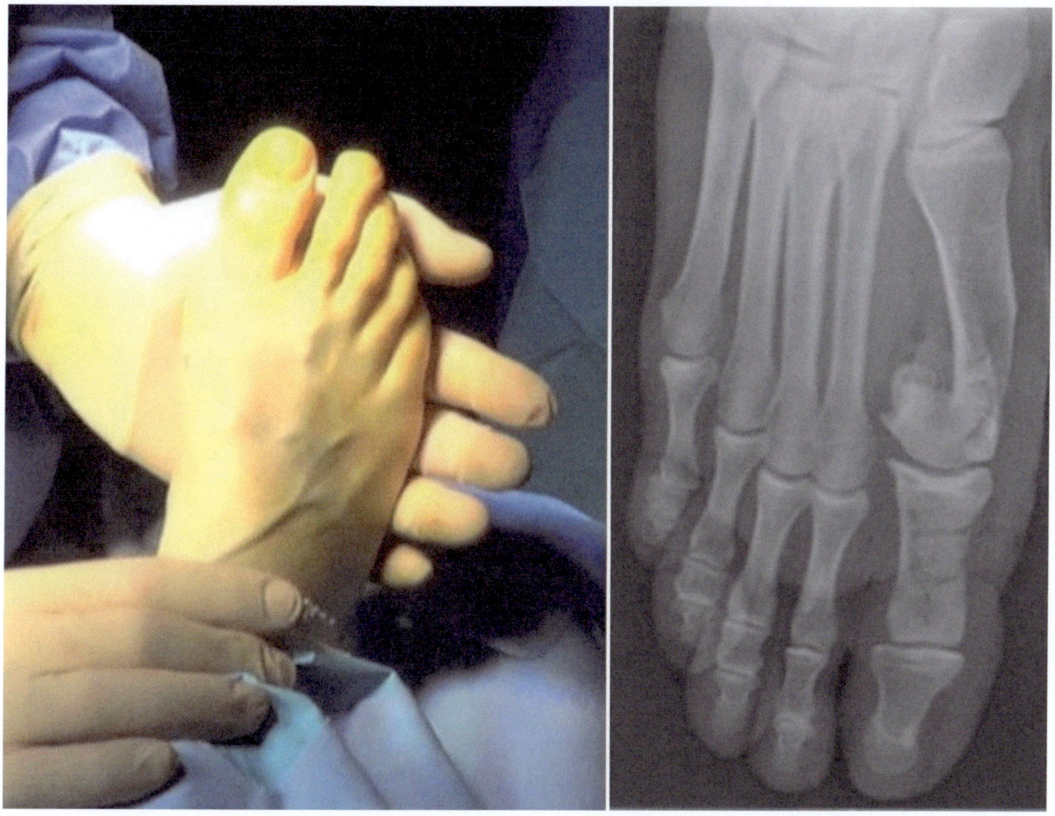

Fig. 13.13 Immediate postoperative appearance. © Michel Benichou 2015. All Rights Reserved

References

1. Donnelly RE, Saltzman CL, Kile TA, Johnson KA. Modified Chevron osteotomy for hallux valgus. Foot Ankle Int. 1994;15:642–5.
2. Elleby DH, Barry LD, Helfman DN. The long plantar wing distal metaphyseal osteotomy. J Am Podiatr Med Assoc. 1992;82:501–6.
3. Benichou M. Traitement chirurgical de l'hallux valgus par mini-abord. Med Chir Pied. 2006;23:140–5.
4. Vienne P, Favre P, Meyer D, Schoeniger R, Wirth S, Espinosa N. Comparative mechanical testing of different geometric designs of distal first metatarsal osteotomies. Foot Ankle Int. 2007;28:232–6.
5. Ravenell RA, Kihm CA, Lin AS, Garing FX. The offset V osteotomy versus the modified Austin with a longer plantar arm: a comparison of mechanical stability. J Foot Ankle Surg. 2011;50:201–6.

14 Percutaneous Correction of Mild to Severe Hallux Valgus Defomity: The Evolution and Current Concepts of the PECA Technique

Peter W. Robinson and Peter Lam

14.1 Introduction

Over the last 30 years, minimally invasive surgery (MIS) has become the gold standard across various orthopaedic subspecialities, including arthroscopic knee, shoulder and ankle surgery. Any MIS approach, with less soft tissue stripping and smaller incisions, has the potential benefit of lower infection rates, fewer wound healing problems, less pain, earlier return to function and lower nonunion rate. MIS or percutaneous hallux valgus surgery has been around for over 50 years [1]. First-generation techniques involve osteotomies with no fixation, relying on meticulous bandaging to maintain the hallux correction. Bosch popularised the approach in the 1980s with the second-generation technique relying on intramedullary K-wires to maintain the correction [2]. However Vernois and Redfern revolutionised MIS hallux valgus correction with the minimally invasive chevron akin (MICA), a third-generation technique combining percutaneous osteotomies with rigid internal fixation [3].

There are over 150 open techniques described for hallux valgus correction. Although the debate continues about the optimum technique, the gold standard now for any osteotomy is widely considered to involve rigid internal fixation. The principles of any corrective osteotomy for hallux valgus are to restore the alignment and rotation of the hallux, which refunctions the medial column, as well as maintaining good first MTPJ motion. At the same time, it is important to avoid shortening or elevation of the metatarsal head to protect against transfer metatarsalgia. We believe these principles should also underpin MIS hallux valgus correction and are only possible to entirely adhere to with third-generation techniques. Despite this first- and second-generation techniques continue to be practised with varying results. A 2019 review including all generations of techniques found a 7.8% recurrence of deformity, 9.8% cases with first MTPJ stiffness and overall complication rate of 13% [4]. Open surgery does not offer the panacea either with mean rates of patient dissatisfaction of 10.6%, recurrence of deformity of 4.9% and removal of hardware in 3.8% (16% in combined shaft and akin osteotomies) [5]. Studies of third-generation techniques report postoperative American Orthopaedic Foot and Ankle Society (AOFAS) scores of 87–97, with patient reported satisfaction of satisfied, good or excellent 87–100% [3, 6–10]. These studies reported complications rates of between 2 and 42%. The majority of complications reported were for removal of metalwork and often included the surgeon's learning curve. The earlier studies

P. W. Robinson
Avon Orthopaedic Centre, Southmead Hospital, Westbury-on-Trym, Bristol, United Kingdom

P. Lam (✉)
Orthopaedic and Arthritis Specialist Centre, Sydney, NSW, Australia
e-mail: admin@peterlam.com.au

C. Cazeau, Y. Stiglitz (eds.), *Percutaneous and Minimally Invasive Foot Surgery*,
https://doi.org/10.1007/978-3-030-98791-6_14

used traditional flat headed screws. The second-generation screws with oblique heads prevent screw head prominence, while maintaining good cortical hold, and should lead to lower rates of screw removal as reflected by more recent third-generation series [10].

14.2 Evolution of the PECA Technique

The percutaneous chevron akin (PECA) technique evolved from the early MICA technique as a third-generation technique. It is an extra-articular osteotomy, which like MICA started with a chevron osteotomy with a small plantar limb. An extra-articular osteotomy minimises capsular contracture and postoperative stiffness, as well as improving the ability to translate the head laterally. The translation is achieved using a flexible translation wire with a 4 mm flair. The flexibility enables the wire to be wrapped under the hallux during translation. This helps when gripping the hallux to correct rotation, but primarily is key to avoid plantar translating or plantar flexing the head. As described in detail below the key to stability of the construct is two-point fixation of the most proximal screw in the metatarsal shaft. This enables the screw to act as a post, preventing loss of reduction through rotation pivoting from the medial cortex. A chevron osteotomy is a relic from open procedures, where it was crucial for stability. Frequently we achieve 100% translation of the metatarsal head; there is no bone contact from a plantar chevron limb and it thus becomes redundant. The PECA technique has evolved to a purely transverse osteotomy in recent years. This gives much greater rotational freedom during translation, enabling easy correction of any first metatarsal and hallux pronation. A transverse osteotomy also makes it easier to establish two-point fixation with the screw in the metatarsal shaft. If the apex of a chevron osteotomy is too dorsal or the screw position too plantar, it is possible that the screw may pass through the lateral cortex at the level of the osteotomy. It is possible, in inexperienced hands, to not appreciate this on the anteroposterior (AP) intraoperative image, thus leaving only a single point of fixation medially and an unstable construct, leading to recurrence of deformity. A transverse osteotomy helps to avoid this pitfall. The entry point of the screws is now much more proximal than in the earlier PECA technique, with the most proximal screw starting right at the first metatarsal base. This enables a larger corner of metatarsal shaft to be removed after screw positioning, giving a smoother medial border and narrower forefoot. The benefits of PECA are listed in Table 14.1. Strict adherence to all aspects of the technique and rehabilitation is crucial for good results and to minimise complications.

Table 14.1 PECA benefits

• A transverse osteotomy gives freedom in 6 planes of motion, allowing the surgeon to easily control the DMMA, rotation, medial/lateral translation, tilt, plantar/dorsal translation and length
• An extra-articular osteotomy facilitates ease of translation, as well as minimising first MTPJ stiffness
• Image-intensifier guidance throughout for complete control of osteotomies, metatarsal head positioning and screw positioning
• Rigid internal fixation maintains the correction achieved and allows early full weight-bearing and range of motion
• Smaller incisions and less soft tissue stripping leads to less postoperative pain and earlier improved satisfaction rates [9]

14.3 Indications

We use the PECA technique for any hallux valgus correction that would be considered for an open distal, shaft or basal osteotomy. Contraindications include first MTPJ arthritis or instability of the first TMTJ, where an arthrodesis procedure is usually preferred. The minimally invasive nature of PECA means that it can be useful for patients with poor skin. As confidence in the technique has grown over the last 5 years so have the indications. The game changing nature of this osteotomy is the ability to translate the metatarsal head 100% or more. This gives huge corrective potential, and thus PECA can be used for patients with severe hallux valgus angles and intermetatarsal angles. In some cases to achieve maximum translation of the head, the proximal metatarsal shaft becomes more medially deviated. This has the added benefit of locking the TMTJ out which helps with stability, decreasing the risk of recurrence and also meaning that PECA can be considered for some cases of first TMTJ instability. We have also found that this technique is powerful for revision cases with previous open metatarsal osteotomies and either recurrence or under correction of the deformity. There is the benefit of avoiding further soft tissue stripping, decreasing the risk of nonunion or avascular necrosis of the metatarsal head. The powerful corrective ability also removes any concerns about narrow or abnormally remodelled metatarsal shafts after previous osteotomies, which would limit the translation achieved in open distal osteotomies. The different orientation of the PECA screw positioning often avoids the need to remove previous screws, although these can usually be removed through small direct incisions if required. We recommend starting with mild to moderate deformities (intermetatarsal angle (IMA) <18°, hallux valgus angle <40°).

14.4 Technique and Concepts

14.4.1 Setup and Imaging

The patient is positioned with the feet hanging off the end of the operating table. This allows the foot to rest freely on the receiver of the image intensifier (Fig. 14.1). We use a thigh tourniquet. The patient is under general anaesthetic with appropriate intravenous antibiotics given on induction. For a right-handed surgeon, we find it easiest to stand on the medial side of the right foot and lean over the left foot from the lateral

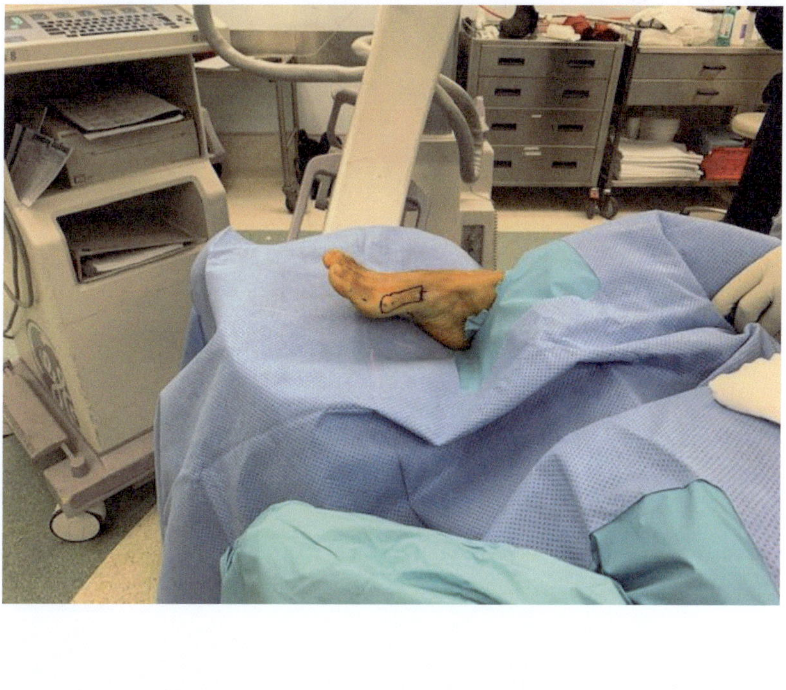

Fig. 14.1 Operative photo showing the patient setup. The foot is off the end of the table resting on the image intensifier receiver, which is tilted 20° cranially. © Peter Lam 2015. All Rights Reserved

side. Therefore the image intensifier is positioned perpendicular to the table approaching from the right hand side. For bilateral cases the right foot is done first, keeping the left covered with a stockinette. The right foot can then be fully bandaged, preserving sterility as the image intensifier is advanced for the left foot. The image intensifier is tilted 20° cranially. This allows the forefoot to rest easily on the receiver, giving a good AP image. The lateral image is achieved by slight flexion of the knee with external rotation at the hip with the help of an assistant. The surgeon then holds the heel and toes, bringing the foot round for a lateral image (Fig. 14.2). It is important that a true lateral is achieved with the metatarsals superimposed over each other. This ensures accurate position of the wires which must be parallel with the first metatarsal in the mid axial line.

An image intensifier is used throughout ensuring precise and reproducible positioning of each osteotomy, positioning of the metatarsal head and the screw placement. We cone the image in to just cover the metatarsal and not the tip of the hallux. The image is then magnified and a low-dose setting is used. This minimises the radiation exposure and ensures that all the positioning of the foot can be achieved without irradiating the surgeon's fingers. The mean radiation dose per foot is less than half that of a single foot xray [10]. The osteotomies are performed using an irrigated burr on a hand piece, which is set at low speed and high torque. This helps to minimise any damage to soft tissues. It is controlled with a foot pedal. The irrigation is key to preventing thermal damage to the skin and soft tissues. Attention must be taken to ensure it runs throughout the case. The hand piece is best held in a pencil grip.

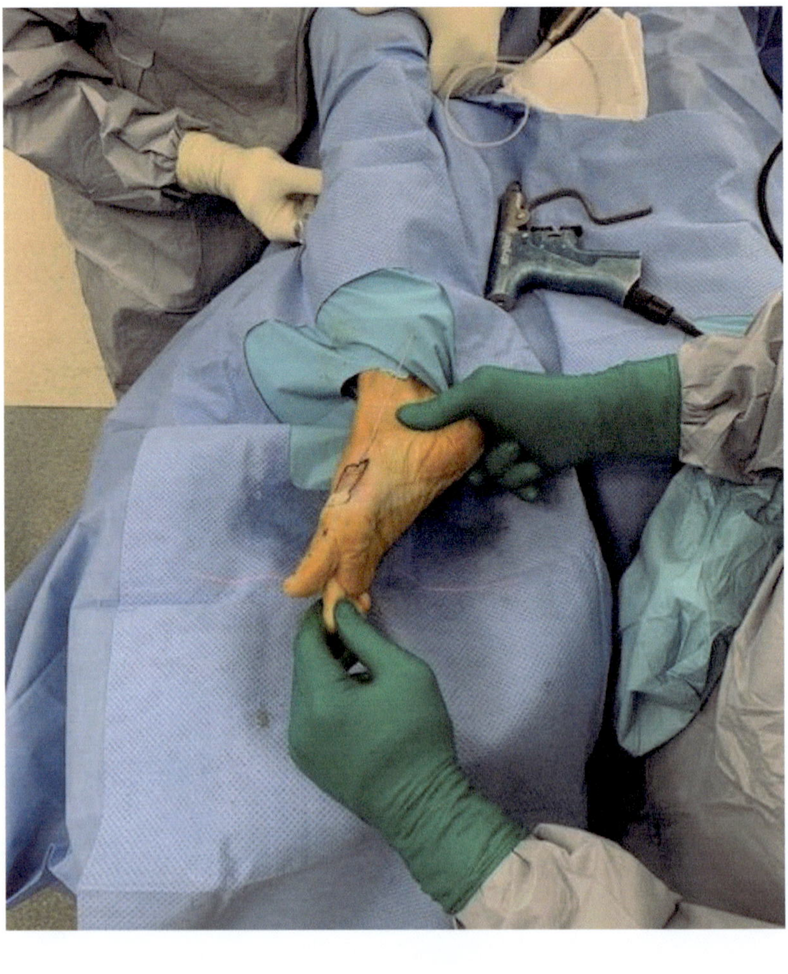

Fig. 14.2 The lateral image is achieved with knee flexion and further external rotation of the foot by gripping the heel and toes. The laser lines help to line up the image and avoid radiation exposure to the surgeon's hands. © Peter Lam 2015. All Rights Reserved

14.4.2 Incisions

We make four incisions at the start of the procedure (Fig. 14.3). It helps to draw the lateral outline of the first metatarsal. Incision 1 is approximately 5 mm long in the mid axial line on the medial side of the first TMTJ. A periosteal elevator is then used to clear the soft tissues along the medial side of the metatarsal towards the neck. Incision 2 is 3–5 mm long at the neck of the metatarsal in line with the incision 1. Here a periosteal elevator is also used to clear soft tissue just at the base of the incision. This helps the burr tip get grip on the bone. It is not necessary to clear tissues around the neck. Incision 3 is at the midpoint of the metatarsal head, half way between the base of the sesamoids and the dorsal part of the head. Incision 4 is in the mid axial line just proximal to the midpoint of the proximal phalanx.

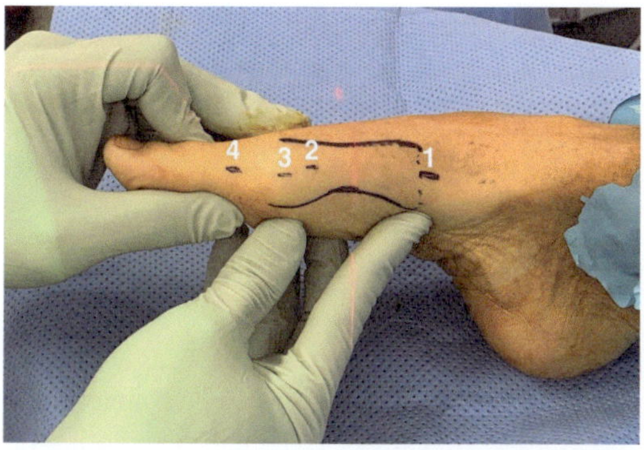

Fig. 14.3 Four incisions are made at the start of the procedure. © Peter Lam 2015. All Rights Reserved

14.4.3 First Metatarsal Osteotomy

Under image-intensifier guidance, the burr (2.2 × 22mm) is positioned at the neck of the first metatarsal. It helps to orientate the image on the screen so that the second metatarsal is vertical, ensuring the starting point is extra capsular. We usually aim just distal of perpendicular to the second metatarsal. A 2-mm burr will remove about 3 mm of bone, so aiming slightly distally helps to maintain metatarsal length. The burr is advanced as far as the lateral cortex aiming slightly plantar. A final X-ray is taken to confirm the position prior to advancing through this cortex (Fig. 14.4).

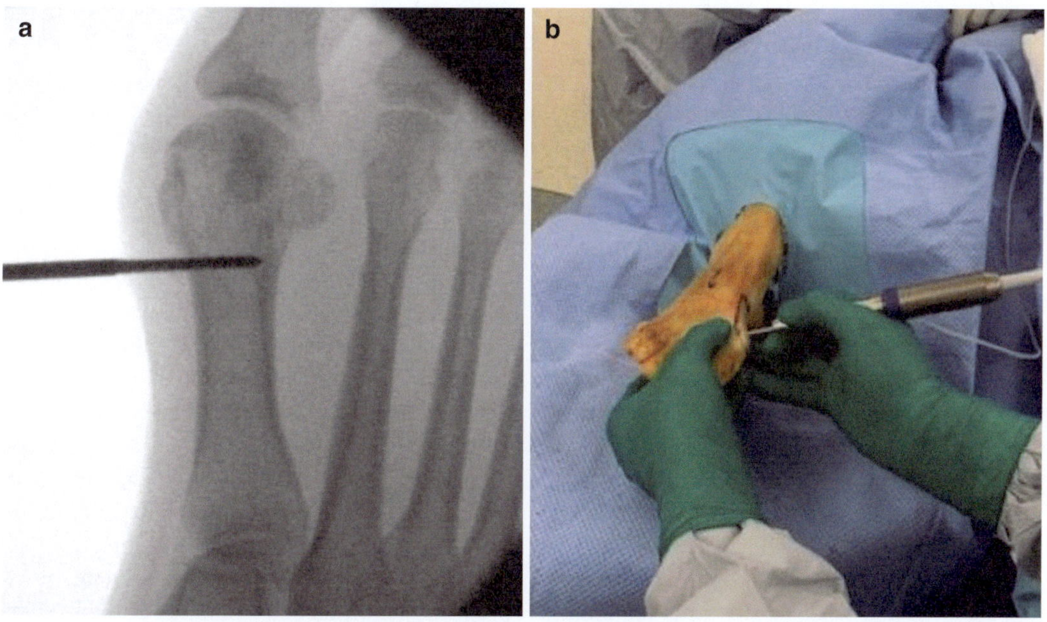

Fig. 14.4 (**a**) Intra-operative image confirming burr alignment prior to penetration of the lateral cortex. Note the osteotomy is extra-capsular and aiming slightly distal of perpendicular to the second metatarsal. (**b**) The irrigated burr and hand piece is held in a pencil grip during the osteotomy. © Peter Lam 2015. All Rights Reserved

The burr is rotated dorsally to complete the dorsal part of the osteotomy. It is important to control the incision during this movement to prevent damage to the surrounding skin. As the burr is rotated dorsally, the skin incision can be rotated in a plantar direction with the thumb and index finger of the other hand. This keeps the burr in the centre of the incision at all times. When the burr reaches the edge of the incision and there is no further option to rotate it is translated dorsally. The skin incision is also then translated with the burr. When the dorsal part of the osteotomy is completed, the burr is returned to the original position in preparation for the plantar limb. This has historically been completed as a small plantar chevron by aiming toward the tip of the heel. Again the skin incision is rotated and then translated around the burr to protect the skin edges. For the last 2 years, we have changed the osteotomy, making it entirely transverse as discussed above.

The surgeon has complete control of the osteotomy direction. For moderate to severe deformity, it can be useful to aim more proximally to build in some shortening of the metatarsal to help with the correction. Equally an already short metatarsal with transfer metatarsalgia can be lengthened by aiming more distally.

When the osteotomy is complete, a reduction tool can be inserted through incision 2 into the metatarsal shaft and used to translate the head laterally. We recommend a flexible reduction tool. We use a 3-mm wire that widens to 4 mm over the last 4 cm (Novastep, Saint-Grégoire, France). This enables adequate lateral translation of the metatarsal head, but also has the added benefit of preventing plantarisation of the head, which can be a problem with more rigid reduction tools. The metatarsal head is gripped between the finger and thumb of 1 hand, while the narrow diameter end of the wire is wrapped under the hallux. Here it can be held by the other hand using the ring and little finger, while the thumb and index finger correct the hallux pronation (Fig. 14.5). The image intensifier is used to confirm the translation achieved and whether any tilt is required to correct the DMMA. It is important to pay attention to the DMMA during lateral translation of the head. It can tip into more valgus at the extremes of translation. This can be countered by applying a varus stress to the hallux, pivoting on the intact lateral ligaments. A lateral view is used to ensure the head remains lined up with the metatarsal shaft, with no plantar angulation or translation. We then relax the reduction for the initial guide wire insertion.

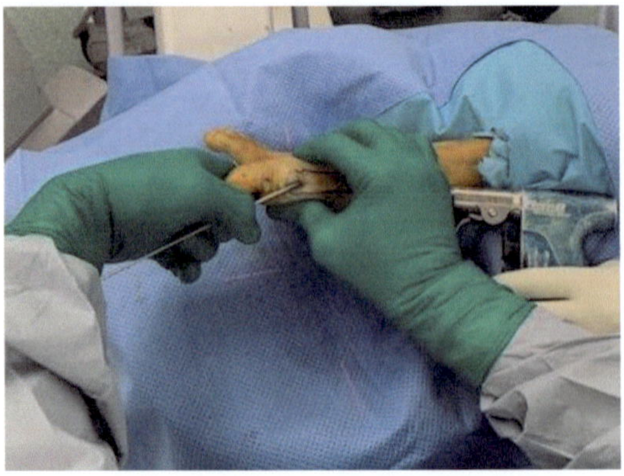

Fig. 14.5 The reduction manoeuvre. Note the dorsal pressure of the thumb on the plantar surface of the metatarsal head to prevent plantar translation. The hallux is gripped by the other hand, correcting the pronation, while translating the head laterally with pressure from the flexible reduction wire. © Peter Lam 2015. All Rights Reserved

14.4.4 Guide Wire and Screw Positioning

We stabilise the construct with two screws. These should be fully threaded (non-compressive) headless cannulated screws. We use 4.0-mm screws with an oblique head (PECA 4 screw, Novastep, Saint-Grégoire, France). In very small metatarsal on occasion, a smaller 3.0-mm screw will be used. The benefit of a 4.0-mm screw is the large 1.4-mm guide wire, which is easier to control and position during insertion. The guide wire is inserted from the base of the first metatarsal through incision 1. We now aim to be as proximal with this entry point as possible. This leaves a larger medial corner of metatarsal shaft for resection at the end, giving a smoother medial

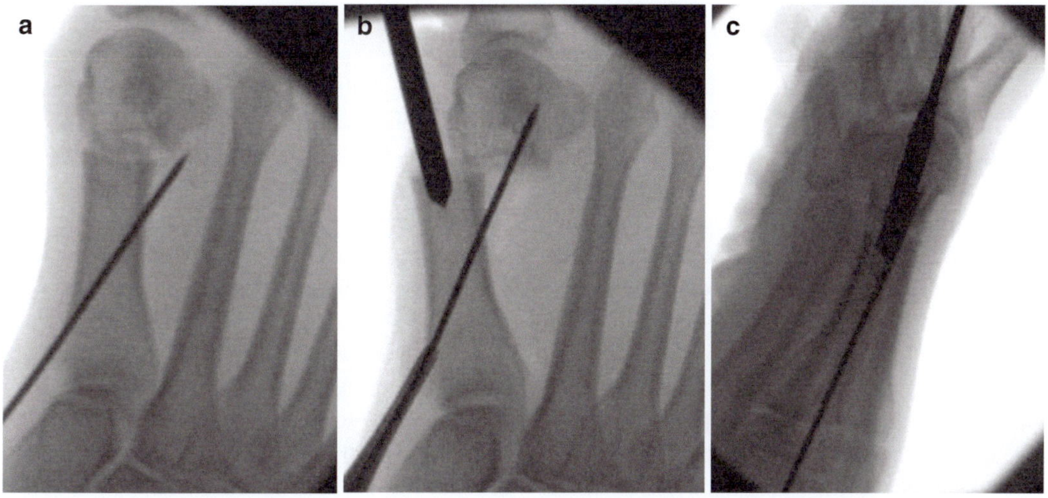

Fig. 14.6 (**a**) Intra-operative image showing initial guide wire position. Note the basal starting point and crossing the lateral cortex approximately 10 mm proximal to the transverse osteotomy to avoid lateral wall fracture into the osteotomy. (**b**) The reduction manoeuvre is then performed and the wire is advanced into the head. The DMMA is checked at this stage. (**c**) A lateral image confirms the alignment with no plantar translation or tilt.

edge and a narrower foot. The guide wire is advanced as far as the lateral cortex, approximately 10 mm proximal to the osteotomy. This distance is important. Too proximal and the screw would miss the head laterally and too distal, and there may be blow out of the lateral cortex with drilling or screw insertion thus losing the vital two-point fixation. We check on the image-intensifier AP view and then on the lateral view, aiming to have the wire parallel with the shaft in the mid axial line. When happy with the position, the wire is advanced through the lateral cortex (Fig. 14.6a). We irrigate the wire during this process to prevent thermal skin damage at incision 1. We apply very little forward pressure, letting the wire drive through slowly. This prevents it from slipping too distally as it passes through the cortex. The reduction manoeuvre is then performed and held, while the assistant advances the wire into the metatarsal head (Figs. 14.6b, c and 14.7). When happy with the position, the wire is measured for screw length, and the near and far cortices are over drilled. There is no need to drill into the metatarsal head. The head is then stabilised, while the screw is

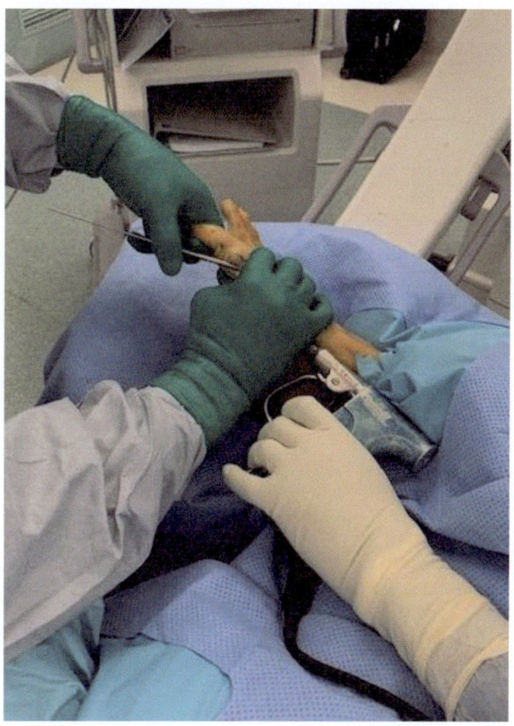

Fig. 14.7 The surgeon holds the reduction as the wire is advanced into the metatarsal head.

inserted usually by the assistant. We take care to protect the skin from the screw as it is inserted. During screw insertion the head can be distracted as the screw initially advances into the head. This can tip the head into varus. This can be corrected by initially backing the screw out of the head, before correcting the head position and holding it firmly reduced as the screw is reinserted. Because the screw threads have already cut a track, further distraction does not occur again.

The oblique head of the second-generation screw should enable it to be completely buried in the cortex and not prominent, while maintaining good hold. Due to the triangular cross-sectional shape of the base of the first metatarsal, we perform an internal rotation X-ray. This brings the medial shaft of the metatarsal perpendicular to the image intensifier to check the screw head is fully buried. If an internal rotation view is not taken, it is possible for the screw to appear fully buried, when in fact it is slightly prominent (Fig. 14.8). This can be a cause for metalwork irritation and the need for removal.

A second wire is then inserted just distally and parallel to the first, but still through incision 1. This can enter the metatarsal head through the osteotomy, acting mainly as an anti-rotation screw (Fig. 14.9). It is important to not try and pass through the lateral cortex as it may compromise the hold of the first screw, by blowing out the lateral cortex distally. The near cortex is then drilled and the second screw inserted. Finger palpation of the screw head under the skin can help provide the surgeon feedback about the screw depth and help minimise unnecessary X-rays. We usually insert the second guide wire and then proceed to the akin osteotomy and akin wire insertion prior to inserting the second screw, which makes the procedure more time efficient.

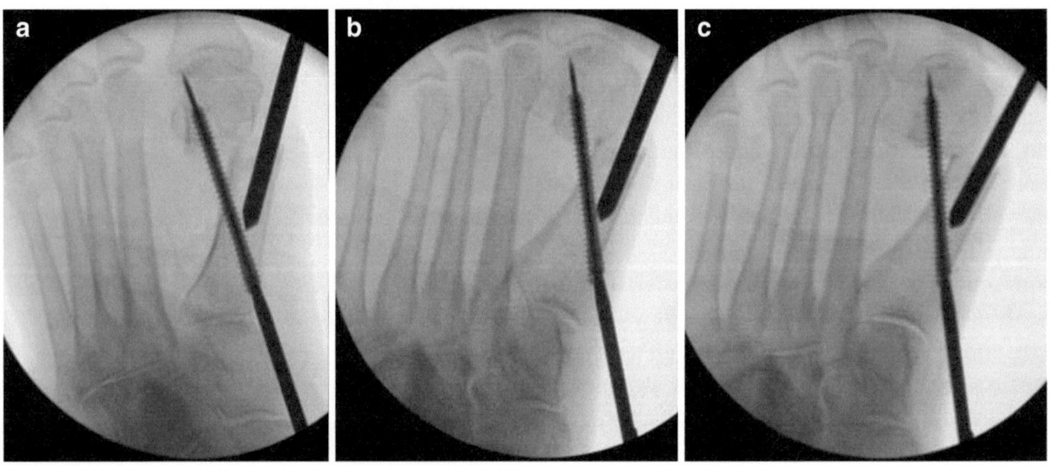

Fig. 14.8 (**a**) AP image showing the oblique headed screw appears buried. (**b**) The internal oblique image shows the screw head is still prominent. (**c**) The internal oblique image subsequently showing the screw head is buried after further insertion.

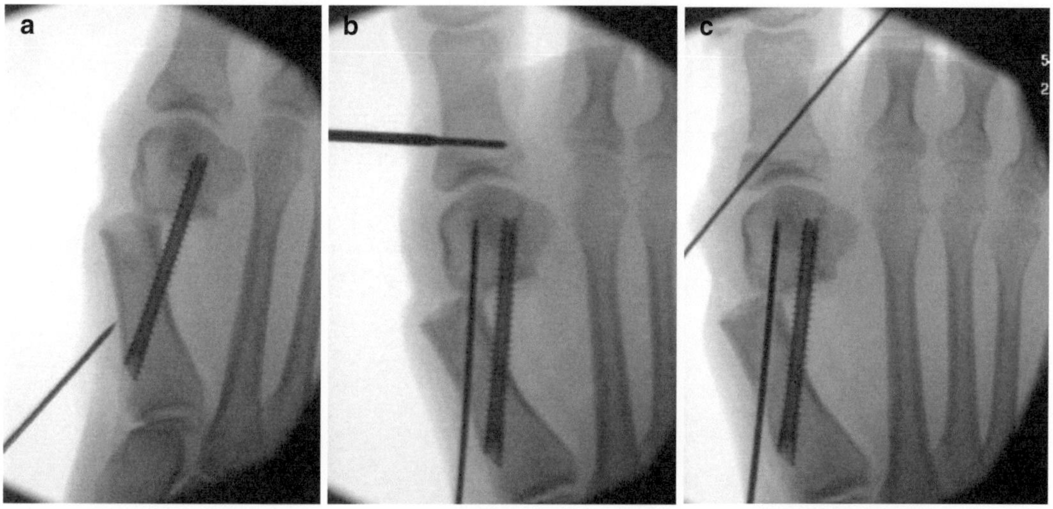

Fig. 14.9 (**a**) The second guide wire is inserted parallel to the first screw. (**b**) Note the second wire must not pass through the lateral cortex so as not to compromise the stability of the first screw. At this stage the akin osteotomy can be performed. (**c**) The akin guide wire is then inserted.

14.4.5 Akin Osteotomy

A 2 × 12-mm burr is used through incision 4. The osteotomy is started in the mid axial line aiming towards the lateral base of the proximal phalanx. This ensures the osteotomy is perpendicular to the screw. We try and keep this osteotomy as metaphyseal as possible to aid bone union. The burr is advanced as far as the far cortex but not through (Fig. 14.9b). It is then rotated dorsally before penetrating the dorsal cortex and sweeping medially again to complete a dorsal osteotomy. It is reinserted in the original direction before penetrating the thick plantar lateral cortex, rotating and pulling medially to complete the plantar cortex. The hallux can be held in flexion to keep the FHL tendon away from the tip of the burr. We aim to leave the lateral cortex intact to act as a hinge from which the osteotomy can be closed down, adding to stability. The osteotomy is then held closed by a small (2.9 mm or equivalent) headless compression screw. The guide wire is inserted from incision 3, entering the proximal phalanx at the medial proximal corner. It should pass perpendicularly across the osteotomy and through the lateral cortex. It is measured and then the screw is inserted. The small guide wire can be passed through the skin laterally and the end clipped which can be helpful, preventing the wire from displacing when the drill is backed out (Fig. 14.9c). As the screw hits the far cortex, the hallux is held medially angulated to help close down the osteotomy (Fig. 14.10a). We take care to measure the screw length accurately, as it can be uncomfortable having a prominent screw end in the first web space particularly with some shoe wear.

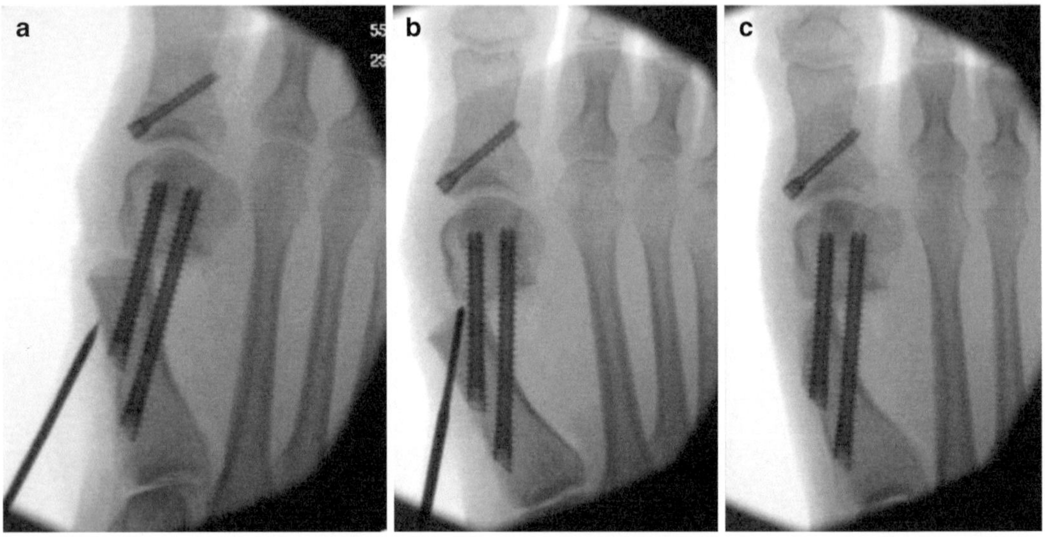

Fig. 14.10 A 2-mm K-wire is inserted initially (**a**) to help direct the 2.2 × 22-mm burr (**b**). After the medial shaft corner is cut off, it is removed, leaving a smooth medial edge to the metatarsal (**c**).

14.4.6 Medial Eminence and Metatarsal Shaft Corner Resection

There is always a medial corner of the metatarsal shaft that needs to be removed as discussed earlier (Fig. 14.10). This can either be burred away with a wedge burr (3.1 × 13 mm) or by cutting it off and removing it directly, which is our preferred technique. First the soft tissues have to be cleared from it using a periosteal elevator. The resection line is parallel and just distal to the more distal screw, again under image guidance. It can help to use a 2-mm K-wire inserted in this line into the metatarsal and then removed (Fig. 14.10a). This leaves a hole through which the burr (2.2 × 22 mm) can be inserted to get started (Figs. 14.10b and 14.11a). Once complete the metatarsal shaft corner can be removed whole through incision 1 or 2. This leaves a smooth medial edge (Fig. 14.10c). The medial eminence is resected using the wedge burr. It helps to insert the burr directly into the part of the eminence to be resected. This resection is done mostly by palpation, as the dorsomedial prominence is most troubling to patients but not clearly seen on the X-ray. We use palpation and X-ray to ensure we know where the tip of the burr is at all times, in order to prevent iatrogenic damage to the first MTPJ (Fig. 14.11b). The burr cuts from right to left more easily. On the right foot, the medial eminence can be removed by starting on the plantar side and creating a groove with a dorsal lip against which the burr can be advanced to prevent it from slipping off. We ensure the dorsomedial eminence is resected by passing over onto the dorsal neck and then sweeping the burr back from dorsal to plantar.

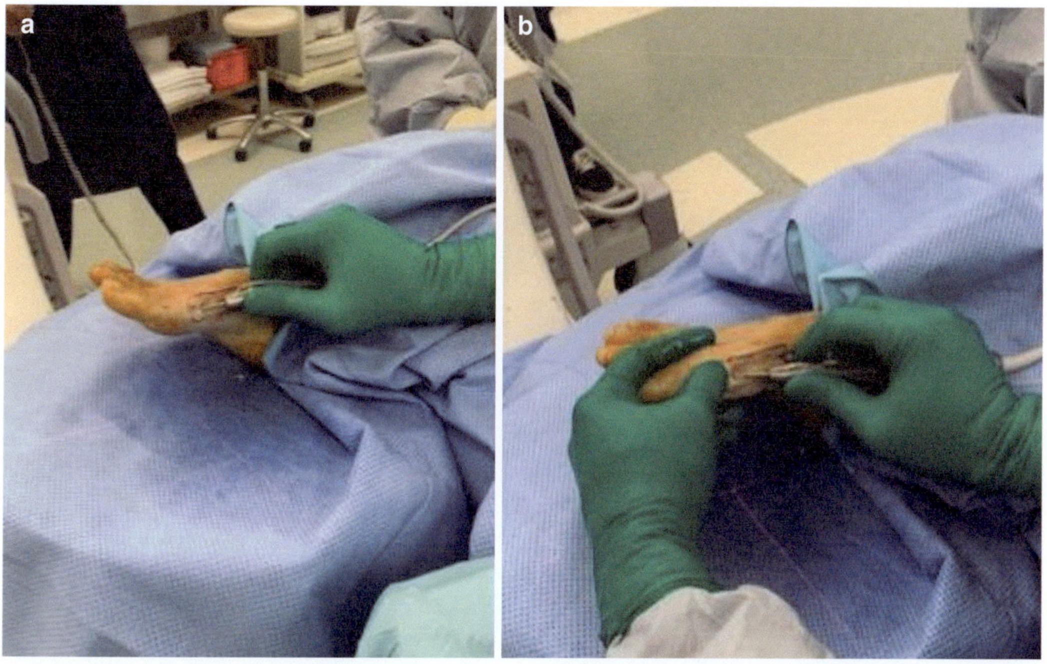

Fig. 14.11 (**a**) Burr positioning to remove the medial metatarsal shaft corner. (**b**) Digital palpation during medial eminence resection. This ensures the surgeon always knows where the tip of the burr is to prevent damage to the joint and helps judge adequacy of dorsal medial eminence resection. © Peter Lam 2015. All Rights Reserved

14.4.7 Lateral Release

This is performed with a small beaver or no. 15 blade. The sulcus of the first MTPJ is palpated and the blade inserted just lateral to the EHL tendon. It is inserted towards the plantar surface of the joint. By holding it perfectly perpendicular to the foot, the risk of FHL damage is lessened (Fig. 14.12). The blade is then rotated laterally and the hallux medially, cutting the plantar lateral capsule and adductor hallucis tendon at the attachment on the base of the proximal phalanx. Care is taken to not cut the collateral ligament, to avoid iatrogenic hallux varus.

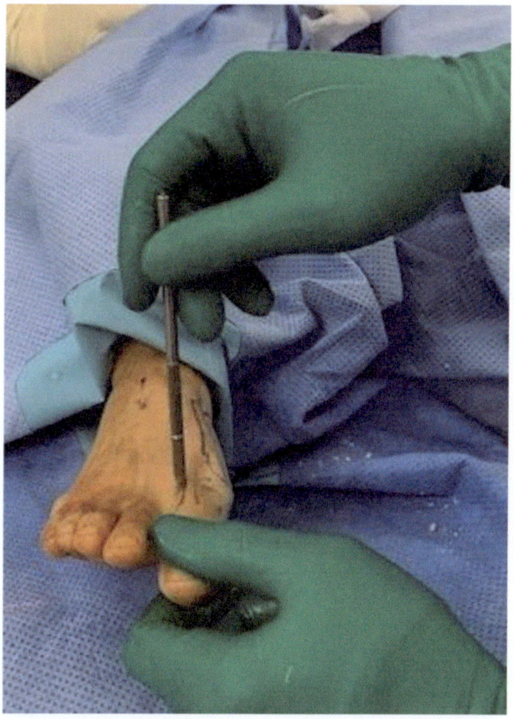

Fig. 14.12 Beaver blade positioning perpendicular to the foot and just lateral to the EHL tendon for the lateral release. © Peter Lam 2015. All Rights Reserved

14.4.8 Wound Closure and Dressings

If there has been any damage to the surrounding skin from screw or wire insertion or the burr, we recommend excising this area of the skin. This is rare, providing care is taken to protect the skin edges, an irrigated burr is used, and the wire is irrigated during insertion. The two proximal inci-

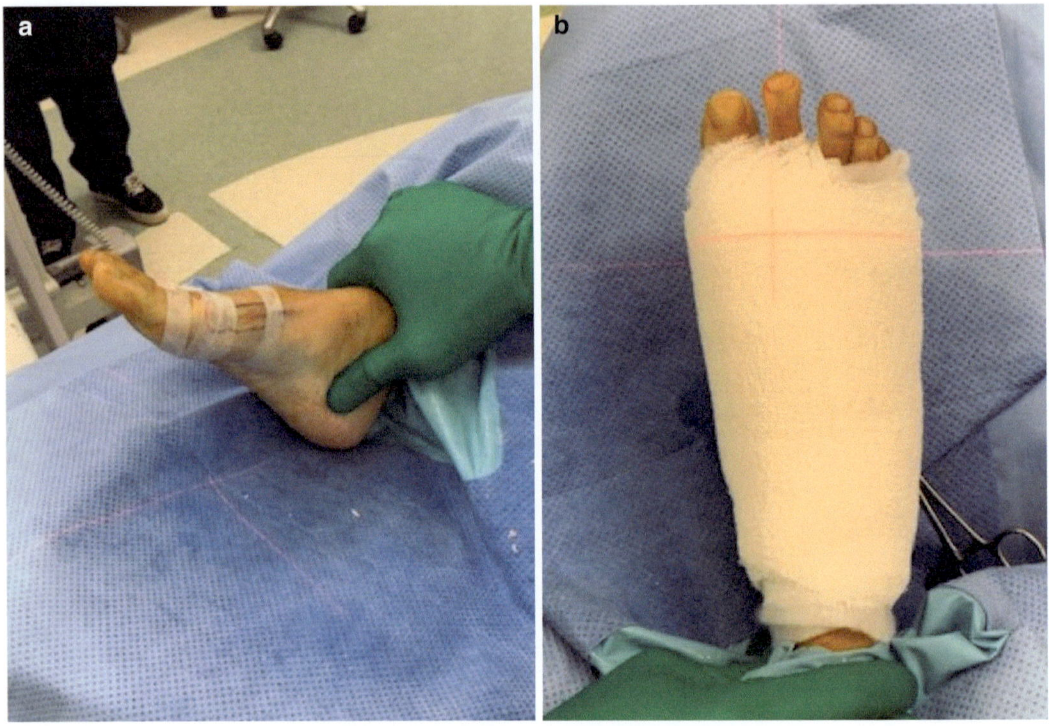

Fig. 14.13 (**a**) SteriStrips to close the wounds. (**b**) Hallux valgus bandage. © Peter Lam 2015. All Rights Reserved

sions are closed with an interrupted subcuticular 4-0 monocryl. SteriStrips are then used for the rest of the wounds (Fig. 14.13a). Local anaesthetic is infiltrated as a medial foot block. A non-adherent dressing is used and then wool and crepe incorporating a standard hallux valgus bandage (Fig. 14.13b).

14.5 Postoperative Instructions

Patients are allowed to fully weight bear in a rigid-soled flat surgical shoe immediately after surgery. Elevation is encouraged over the first 2 weeks. At the 2-week follow-up, the bandages are all removed. A bunion sleeve is then used as support for the next 4 weeks. This is a thin bunion splint made of firm elastic stocking material (Fig. 14.14). It can be quite powerful, and to avoid overcorrection, we advise wearing it in combination with a new tight sports sock. This is worn throughout the day but removed at night time. At 2 weeks patients can transition back into a pair of trainers or running shoes. The only requirement here is that the medial side of the shoe is straight and does not curve in too much onto the hallux. Patients are shown exercises to perform twice daily. These help to restore early range of motion. The hallux is held for 20 s in plantar flexion while pushing dorsally on the plantar side of the metatarsal head. Then repeated 10 times. Next, the hallux is pushed into a varus position to keep a stretch on the lateral ligaments and held for 20 s, repeated 10 times. The patient then scrunches all the toes up, as if they were to pick up a towel with their toes. This is repeated 10 times. By walking normally in a pair of trainers, dorsiflexion is quickly restored. Twice daily wound moisturising is started and then from week 3, deep massage to all wounds. Usually at the 6-week stage, after a check X-ray, the bunion sleeve can be discarded. Most patients do not require physiotherapy unless stiff at the 6-week follow-up.

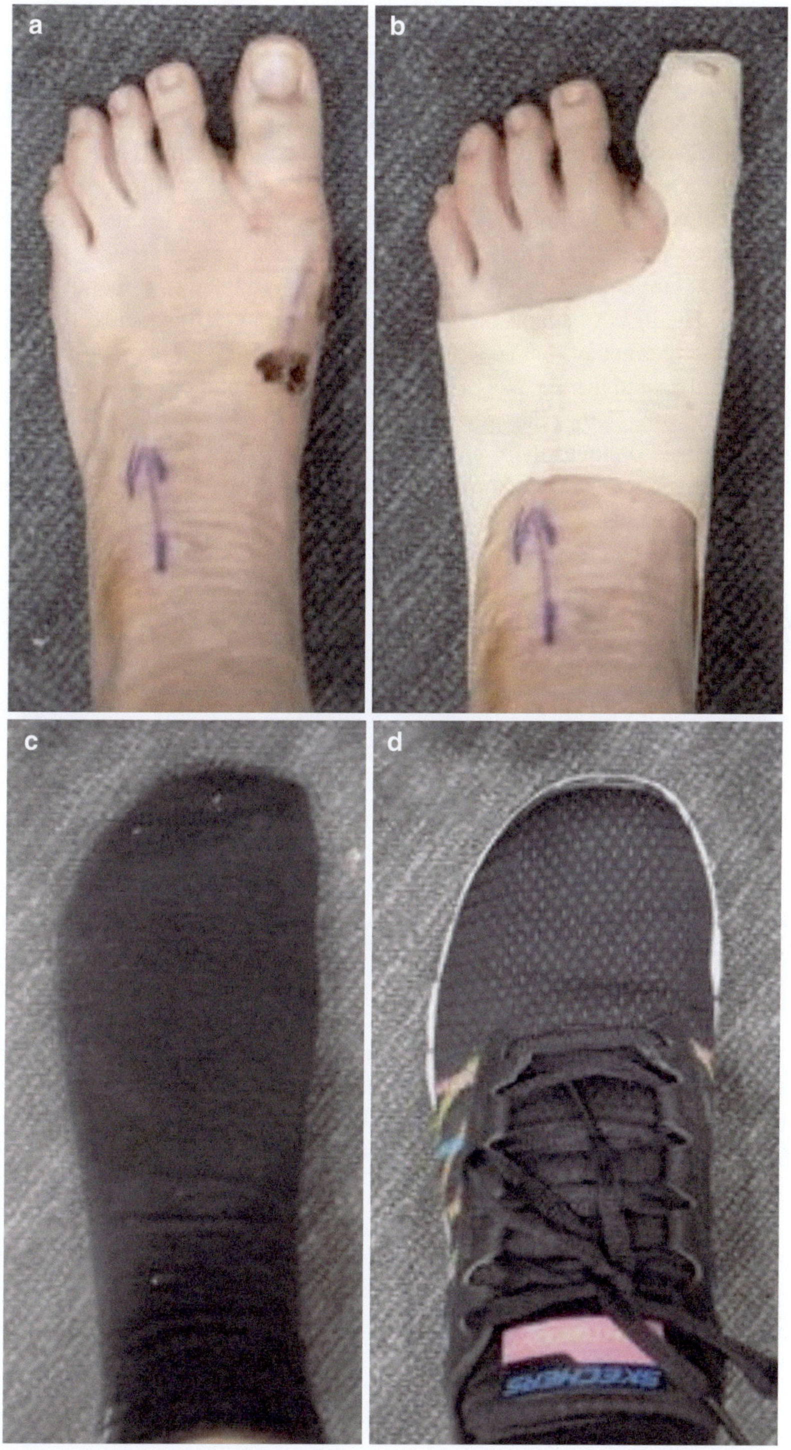

Fig. 14.14 (**a**) 2-week clinical photograph showing the foot after bandage removal. (**b**) After application of the bunion sleeve. Note in this case there was a slight over correction into varus; however a firm sports sock over the top (**c**) overcomes this and supports the toe in normal alignment. (**d**) The patient can mobilise fully weight-bearing in a pair of trainers with a straight medial last.

14.6 Outcomes

We find at 6 weeks there is very minimal swelling, little discomfort and excellent movement. Patients usually walk in comfortably in their own shoes. An RCT has compared open scarf/akin osteotomies with PECA osteotomies [9]. At 6 months the correction achieved and the AOFAS Hallux-Metatarsophalangeal-Interphalangeal Scores were similar. The PECA patients had significantly lower pain scores at day 1 and 6 weeks, shorter scar length and operative time. No serious complications were seen. Now the second-generation screw head is oblique; there are no problems with prominent metalwork. In the early series with traditional screws, some had to be removed for prominence. A retrospective review of the senior author's (PL) cases revealed removal of screws in 3.9% (5/127 cases) at a mean follow-up of 69 ± 7 months. At 6 weeks the X-rays may show some new bone formation medially, but frequently this is not seen until later. By 6–12 months extensive remodelling is seen. This is possible due to the limited soft tissue stripping through the percutaneous approach.

14.7 Cases

Figure 14.15 shows the preoperative and postoperative clinical photograph for the case shown in the previous figures.

Figure 14.16 shows preoperative and postoperative radiographs of another PECA correction. This case highlights the importance of taking an internal rotation X-ray intraoperatively. Note in Fig. 14.16b at 6 weeks, the screws look over buried in the metatarsal; however the internal oblique X-ray shows the screw heads are only just buried in the medial cortex. Had an internal oblique view not been taken intra-operatively, the screws may not have been inserted as far, which could have led to prominence requiring removal. Figure 14.16d shows 6-month radiographs with extensive remodelling across the osteotomy.

Figure 14.17 shows preoperative and 6-month postoperative radiographs of a case with additional preoperative transfer metatarsalgia. The first metatarsal was lengthened through the osteotomy in order to off load the second metatarsal head.

Figure 14.18 shows clinical photographs and radiographs preoperatively, at 6 weeks and 6 months. By 6 months an extensive new bone has formed medially across the osteotomy site.

Figures 14.19 and 14.20 show a patient with bilateral severe hallux valgus. Additionally there was a hammer second toe, which was corrected with percutaneous PIPJ fusion and proximal phalanx plantar closing wedge osteotomy.

Figure 14.21 shows how PECA can be used for revision hallux valgus correction. The old screw is removed through a small incision directly over it. The PECA technique can then be performed. This patient had a symptomatic hammer toe so also underwent a percutaneous PIPJ fusion, stabilised with a screw, as well as a proximal phalanx percutaneous proximal plantar closing wedge osteotomy. Minimal swelling is noted at 6 weeks.

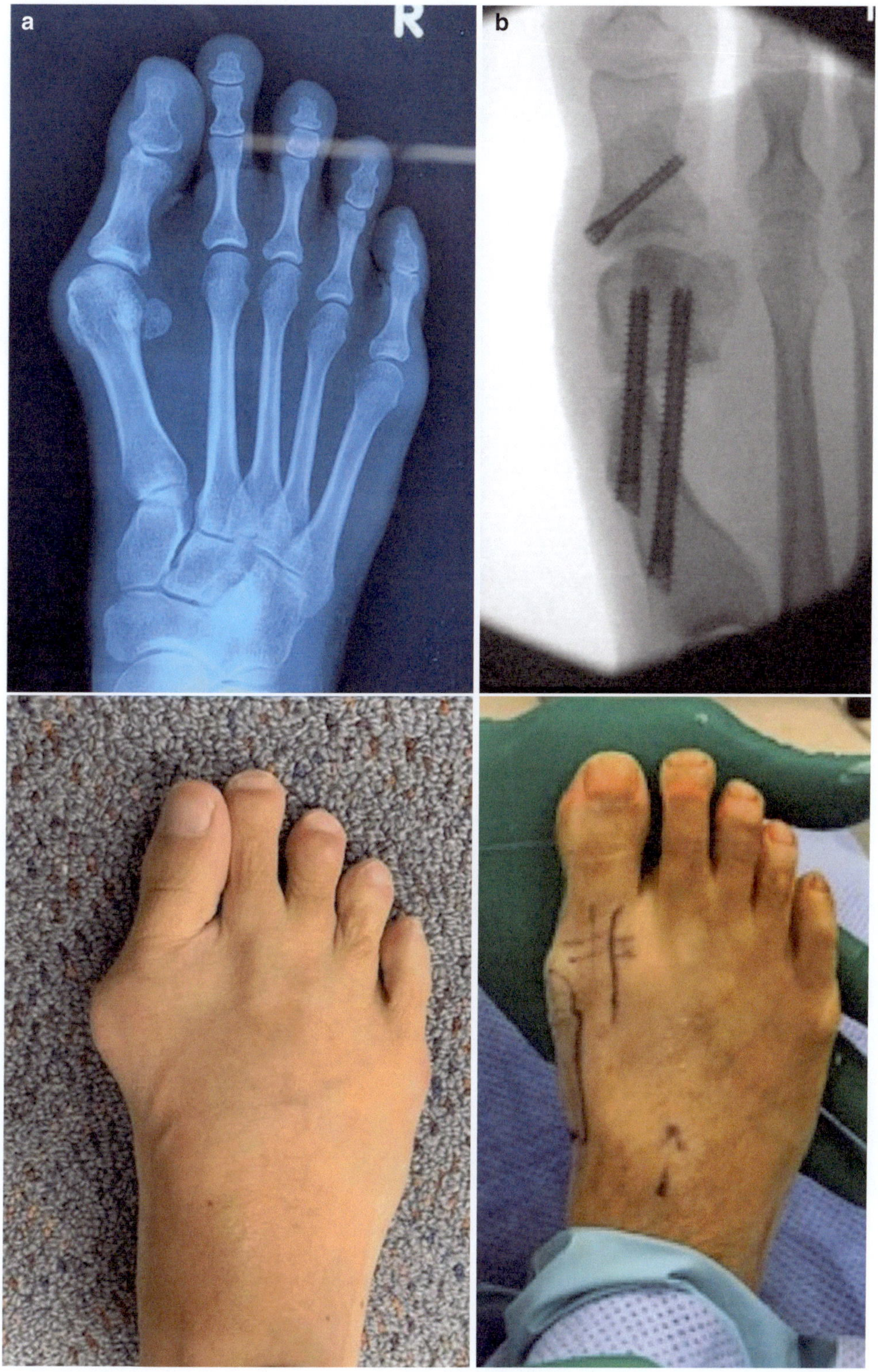

Fig. 14.15 (**a**) Preoperative clinical photo and radiograph. (**b**) Intraoperative image-intensifier film and clinical photograph showing the correction achieved.

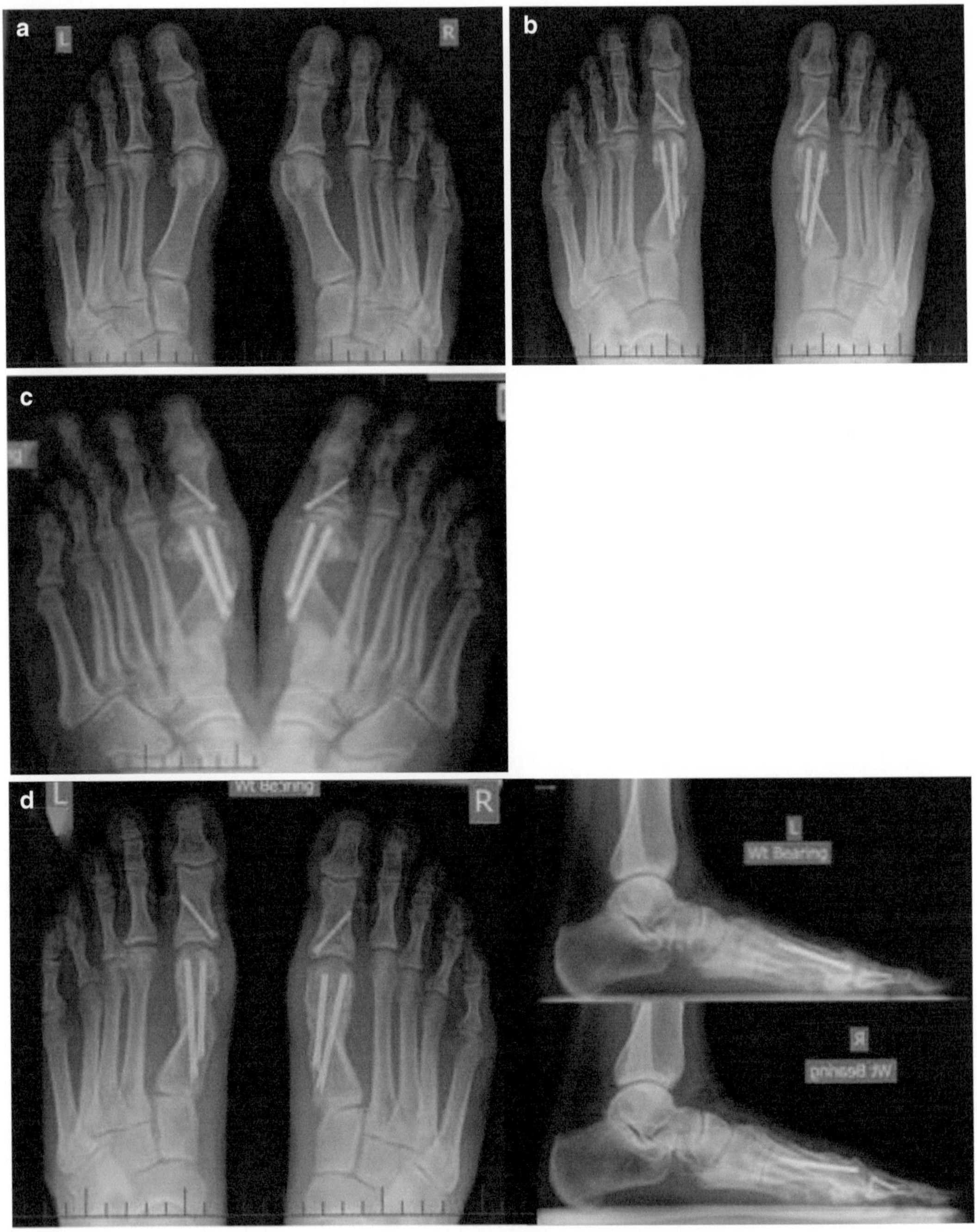

Fig. 14.16 (**a**) Preoperative standing radiographs. (**b**) 6-week postoperative radiographs. (**c**) Internal oblique radiographs showing the screw heads are only just buried in the medial cortex. (**d**) 6 months postoperative radiographs showing remodelling across the osteotomy.

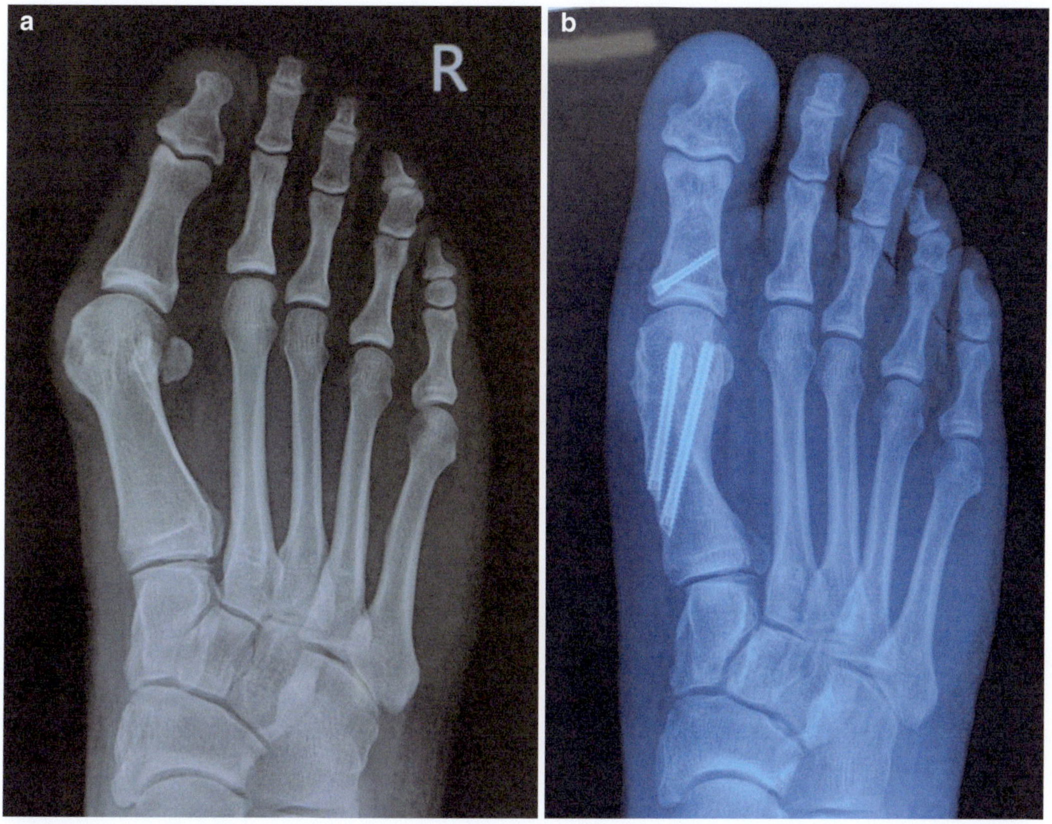

Fig. 14.17 (**a**) Preoperative radiographs. (**b**) 6-month postoperative radiographs showing a lengthened first metatarsal in order to offload the second metatarsal. Note the rotational correction through the osteotomy reducing the position of the seasamoids.

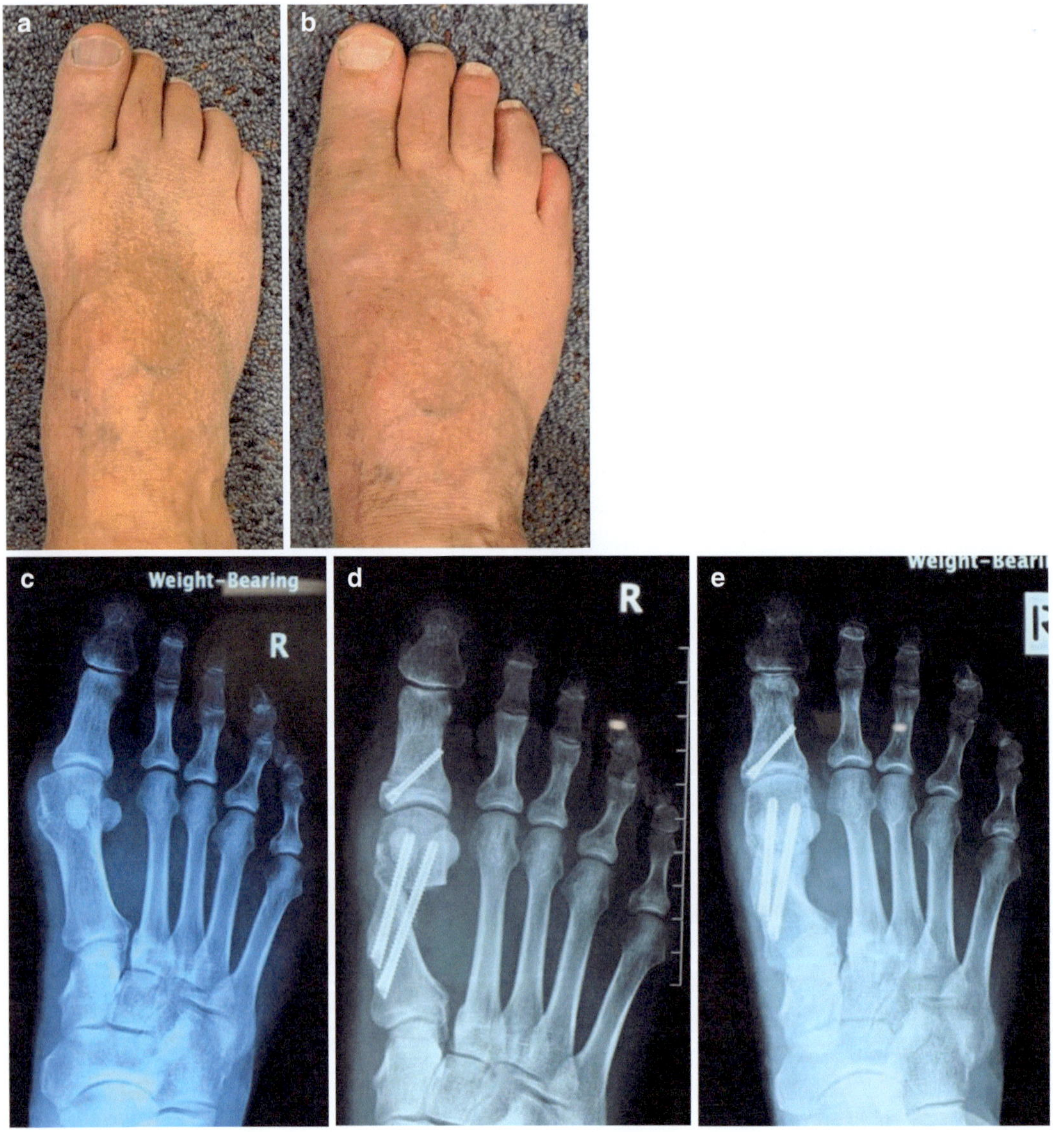

Fig. 14.18 Clinical photographs preoperatively (**a**) and at 6 months (**b**). Standing radiographs preoperatively (**c**), at 6 weeks (**d**) and at 6 months (**e**).

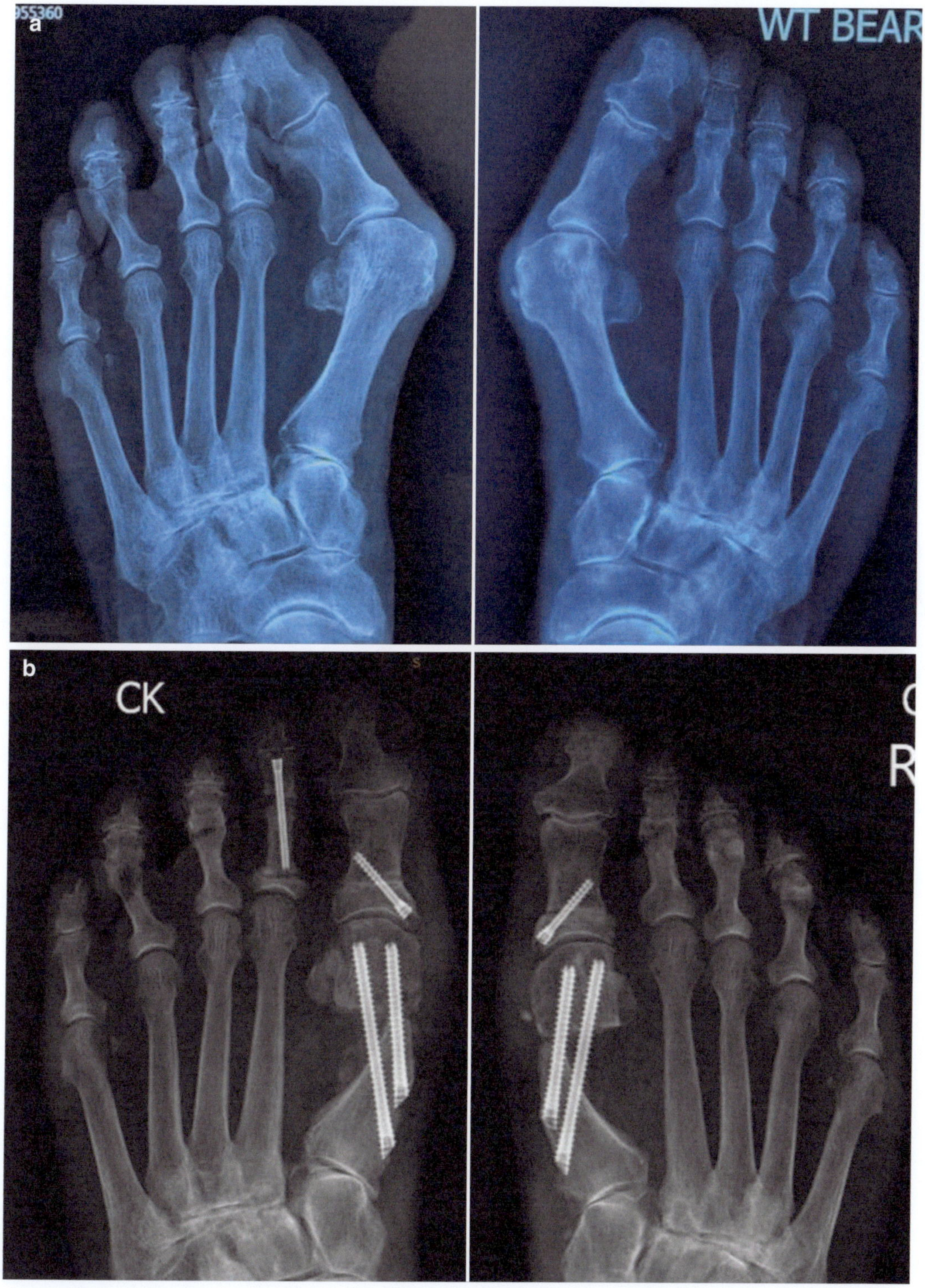

Fig. 14.19 (**a**) Preoperative radiographs of severe hallux valgus. (**b**) 6 weeks post PECA correction. (**c**) 6 months post PECA correction showing completely united osteotomies. © Peter Lam 2015. All Rights Reserved

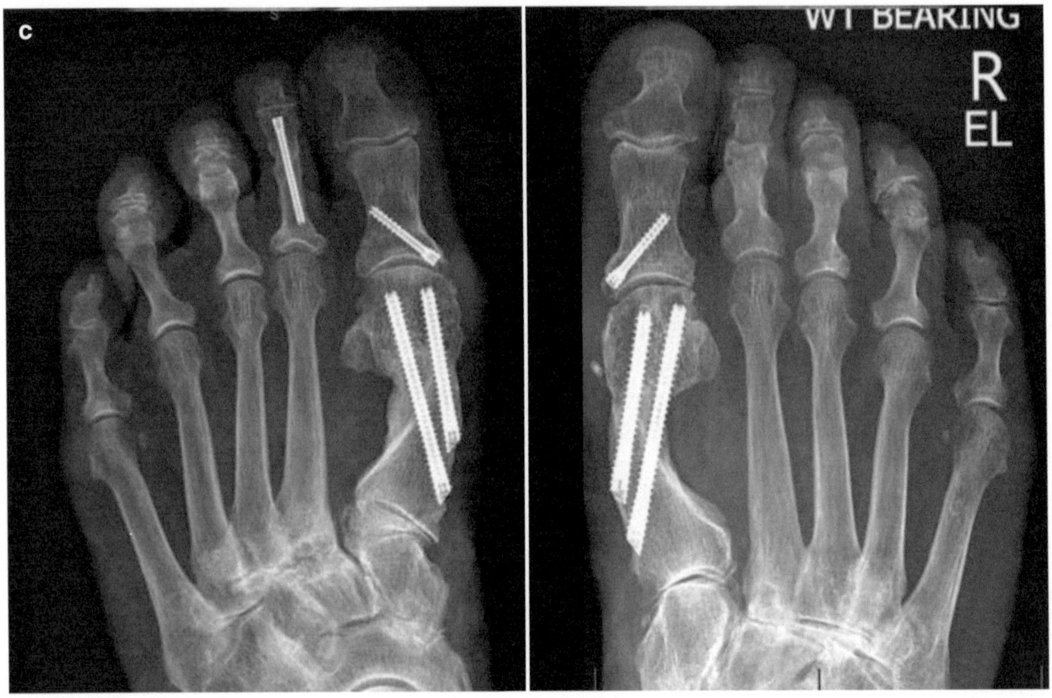

Fig. 14.19 (continued)

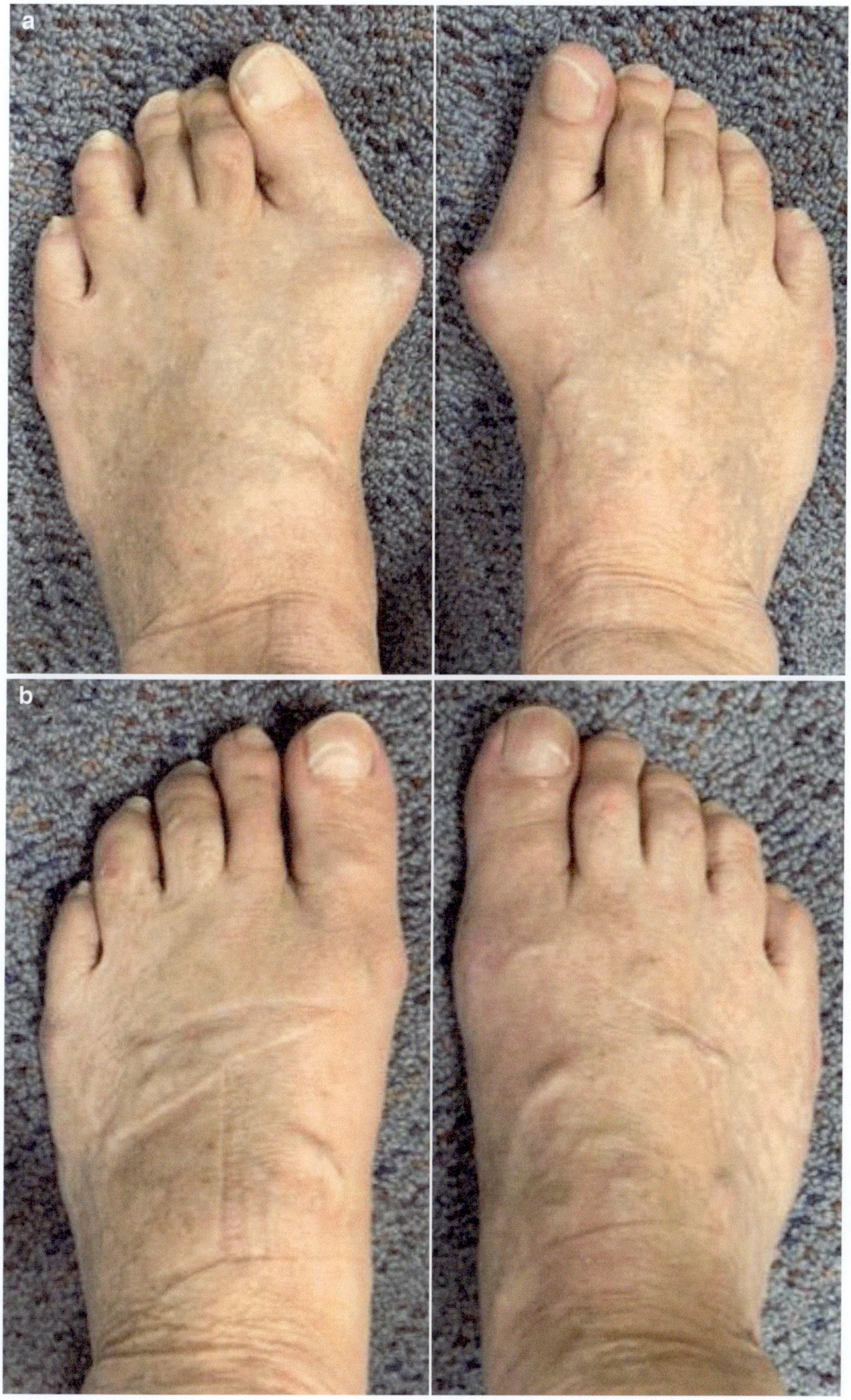

Fig. 14.20 (**a**) Preoperative clinical photographs of the case from Fig. 14.19 with severe hallux valgus. (**b**) Clinical photographs 6 months after PECA correction.

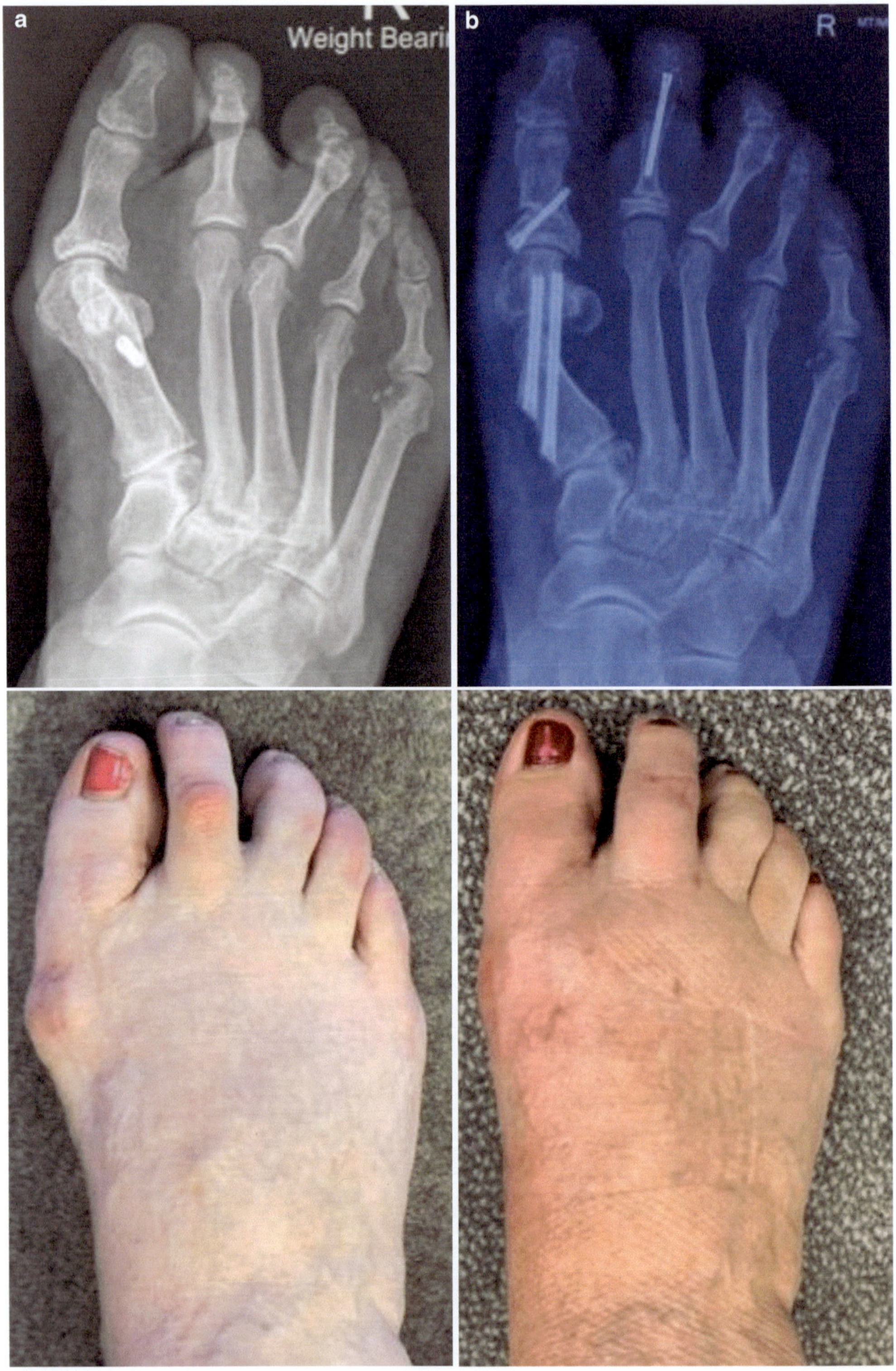

Fig. 14.21 (**a**) Preoperative radiographs and clinical photographs of a recurrent hallux valgus after previous open osteotomy. (**b**) 6-week radiograph and clinical photograph after PECA correction.

Table 14.2 Key steps of PECA technique

• Direction of the metatarsal osteotomy controls direction of translation. It is key to avoid significantly shortening the metatarsal
• Initial guide wire position is crucial to ensure two-point fixation in the metatarsal shaft. Ensure the second wire does not pass through the lateral cortex as this could compromise stability of the first screw
• Pay particular attention to the DMMA after translation
• Use oblique headed screws, and check they are fully buried on an internal rotation image
• Resection of the medial corner of the metatarsal shaft and the dorsomedial part of the medial eminence ensures all bony prominences are resected. If not these can be troublesome to patients
• Perform a limited lateral release. Only aim to divide the plantar lateral first MTPJ capsule and the distal attachment of the adductor hallucis tendon to avoid iatrogenic hallux varus
• Postoperative care, involving full weight-bearing, hallux exercises and a hallux toe holding splint are part of the technique and key to good results

14.8 Summary

Table 14.2 summarises the most important parts of the technique. The PECA third-generation hallux valgus correction offers greater corrective ability than open distal or shaft osteotomies. The transverse osteotomy allows for complete control of metatarsal head positioning under image guidance. Rigid internal fixation maintains the correction achieved and allows immediate full weight-bearing. The technique is reliable and reproducible. Strict adherence to all aspects of the technique is crucial. We don't believe it is possible to learn this technique from a single cadaveric course and surgeon visits to observe cases, with ongoing mentorship for critical analysis of cases during the learning curve is of benefit. Ideally we advocate fellowship training in the technique.

References

1. Trnka HJ, Krenn S, Schuh R. Minimally invasive hallux valgus surgery: a critical review of the evidence. Int Orthop. 2013;37(9):1731–5.
2. Bösch P, Wanke S, Legenstein R. Hallux valgus correction by the method of Bösch: a new technique with a seven to ten year follow-up. Foot Ankle Clin. 2000;5:485–98.
3. Vernois J, Redfern D. Percutaneous chevron; the union of classic stable fixed approach and percutaneous technique. Fuß Sprunggelenk. 2013;11(2):70–5.
4. Malagelada F, Sahirad C, Dalmau-Pastor M, Vega J, Bhumbra R, Manzanares-Cespedes MC, Laffenetre O. Minimally invasive surgery for hallux valgus: a systematic review of current surgical techniques. Int Orthop. 2019;43:625–37.
5. Barg A, Harmer J, Presson A, Zhang C, Lackey M, Saltzman CL. Unfavourable outcomes following surgical treatment of hallux valgus deformity: a systematic literature review. JBJS. 2018;100:1563–73.
6. Lam KLK, Kong SW, Chow YH. Percutaneous chevron osteotomy in treating hallux valgus: Hong Kong experience and mid-term results. J Orthop Trauma Rehabil. 2015;19(1):25–30.
7. Hernandez JLY, Golanó P, Roshan-Zamir S, Darcel V, Chauveaux D, Laffenêtre O. Treatment of moderate hallux valgus by percutaneous, extra-articular reverse-L chevron (PERC) osteotomy. Bone Joint J. 2016;98-B(3):365–73.
8. Jowett C, Bedi H. Preliminary results and learning curve of the minimally invasive chevron akin operation for hallux valgus. J Foot Ankle Surg. 2017;56:445–52.
9. Lee M, Walsh J, Smith M, Ling J, Wines A, Lam P. Hallux valgus correction comparing percutaneous chevron/akin (PECA) and open scarf/akin osteotomies. Foot Ankle Int. 2017;38:838–46.
10. Holme TJ, Sivaloganathan SS, Patel B, Kunasingam K. Third-generation minimally invasive Chevron akin osteotomy for hallux valgus. Foot Ankle Int. 2020;41(1):50–6.

Percutaneous Extra-Articular Reverse-L Chevron (PERC)

15

Olivier Laffenêtre and Julien Lucas Y. Hernandez

15.1 Introduction

Percutaneous distal chevron osteotomy of the first ray differs from its minimally invasive or even conventional cousins in a few notable ways, even though the goals are the same, namely, three-dimensional displacement of the head to correct minor to moderate hallux valgus:

- The medial exostosis is preserved. It serves as a support point for the displacement and avoids leaving bone paste in the joint, which some think is the reason why joint stiffness occurs after percutaneous Isham osteotomy [1, 2].
- This chevron osteotomy has an L-shape, is more proximal, and most importantly, is extra-articular.
- Lateral metatarsophalangeal release is optional. Like in conventional surgery, the aim is to make the distal articular surfaces of the first and second metatarsals parallel.
- A phalangeal osteotomy can be added as needed, depending on whether hallux valgus interphalangeus or hallux pronation is present and/or on the foot shape.

15.2 Surgical Technique

15.2.1 Materials

- Non-specific: Beaver blade, 3-mm saw, elevator, rasps, powered surgical instrument with speed limiter, mini-C-arm fluoroscopy.
- Specific: Osteotomy bone lever that is used to push laterally on the M1 head through a percutaneous approach. Its shape allows it to fit inside the medullary canal and to hold the correction until bone fixation is added (Fig. 15.1).
- Burrs: A 20 mm-long burr makes it easier to perform the cuts; a 3-mm -ide burr simplifies the shortening in the superior cut, while a 2 mm-wide burr (extra-long Shannon burr) is used solely to make the two cuts. A long Shannon burr (2 × 12 mm) is used for the plantar cut (when a 3 × 20 mm burr is used for the superior cut) and the Akin osteotomy. In certain cases, a 4.1-mm wedge burr is used for exostectomy at the head.

O. Laffenêtre (✉)
Institut de la Cheville et du Pied, Paris, France

J. L. Y. Hernandez
Orthopedic Department, Bordeaux University Hospital, Bordeaux, France

C. Cazeau, Y. Stiglitz (eds.), *Percutaneous and Minimally Invasive Foot Surgery*,
https://doi.org/10.1007/978-3-030-98791-6_15

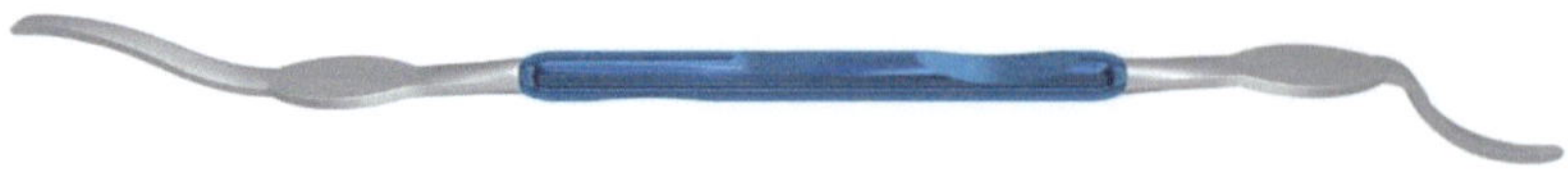

Fig. 15.1 Osteotomy bone lever that is used to translate the M1 head and maintain the reduction.

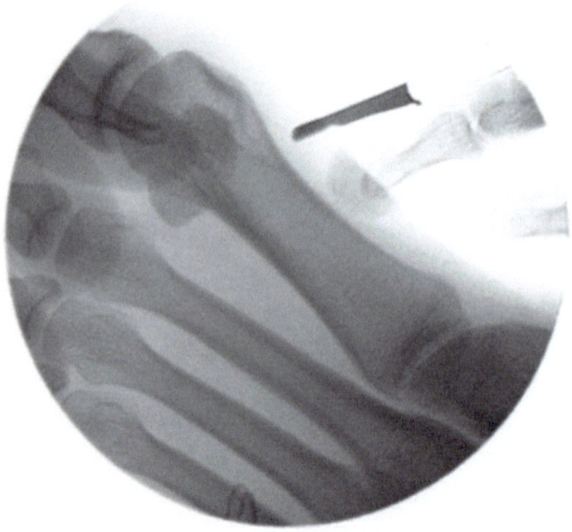

Fig. 15.2 Fluoroscopy view of the approach for the metatarsal osteotomy.

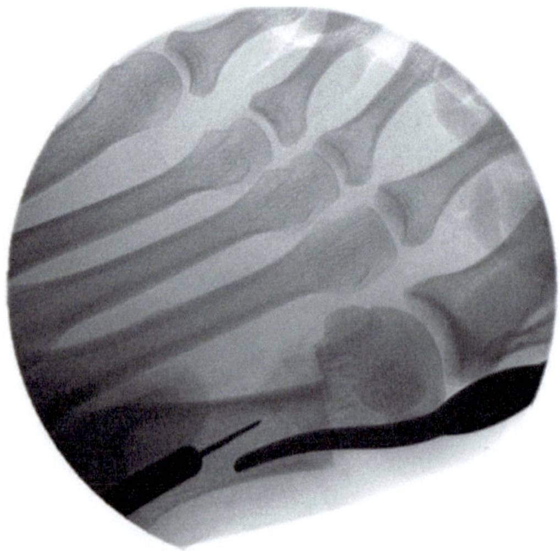

Fig. 15.3 Fluoroscopy view of the approach used to insert the main metatarsal fixation screw.

15.2.2 Surgical Approaches

Each approach is associated with a specific procedure.

15.2.2.1 First Approach

The first approach is used to carry out the chevron osteotomy. Its location is crucial since; unlike in open techniques, it serves as the burr's rotation point, which determines the position of the two cuts, not the junction of the two cuts. It consists of a medial incision behind the M1 head at the 1/3 superior and 2/3 inferior junction and is located extra-articular (Fig. 15.2). When a 2 mm-diameter burr is used and no shortening is desired (index-minus foot), it can be shifted 2 or 3 mm more proximal to allow the burr to be angled 10° or so from proximal to distal in the horizontal plane to cancel out the shortening induced by the cut.

Exceptionally, the medial and especially superior volume of the M1 head can be reduced slightly through an intra-articular approach as described in Chap. 7. In this scenario, it is preferable to perform the exostectomy first.

15.2.2.2 Second Approach

The second approach is done on the dorsal side of the metatarsal, 2 cm proximal to the osteotomy between the lateral side of the extensor hallucis longus and that of the brevis tendons (Fig. 15.3).

15.2.2.3 Third Approach

The third approach is located over the lateral portion of the metatarsophalangeal joint. It can be used to perform lateral release, as needed. Lastly, one or two additional stab incisions can be made to perform a phalangeal osteotomy (if needed) (Fig. 15.4a) and to fix it (Fig. 15.4b).

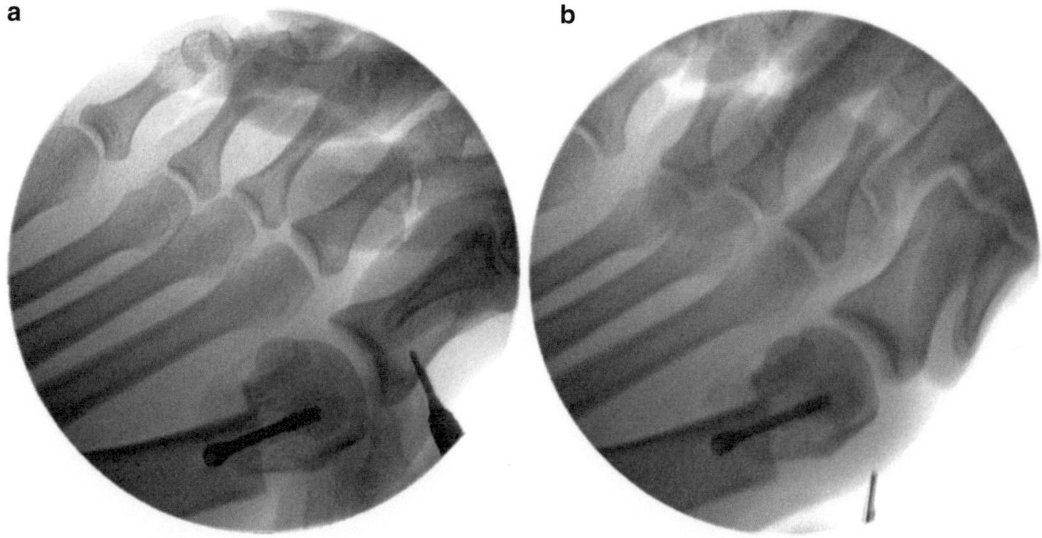

Fig. 15.4 Fluoroscopy view of the surgical approaches used for the proximal phalanx. (**a**) Osteotomy. (**b**) Fixation.

Throughout these procedures, the various steps are verified using fluoroscopy and by manually palpating the bone landmarks through the skin.

15.2.3 Patient Positioning

The patient is supine with the operated foot extending beyond the surgical table and resting on an X-ray detector. The contralateral leg is flexed 90° to remove it from the surgical field. This technique is performed without a tourniquet.

15.2.3.1 First Step: Metatarsal Osteotomy

The first medial incision behind the M1 head is carried out as described above. The blade goes straight down to the bone, without tissue detachment. The type of burr is selected based on the metatarsal index, whether shortening is needed and how it will be done.

- In an index-plus or plus-minus foot, a 3 × 20-mm burr applied parallel to the articular surface will provide shortening of 3 mm or more automatically while increasing the width of the cut in the proximal portion of M1.
- For an index-minus foot, a thinner 2 × 20-mm burr is used instead; it is angled forward to offset the shortening effect of the bone cut by a lengthening effect during lateral translation.
- When shortening is needed, the opposite can also be done: The burr is angled backward from distal to proximal. But one must remember that the decision to shorten or lower depends more on the clinical findings (e.g., load transfer or joint stiffness) than on how the foot looks visually or radiologically.

Across from the incision, the burr is used to make a bicortical tunnel positioned in the horizontal plane as described previously, according to its diameter and the preoperative plan (Fig. 15.5). In the frontal plane, it remains parallel to the inferior cortex of M1 just like a saw blade would in the open techniques, to combine the usual lowering with the desired translation.

By staying perpendicular to the diaphysis and by lifting the hand, the superior chevron cut is made from the tunnel that was created.

Depending on how much DMAA correction is needed, the medial border can be resected more to achieve a DM2A of 0.

The plantar cut is then made, switching the 3 mm burr to a 2 × 12 or 2 × 20 mm Shannon burr, or using the same burr if a 2-mm wide one was used previously.

The burr is inserted in the starting tunnel to locate the chevron's center of rotation again. The oblique plantar cut is made downward and backward by rotating the wrist while staying parallel to the sole of the foot (Fig. 15.6).

Once the osteotomy is completed, the head is translated by inserting the osteotomy bone lever into the diaphysis, with its flat portion resting against the medial side of the head (Fig. 15.7).

The M1 head must be impacted fully against the diaphysis, lowered, and then its position verified with fluoroscopy (DMAA correction). For this reason, lateral release must be not performed beforehand, as it destabilizes the joint and makes it harder to mobilize the head.

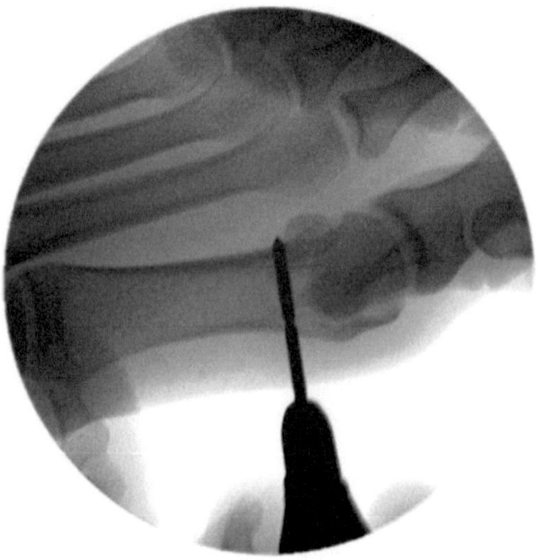

Fig. 15.5 Positioning of the 3 × 20-mm burr parallel to the joint line in an index-plus foot that requires shortening, lowering, and translation. © Olivier Laffenêtre 2015. All Rights Reserved

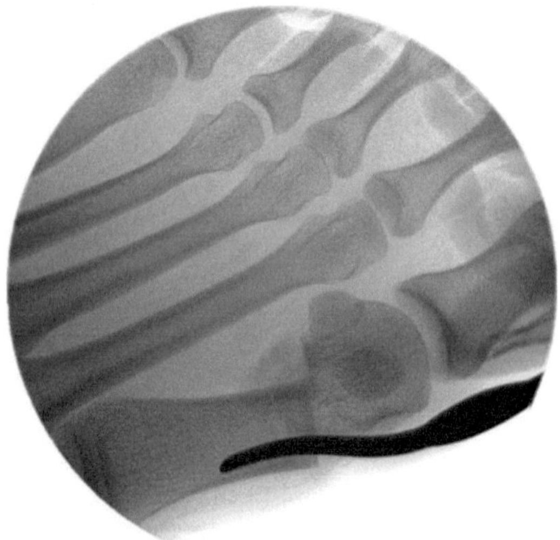

Fig. 15.7 Osteotomy bone lever is inserted to help translate the head. © Olivier Laffenêtre 2015. All Rights Reserved

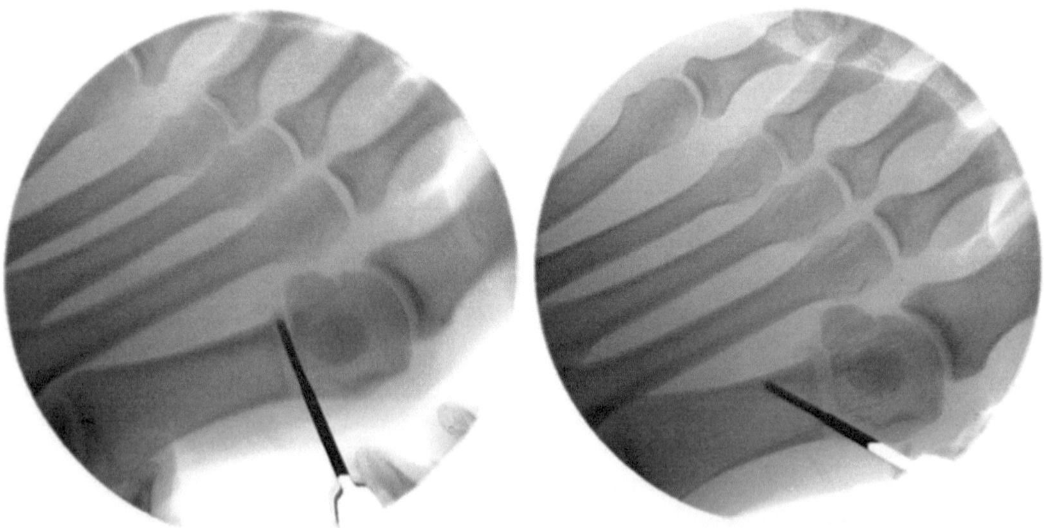

Fig. 15.6 Plantar cut made with a 2-mm-diameter burr. © Olivier Laffenêtre 2015. All Rights Reserved

Once the desired displacement has been achieved and maintained, the second incision is made with the beaver blade along the lateral edge of the extensor hallucis longus tendon, as described previously (Fig. 15.3). The subcutaneous plane is carefully dissected to expose the periosteum, which is released in the area where the screw will be introduced.

A K-wire is inserted proximal to distal and lateral to medial to help the screw's compression achieve the desired lateral displacement (Fig. 15.8). At the very worst, it must be axial to neutralize the displacement. A 3-mm-diameter compression screw is used; its head must be thick enough to get good purchase on the superior cortex of M1 (Fig. 15.9).

In a foot with a large initial deformity that requires a larger displacement, two screws can be used to stabilize the site. In this scenario, a second K-wire is inserted medial to lateral and proximal to distal, crossing under the first one; this allows a 3-mm-diameter beveled screw to be added (Fig. 15.10).

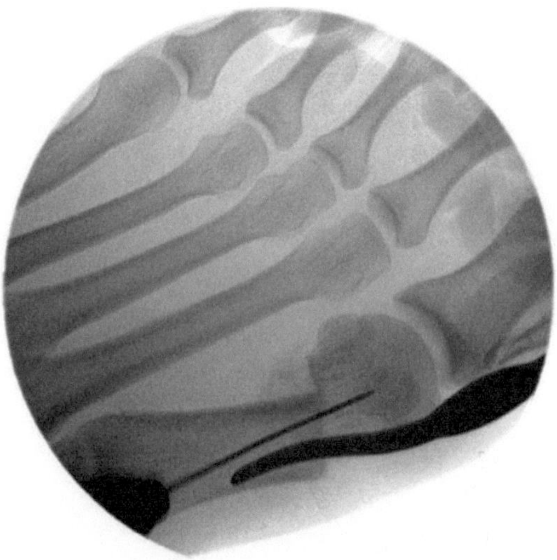

Fig. 15.8 Neutral positioning of K-wire.

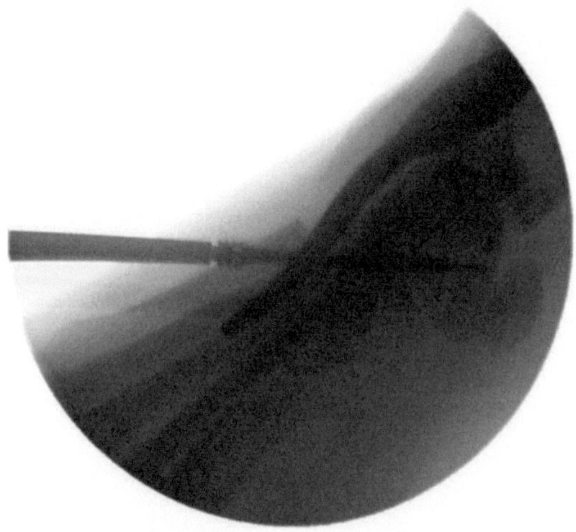

Fig. 15.9 Positioning of screw on lateral view. The screw head must not be too close to the osteotomy cut and must catch the entire thickness of the superior cortex. M1 head lowering can be checked on this view.

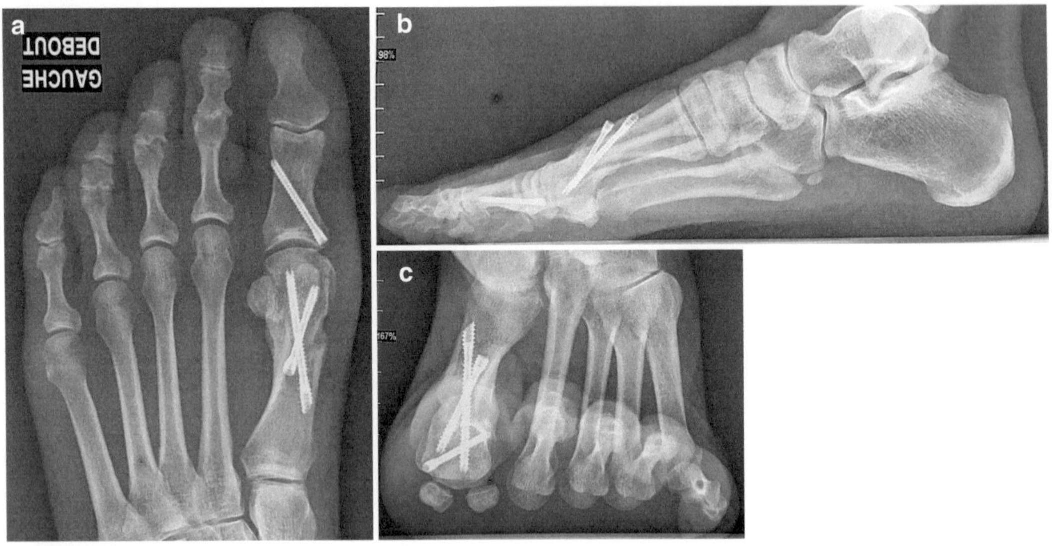

Fig. 15.10 Double screw fixation of osteotomy (modified PERC) on AP view (**a**) lateral view (**b**) and sesamoid view (**c**) at 6 months postoperative that stabilizes the metatarsal head after it was lowered and translated by 50%.

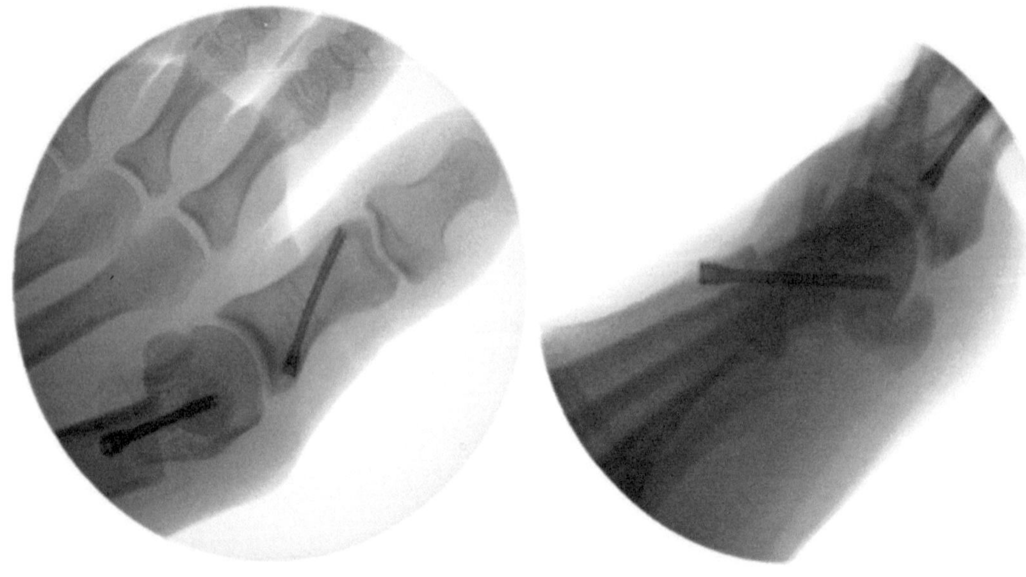

Fig. 15.11 Procedure supplemented by an Akin osteotomy with screw fixation but without release because of the satisfactory joint congruency.

15.2.3.2 Second Step: Lateral Release (Optional)

Once the metatarsal osteotomy has been secured, the surgeon makes sure no residual joint incongruency due lateral ligament contracture remains, which is typically the case for advanced, chronic deformities. If this is the case, a third dorsolateral incision is made above the joint line. A 1-mm beaver blade is used to cut the sesamoid suspensory ligament on the lateral side of the M1 head, then if needed, the extension of the transverse adductor hallucis to the phalangeal base.

15.2.3.3 Third Step: Proximal Phalanx Osteotomy (Optional)

Depending on the forefoot morphotype and whether or not hallux valgus interphalangeus or residual hallux pronation is present, a percutaneous Akin osteotomy (Fig. 15.11) can be done in addition.

15.2.4 Exostectomy (Rarely Done)

Resection of the medial and superior bone bump on the M1 head is not performed in every case; it depends on whether the displacement induced is able to eliminate it without having to perform an intra-articular procedure that may contribute to stiffness. Since it may reduce the stability when performed after the bone fixation, it should be done before the chevron osteotomy when it is required. Exostectomy is performed using a wedge burr [1, 4].

15.3 Postoperative Course

Immediate weight-bearing is allowed with the patient wearing a flat postoperative shoe for the first 3 weeks after the procedure, which allows the patient to move around while protecting the construct. Antithrombotic prophylaxis with low-molecular-weight heparin is not necessary except in patients with specific risk factors identified by the anesthesiologist (prophylaxis prescribed for a few days if needed). The first dressing is changed after 15 days. If the proximal phalanx osteotomy was not fixed, a custom toe spacer is added to the initial dressing to hold the correction for an additional 8–15 days. In more extensive forefoot surgery cases, another option is to use small strips to hold the reduction. Rehabilitation based on a set protocol is generally prescribed and starts after the third week.

15.4 Complications

The main risk is secondary displacement due to poor fixation, either because the fixation was inadequate for the large displacement required or because the screw used was not appropriate, typically with the head being too small to lock itself into the superior cortex. The osteotomy site must be secured either with a second screw or by doing the MICA variation described by Vernois [3, 4].

Indicated for minor or moderate hallux valgus, percutaneous chevron osteotomy provides the same results as other procedures, with the advantages of a percutaneous technique in terms of the postoperative course and lower morbidity of the surgical approaches [5, 6].

15.5 Conclusion

A chevron osteotomy can be done percutaneously. It offers all the benefits of percutaneous surgery—simple postoperative course, less pain, and excellent mobility because of its extra-articular nature—while still being a reliable osteotomy that was proven effective many years ago.

Editors' Point of View

The percutaneous extra-articular reverse-L chevron osteotomy of M1 is a difficult technique that should not be attempted early in one's learning curve. In terms of geometric correction, the pitfall of automatic shortening needs to be avoided, generated by the burr's width. The other corrections (lowering; rotation in the frontal and horizontal planes) are harder to control. Almost all the articles published describe the technique, but very few describe the geometric corrections achieved.

References

1. Bauer T, de Lavigne C, Biau D, De Prado M, Isham S, Laffenêtre O. Percutaneous hallux valgus surgery: a prospective multicenter study of 189 cases. Orthop Clin North Am. 2009;40:505–14.
2. Bauer T, Biau D, Lortat-Jacob A, Hardy P. Percutaneous hallux valgus correction using the Reverdin-Isham osteotomy. Orthop Traumatol Surg Res. 2010;964:407–16.

3. Vernois J. The treatment of the hallux valgus with a percutaneous chevron osteotomy. Orthop Proc. 2011;93B Suppl IV:482.
4. Vernois J, Redfern D. Percutaneous Chevron; the union of classic stable fixed approach and percutaneous technique. Fuß & Sprunggelenk. 2013;11:70–5.
5. Laffenêtre O, Golano P, GRECMIP. Evolution de la chirurgie percutanée du 1er rayon en 2013. Académie Chir, E-mémoire. 2014;13:42–9.
6. Lucas J, Hernandez Y, Golanó P, Roshan-Zamir S, Darcel V, Chauveaux D, Laffenetre O. Treatment of moderate hallux valgus by Percutaneous, Extra-articular, Reverse-L Chevron (PERC) osteotomy. Bone Joint J. 2016:365–73. https://doi.org/10.1302/0301-620X.98B3.

Percutaneous Osteotomy of the First Metatarsal Base

16

Christophe de Lavigne and Thomas Bauer

16.1 Introduction

In certain cases of first ray deformity with significant metatarsus adductus (>18°), it may be necessary to a perform a proximal osteotomy of the first metatarsal (M1) to reduce the M1–M2 angle. In fact, distal or diaphyseal metatarsal osteotomies have a limited ability to correct this angle, whereas proximal first metatarsal osteotomy can achieve larger corrections (more than 10°) [1–4]. This proximal M1 osteotomy has two important principles:

- Since the M1–M2 angle is corrected by externally rotating M1, the risk of increasing the angle of the M1 articular surface (DMAA) is greater. Consequently, in some cases, a distal osteotomy must be added to this proximal osteotomy to correct the DMAA.
- The intrinsic stability of this proximal M1 osteotomy is low; thus, there is a considerable risk of secondary displacement into metatarsus elevatus. Fixation is needed to ensure primary stability.

C. de Lavigne (✉)
Clinique du Sport, Merignac, France
e-mail: secdrdelavigne@gmail.com

T. Bauer
Orthopedic Department, Ambroise Paré University Hospital, Boulogne-Billancourt, France
e-mail: thomas.bauer@aphp.fr

16.2 Surgical Technique

This osteotomy is performed through a lateral incision over the hallucis extensor tendon by placing the burr on the lateral side of M1 at its proximal third.

This is a planar oblique osteotomy-oriented lateral distal to medial proximal while preserving a superomedial hinge. On a cross-section, the first metatarsal has a triangular shape with plantar base. The proximal M1 osteotomy must preserve the superomedial cortex, which after the lateral closing wedge osteoclasis, makes it possible to lower the metatarsal diaphysis and reduces the possibility of metatarsus elevatus (Fig. 16.1).

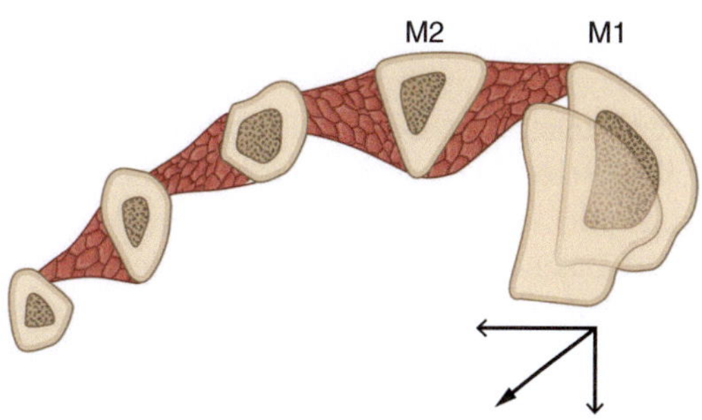

Fig. 16.1 Triangular shape of M1 cross-section. The superomedial hinge (blue dotted line) must be preserved to achieve lowering and prevent metatarsus elevatus. © Christophe de Lavigne 2015. All Rights Reserved

C. Cazeau, Y. Stiglitz (eds.), *Percutaneous and Minimally Invasive Foot Surgery*,
https://doi.org/10.1007/978-3-030-98791-6_16

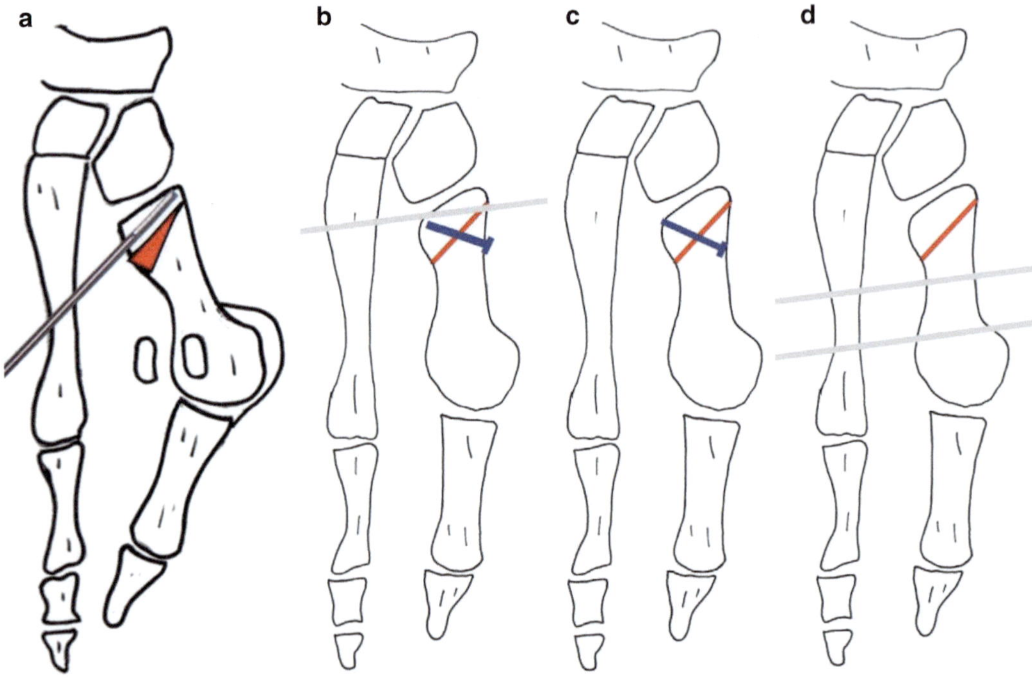

Fig. 16.2 (**a**) Osteotomy cut. (**b**) K-wire added between M1 and M2 to hold correction. (**c**) Cannulated screw inserted perpendicular to osteotomy cut. (**d**) Supplemental fixation with intermetatarsal pinning.

The burr is positioned on the lateral edge of M1 on its proximal third starting at the lateral cortex. The osteotomy is performed from distal lateral to proximal medial, and the burr is directed from plantar distal to dorsal proximal, while preserving the superomedial cortex (Fig. 16.2a).

This osteotomy is verified with fluoroscopy. The angular correction is achieved by the surgeon shifting the M1 head outward; this closes the metatarsal osteotomy and reduces the M1–M2 angle. Lateral metatarsophalangeal joint release is carried out before correcting the metatarsus adductus.

Before fixation, the correction can be maintained by placing an intermetatarsal K-wire (between M1 and M2), which prevents any movement of the cuneometatarsal joint and especially displacement into metatarsus elevatus (Fig. 16.2b). A second K-wire is inserted with fluoroscopy guidance to allow placement of a cannulated screw. The screw will be inserted medial distal to lateral proximal, perpendicular to the osteotomy cut, to ensure the best compression (Fig. 16.2c).

If residual instability is present (osteoporosis, persistent motion), this fixation can be supplemented by intermetatarsal pinning for 4–6 weeks (Fig. 16.2d).

16.3 Postoperative Course

Immediate full weight-bearing is allowed with a rigid-soled, flat postoperative shoe. The initial dressing is left in place for 10–15 days. Obviously, the biggest risk of this proximal metatarsal osteotomy is displacement into elevatus, especially since minimal fixation is used. For this reason, true full-plantar weight-bearing is not allowed right away.

Editors' Point of View

As a percutaneous osteotomy, this procedure is easy and has spectacular results. Nevertheless, it does not get around the typical problem of postoperative elevatus, and surgeons always need to ask themselves if immediate full weight-bearing will be possible.

References

1. Lutonsky M, Sponer P. Personal experience with the basal wedge closed osteotomy of the first metatarsus in hallux valgus. Acta Chir Orthop Traumatol Cechoslov. 2002;69:45–8.
2. Seiberg M, Felson S, Colson JP, Barth AH, Green RM, Green DR. Closing base wedge versus Austin bunionectomies for metatarsus primus adductus. J Am Podiatr Med Assoc. 1994;84:548–63.
3. Pontious J, Marcoux JT. Autogenous calcaneal bone graft repair of a closing base wedge osteotomy nonunion. J Am Podiatr Med Assoc. 1996;86:25–32.
4. Banks AS, Cargill RS, Carter S, Ruch JA. Shortening of the first metatarsal following closing base wedge osteotomy. J Am Podiatr Med Assoc. 1997;87:199–208.

Conservative Surgical Treatment of First Metatarsophalangeal Joint Arthritis

17

Christophe Cermolacce

17.1 Cheilectomy

17.1.1 Definition and Indications

Cheilectomy consists in resecting the osteophytes along the head of the first metatarsal (M1) in the context of first ray osteoarthritis. Cheilectomy is indicated for treating hallux rigidus, no matter its stage. It can be performed alone, typically using a percutaneous technique (Fig. 17.1) in patients with osteoarthritis who have osteophytic growths that rubs in shoes, or in combination with other procedures, often open ones (metatarsal or phalangeal osteotomy, arthrodesis, resection arthroplasty).

In every case, the indication is made because the patient has problems wearing shoes due to the presence of large osteophytes on the superior, medial, and lateral sides of the M1 head (Fig. 17.2).

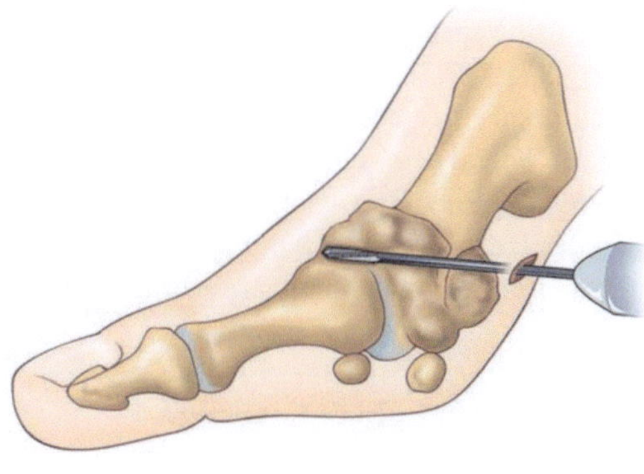

Fig. 17.1 Percutaneous cheilectomy. © Christophe Cermolacce 2015. All Rights Reserved

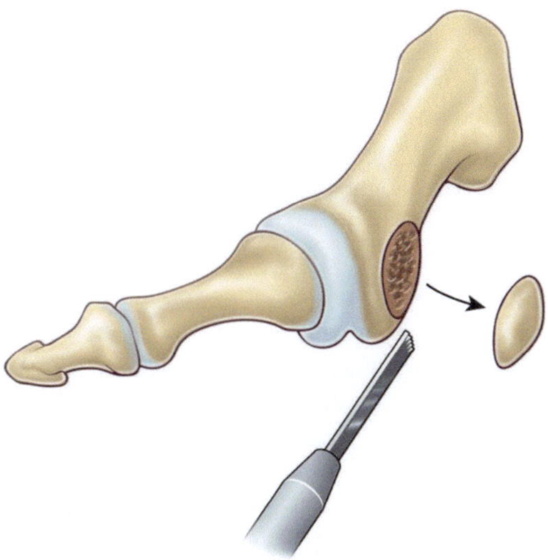

Fig. 17.2 Medial cheilectomy. © Christophe Cermolacce 2015. All Rights Reserved

17.1.2 Percutaneous Surgical Technique

17.1.2.1 Surgical Approaches

- The primary approach is medial and plantar, behind the metatarsal head. This is the exact

C. Cermolacce (✉)
Institut de Chirurgie Orthopédique et Sportive, Marseille, France

C. Cazeau, Y. Stiglitz (eds.), *Percutaneous and Minimally Invasive Foot Surgery*,
https://doi.org/10.1007/978-3-030-98791-6_17

same approach used for medial resection of the M1 head during percutaneous treatment of hallux valgus.

- An accessory lateral and dorsal approach can also be used in cases of dorsolateral osteophytosis. This second approach can be placed in the same location as the approach used for lateral release or can be more distal, over the base of the first phalanx, depending on the volume of the dorsal osteophytes and whether lateral contracture is present.

17.1.2.2 Creation of Working Space

A working space is created around all the osteophytes using specific instruments (raspatory, elevator) (Fig. 17.3). This step is essential but sometimes tricky since adhesions may be present or the collateral nerves and extensor hallucis tendon may be in contact with the osteophytes. In addition, creating this working space allows the surgeon to use burrs without stress or traction on the skin.

17.1.2.3 Osteophyte Resection

The osteophytes are resected using a conical burr (often 4.1-mm Wedge® burr but sometimes a larger-diameter Brophy® burr). Medial and dorsomedial osteophytes are removed first through the medial incision. The excision is verified by palpation and with fluoroscopy to assess how much bone still needs to be removed and how good the resection is. The goal is a flat, even surface without potential areas of impingement.

The excision continues on the dorsolateral Side (Fig. 17.4) through the dorsal and lateral incision. The burr is set parallel to the extensor tendon and the resection performed with the ankle in slight dorsiflexion to release the dorsal soft tissue and prevent damaging tendon, nerve, and vascular structures. This procedure allows dorsal and lateral osteophytes (Fig. 17.5) on the metatarsal head and phalanx base to be removed.

The abundant bone debris that is generated must be removed by applying manual pressure with copious saline lavage of the working space, or by using specific rasps. This will help prevent continued inflammation or secondary ossification.

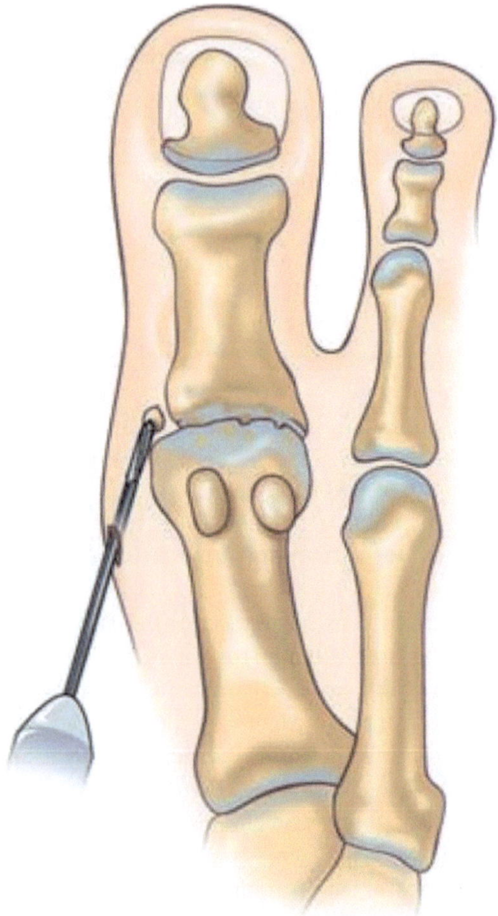

Fig. 17.3 Percutaneous dorsolateral approach. © Christophe Cermolacce 2015. All Rights Reserved

17.1.3 Postoperative Course

The postoperative course is very simple. If a percutaneous technique was used, the dressing is replaced every day until the site is completely healed (about 8 days). Immediate weight-bearing in rigid shoes is allowed. More flexible shoes can be worn soon after in cases of isolated cheilectomy to avoid stiffening in dorsiflexion.

Optional rehabilitation focused on cutaneous viability and gentle joint mobilization can be prescribed; however, we feel it is best to wait 4 or 5 weeks. The patient must be warned that the edema and joint sensitivity will persist for a few weeks.

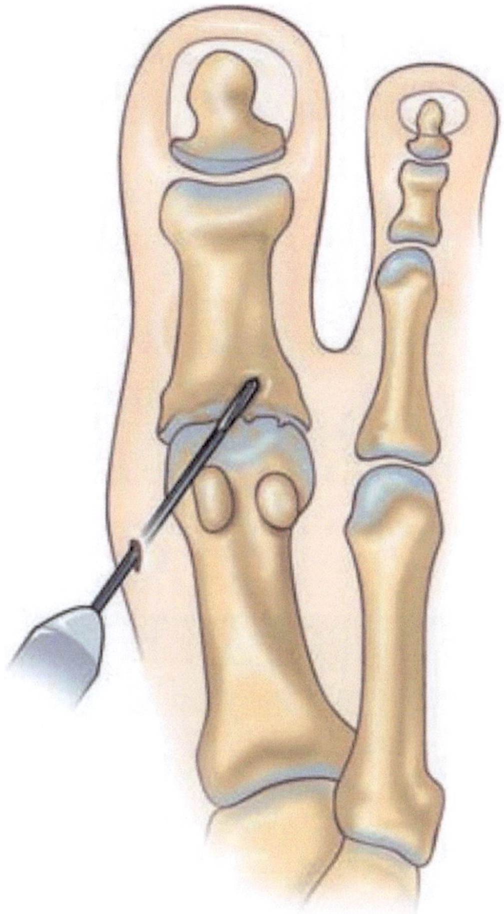

Fig. 17.4 Dorsal view of dorsolateral osteophyte resection. © Christophe Cermolacce 2015. All Rights Reserved

17.1.4 Complications

The main complication is prolonged inflammation and edema, which contribute to pain and stiffness. This inflammation is related to residual bone debris that can be expulsed secondarily and resemble an infection. This risk can be reduced by copious lavage of the working space.

The second risk is rapid deterioration of the joint, accompanied by increased pain, which may require MTP1 arthrodesis. The patient must be warned of this potential progression before undergoing this surgery.

17.1.5 Results and Conclusion

Percutaneous cheilectomy allows for rapid reduction of impingement symptoms due to the osteophytes rubbing in shoes. The resulting joint mobility is less predictable and mainly depends on how stiff the joint was preoperatively, how much osteoarthritis is present, and whether other procedures were done. It is contraindicated in cases of MTP1 inflammatory arthritis. Isolated cheilectomy can be combined with a phalangeal shortening or Moberg osteotomy.

This procedure is very useful in cases of chronic MTP1 osteoarthritis in which there is nearly no movement or pain, only large uncomfortable

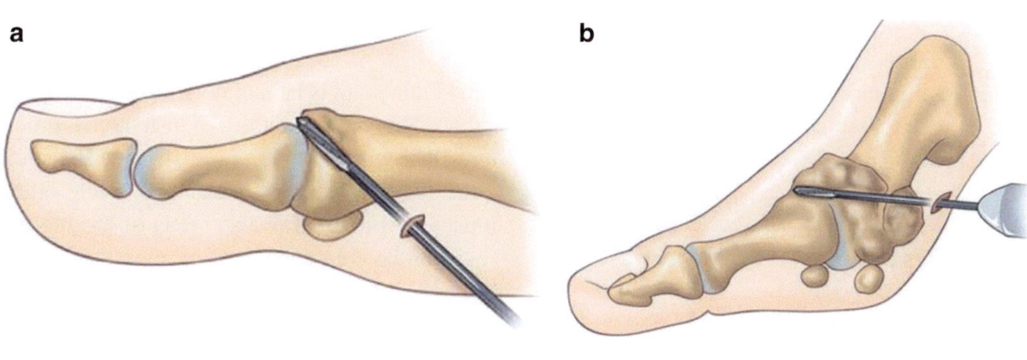

Fig. 17.5 Dorsal osteophyte resection on the proximal phalanx (a) and metatarsal head (b). © Christophe Cermolacce 2015. All Rights Reserved

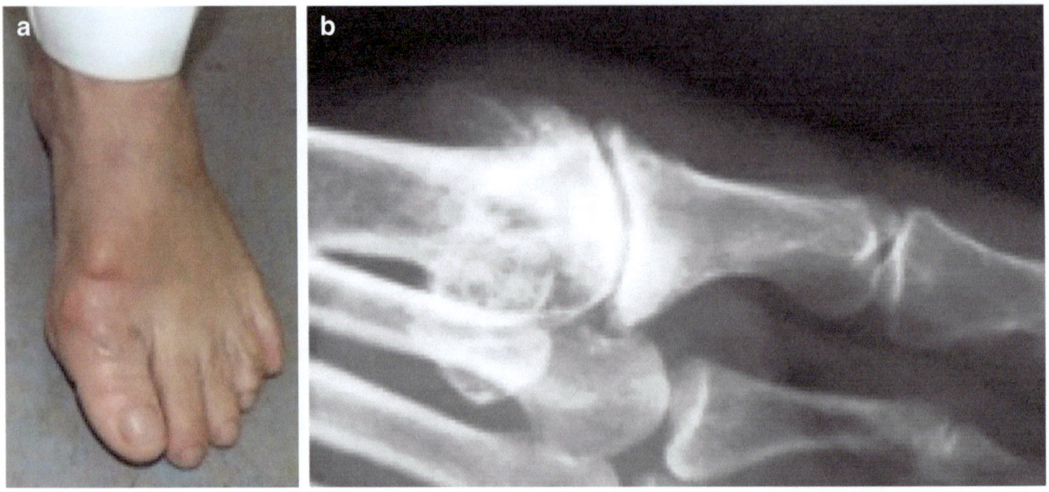

Fig. 17.6 Osteophytes responsible for dorsal rubbing (**a**) and appearance on radiographs (**b**).

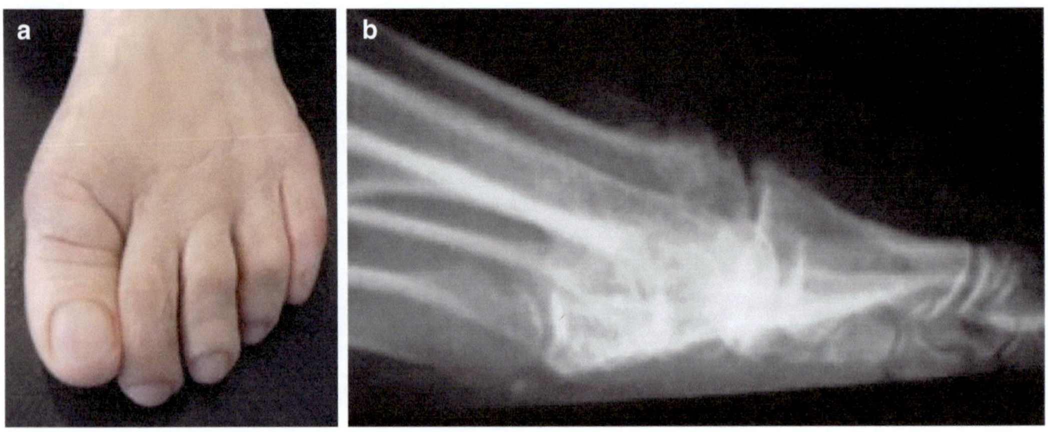

Fig. 17.7 Postoperative result after cheilectomy (**a**) and on radiographs (**b**).

osteophytes. In most cases, this is a palliative surgical procedure, which must be explained to the patient beforehand (Figs. 17.6 and 17.7).

17.2 First Ray MTP Osteotomy

17.2.1 Definition

In the early stages of hallux rigidus, surgery can be performed to eliminate the painful stimulus and to slow the osteoarthritis progression. Early on, patients have symptoms during sports activities; not long after, wearing shoes becomes problematic, including heels in women. The main cause of pain at this point is lack of dorsiflexion. There are a few extra- or intra-articular osteotomy procedures that will preserve the existing MTP1 joint. Some focus on the first metatarsal, while others impact the proximal phalanx (P1) of the big toe. They can be combined and are often paired with the cheilectomy described earlier in this chapter.

17.2.2 Indication

These osteotomy procedures are indicated for treating early stage hallux rigidus. This is one situation in which bone scan and MRI contribute important information (Fig. 17.8).

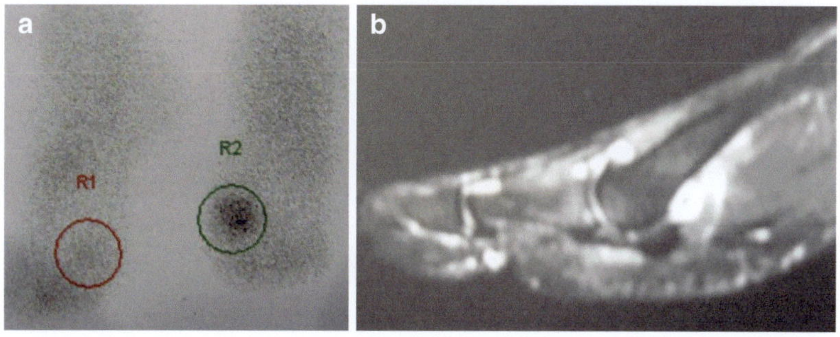

Fig. 17.8 Bone scan (**a**) and MRI (**b**) in early stage hallux rigidus. © Christophe Cermolacce 2015. All Rights Reserved

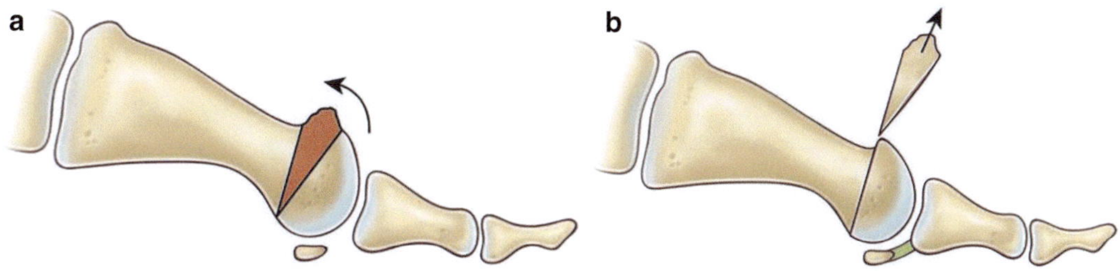

Fig. 17.9 Waterman metatarsal osteotomy: a dorsal closing wedge osteotomy (**a**) will bring the plantar articular surface to a more central position (**b**). © Christophe Cermolacce 2015. All Rights Reserved

This surgery can be performed when there are no large necrotic lesions on the articular surfaces, when inflammation does not envelop the entire joint and when a lack of dorsiflexion appears to be the main cause of the discomfort.

17.2.3 Metatarsal Osteotomies

17.2.3.1 Waterman Procedure

The aim of the Waterman procedure is to reposition better-quality cartilage in the MTP1 joint in the context of central osteoarthritis (Fig. 17.9). This is the parallel procedure to a Gauthier osteotomy at M2 for Freiberg's disease.

The secondary effect of this osteotomy is slight elevation of the head—and thus its center of rotation—which means this procedure is contraindicated in cases of first metatarsus elevatus with load transfer.

Nevertheless, osteoarthritis is often present on the head over the sesamoids; thus the quality of the new articular surface may not be very good. However, the shortening effect is undeniable. Fixation may or may not be used with this osteotomy, depending on whether an open or percutaneous surgery is done.

17.2.3.2 Valenti Procedure

The Valenti procedure consists of wide arthroplasty without interposition of an implant, which allows recovery of dorsiflexion after bone resection (Fig. 17.10). This procedure is rarely used in France and is very damaging to the joint. It can be done either open or percutaneously. There is a risk of triggering arthritis with this osteotomy, and it is difficult to perform secondary MTP fusion if the initial osteotomy is not successful. This procedure is not recommended for treating hallux rigidus in young, athletic patients. It is mostly used in the context of stage IV hallux rigidus.

17.2.3.3 Weil Procedure (Fig. 17.11)

Weil described three procedures for hallux rigidus:

- Weil dorsal flexion osteotomy (WDO) which is nearly identical to the Waterman procedure but is slightly more oblique to make fixation easier.
- Vertical L osteotomy (VLO) for cases where substantial lowering is needed; however, the fixation is difficult, and the neurovascular bundle at the M1 head can get damaged.
- Weil subcapital osteotomy for the first ray.

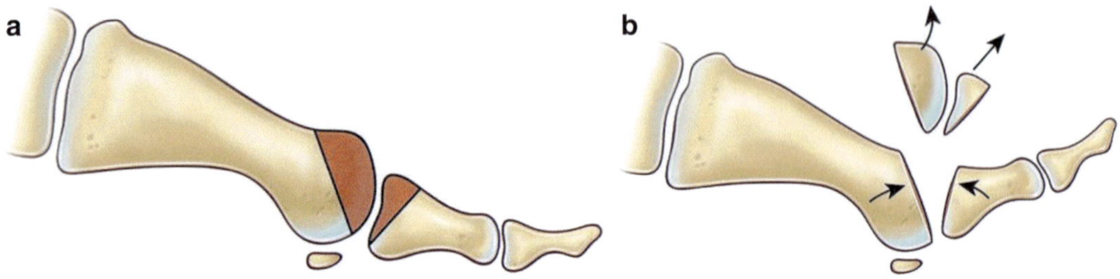

Fig. 17.10 Valenti procedure (**a**) with resection of both sides of the joint (**b**).

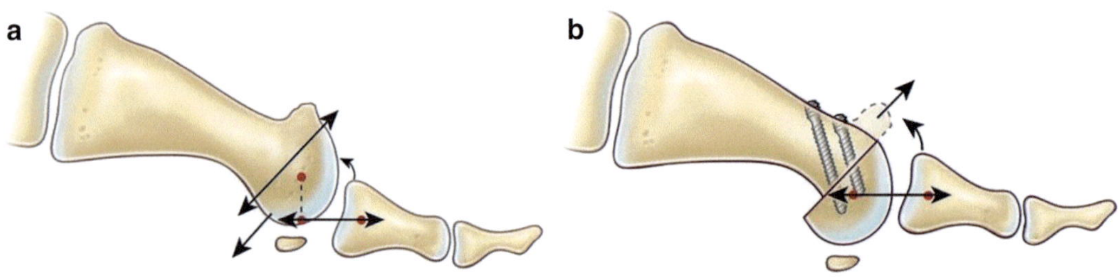

Fig. 17.11 Weil subcapital osteotomy (**a**) with osteophyte removal and double-screw fixation (**b**).

- The latter is our preferred procedure. It is the only one that provides true lowering of the metatarsal head, which makes it especially useful in primus elevatus or secondary elevation of M1 in cases of MTP1 osteoarthritis.
- Also, depending on the chosen angle of the cut, the desired shortening can be achieved based on the preoperative index. Since the cut is planar, two screws are needed to stabilize this osteotomy securely; it is also possible to translate the head laterally to correct any associated hallux valgus.

Because M1 is lowered, the center of rotation between the M1 head and P1 base is reestablished, which results in better joint rotation and thereby MTP1 dorsiflexion. It stops the MTP1 osteoarthritis from getting worse.

17.2.4 Phalangeal Osteotomies

17.2.4.1 Moberg Procedure (Initially Described by Bonney)

The Moberg osteotomy is a surgical technique at the phalanx that aims to create dorsiflexion in P1 of the big toe in order to improve the gait pattern (Fig. 17.12). Fixation can be added as desired.

17.2.4.2 P1 Diaphyseal Shortening

P1 diaphyseal shortening osteotomy is the most commonly used osteotomy as it releases the tension on the first ray present in hallux rigidus cases (Fig. 17.13). Fixation can be added as desired.

17.2.4.3 Keller Procedure

The Keller procedure was extremely popular about 40 years ago but has since been abandoned. Harmful side effects and systematic sesamoid retraction lead to typical complications on the lateral metatarsals (overloading, MP dislocation, etc.) (Fig. 17.14).

Reconstruction by arthrodesis is also very complicated because of the bone defects and the gradual destruction of the phalangeal base.

17.2.5 Combinations

Not surprisingly, the ideal solution involves combining these various metatarsal and phalangeal osteotomies (Fig. 17.15). These combinations depend on the type of hallux rigidus to treat, foot shape (metatarsal index), extent of osteoarthritis,

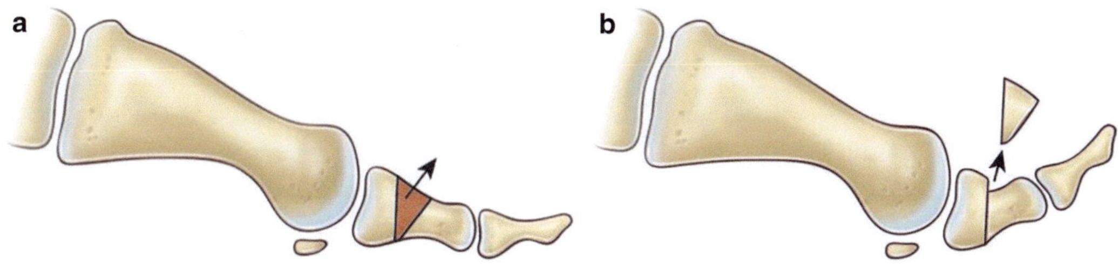

Fig. 17.12 Moberg dorsal closing wedge phalangeal osteotomy (**a**) used to create dorsiflexion at P1 (**b**).

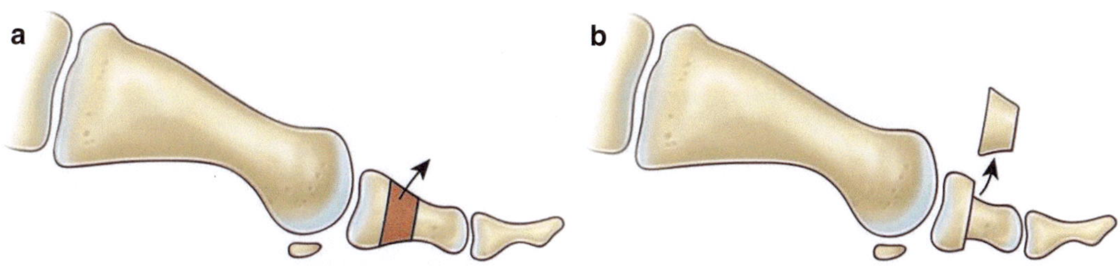

Fig. 17.13 P1 diaphyseal shortening osteotomy (**a**) to remove tension on the first ray (**b**).

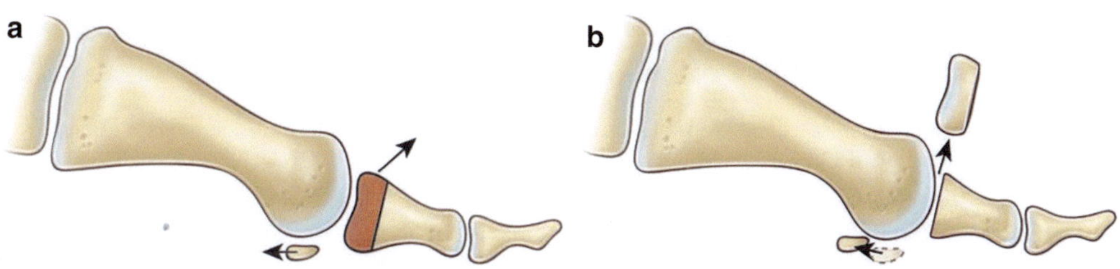

Fig. 17.14 Keller procedure: P1 base resection (**a**) acts as an arthroplasty and reduces tension on the first ray (**b**).

etc. The Valenti and Keller procedures are no longer recommended. The most common combination are as follows:

- Weil M1 + P1 shortening (or Moberg) for hallux rigidus with first metatarsal elevatus.
- Waterman M1 + P1 shortening (or Moberg) for centered hallux rigidus.
- Weil M1 + shortening Akin for hallux valgus with rigidus.

All of these procedures can be performed open or percutaneously; however, we prefer to use mini-incisions for the M1 head as this provides better control over the shortening and the joint lavage. Bone fixation is also useful in our experience as this allows for early mobilization and ensures a better outcome in terms of mobility.

17.2.6 Postoperative Course

The postoperative course is very simple, like for hallux valgus. Immediate weight-bearing is prescribed with a rigid shoe. The dressing is changed on day 8, no matter which technique is used. The patient is allowed to wear flexible shoes fairly soon afterwards.

A few optional rehabilitation sessions focused on cutaneous viability, and gentle joint mobilization can be prescribed; however, we feel it is best to wait 4 weeks since the initial rehabilitation is self-directed. The patient must be warned that edema or joint pain can persist for a few weeks.

Removing the fixation devices after this type of surgery seems preferable to us after about 8 months, in order to perform arthrolysis that will improve the final outcomes in most cases.

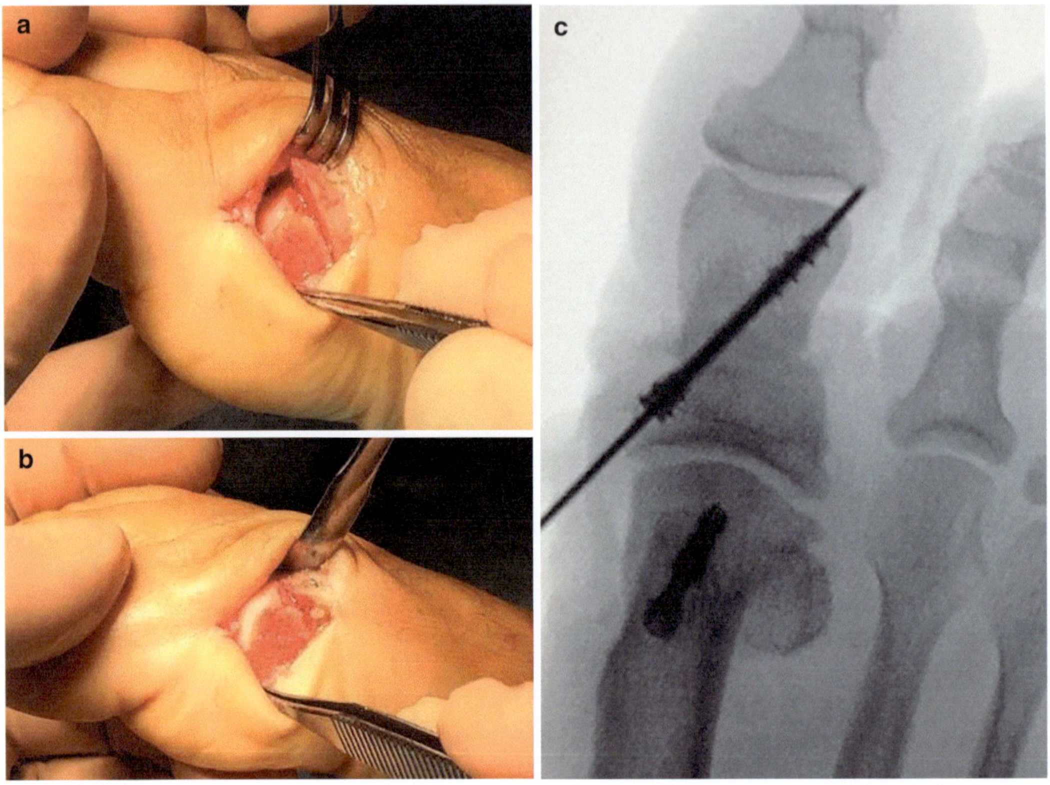

Fig. 17.15 Shortening effect (**a**) of a Weil M1 osteotomy (**b**) followed by an Akin shortening osteotomy (**c**).

A protective insole with arch support and midline pad behind the metatarsal heads appears to be beneficial during the first 8 months postoperative.

17.2.7 Complications

The primary complication is prolonged edema and inflammation, which contribute to pain and stiffness. The second risk is rapid deterioration of the joint, which contributes to pain and may require MTP1 arthrodesis. Patients must be informed of this potential progression before this surgery is performed. Nevertheless, it is rare when the preoperative assessment based on bone scan and MRI is reassuring before the surgery.

There are no specific skin problems as long as the incision is not too long. Complex regional pain syndrome has not been reported often for this type of arthritis surgery, likely due to the joint decompression, which is essential and beneficial.

Lastly, it is not unusual to observe load transfer under the lateral metatarsal heads, especially if the initial foot shape was index minus, hence the need to inform patients of this possibility before surgery.

17.2.8 Outcomes

The long-term outcomes of this type of conservative surgery are surprisingly good when the initial indication is correct. We have more than 23 years' follow-up in our practice and have not needed to perform arthrodesis. Return to the same level of sports participation is possible in two-thirds of cases, and the patient satisfaction rate is near that of hallux valgus surgery (Fig. 17.16).

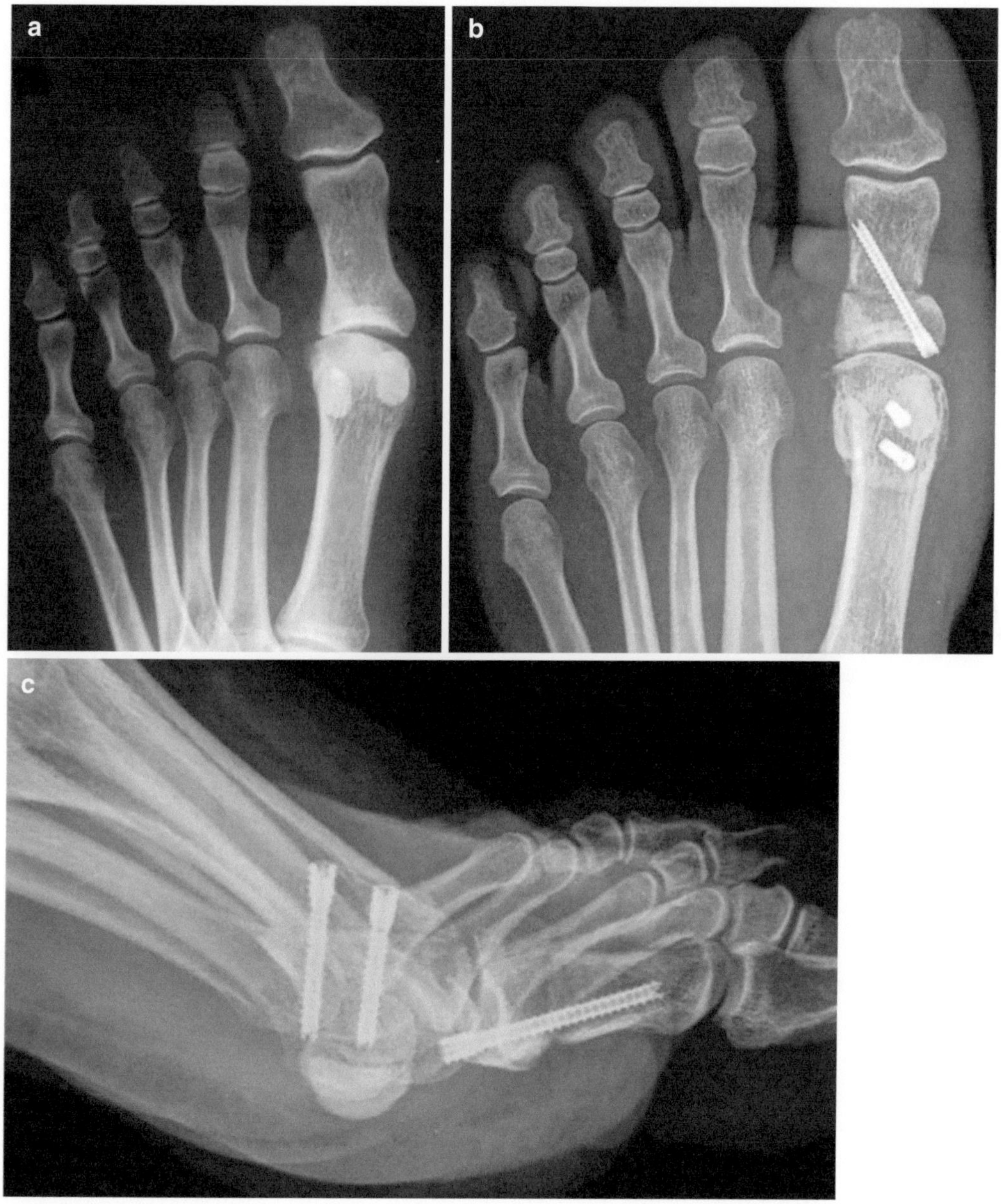

Fig. 17.16 Weil M1 and Akin osteotomies for moderate hallux rigidus: preoperative (**a**), postoperative AP (**b**), and ML views (**c**). © Christophe Cermolacce 2015. All Rights Reserved

17.3 Conclusion

This simple joint-preserving surgery must be performed early on in the context of hallux rigidus. In the advanced stage, the indication will depend on how much inflammation is present in the MTP1 joint (benefit of additional examinations) and must take into consideration the higher likelihood of failure. This alternative means that practicing dynamic sports is still possible and that female patients can still wear heels.

Editors' Point of View
Even though the indications for cheilectomy are rare, this is an especially useful technique to have in one's arsenal. In some ways, it is "the" original percutaneous technique. Compensatory osteotomies of the first ray must be highly accurate to correct the mechanical factors that hinder MTP1 function. For this reason, MIS (not percutaneous) techniques appear to be essential.

18 Minimally Invasive Nonconservative Surgery of the First Metatarsophalangeal Joint

Christophe Cermolacce

18.1 First Metatarsophalangeal Joint Arthrodesis

Arthrodesis of the first metatarsophalangeal (MTP1) joint still has a significant role in forefoot surgery and is the gold standard procedure for treating advanced, painful hallux rigidus. Walking and running can be resumed normally after MTP1 fusion. The mobility mainly occurs in the articular chain, on either side of the first cuneiform, and at the interphalangeal joint with compensatory hypermobility in dorsiflexion.

The main challenge with this procedure is setting the arthrodesis position in the three anatomical planes, which must be adjusted to each patient's specific anatomy, activity level, and preferred footwear. Another challenge, which is not specific to MTP1 fusion, is ensuring the primary stability of the arthrodesis, which is a function of the technique used to prepare the bone surfaces and the type of fixation.

Several open, percutaneous, and arthroscopic techniques have been described with reported fusion rates of 90–100%, depending on the study. We perform MTP1 arthrodesis using both open and percutaneous techniques with fixation in our practice. The minimally invasive technique will be described here and the percutaneous one in another chapter.

18.1.1 Minimally Invasive Technique

18.1.1.1 Instrumentation

The same instrumentation is needed to perform percutaneous MTP1 arthrodesis as for every forefoot surgery, including a fluoroscopy system. The fixation device consists of a plate with self-locking screws, combined with a plantar neutralization screw. While other fixation systems can be used, the locking plate system appears to be the most reliable, especially in patients with severe osteoporosis.

18.1.1.2 Patient Positioning

The patient is positioned supine. The procedure is typically performed under regional anesthesia with a tourniquet.

18.1.1.3 Surgical Approach

The arthrodesis is performed through a standard medial or S-shaped incision over the metatarsophalangeal joint line (Fig. 18.1).

18.1.1.4 Bone Surface Preparation

Resection of the dorsal and lateral metatarsal osteophytes along with release of the lateral capsule and ligament at the MTP1 joint are per-

C. Cermolacce (✉)
Institut de Chirurgie Orthopédique et Sportive, Marseille, France

C. Cazeau, Y. Stiglitz (eds.), *Percutaneous and Minimally Invasive Foot Surgery*,
https://doi.org/10.1007/978-3-030-98791-6_18

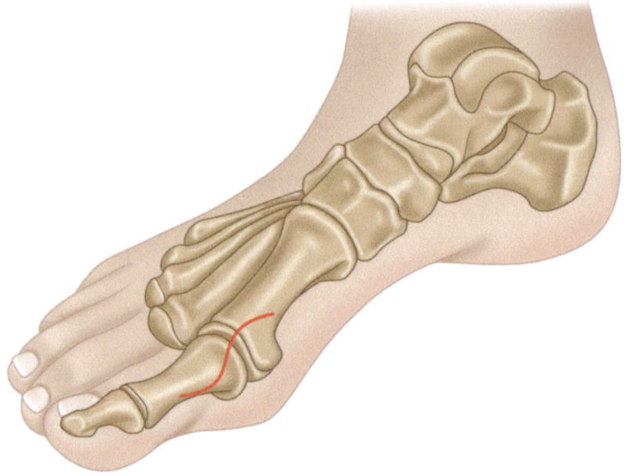

Fig. 18.1 S-shaped dorsomedial incision.

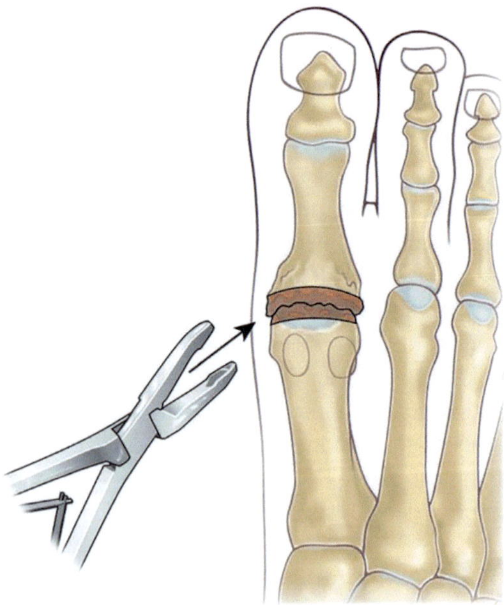

Fig. 18.2 Rongeur used to prepare bone surfaces.

formed first, followed by resection of phalangeal osteophytes as needed. These procedures are performed using a rongeur and a set of large scissors (Fig. 18.2). The bone surfaces are prepared with a rongeur instead of a motorized burr to avoid burning the bone. If a motorized tool is used, the rotation speed must be slow.

The process starts at the metatarsal head; this is a simple and minimal osteophyte removal procedure in which as much bone stock as possible is preserved. The denser P1 base is next; a 2.5-mm drill bit can be used to make a few holes in the articular surface to provide better hold for the rongeur and make it easier to remove the entire articular surface. These holes in the epiphysis also help drive bone marrow into the arthrodesis site. Lastly, the lower portion of M1 is prepared by removing the middle groove and any excising any excess bone from the arthritic sesamoids.

The two prepared surfaces will make a convex/concave pair, but they should not be completely smooth as some roughness is needed to counter the micromovements that could slow down bone fusion. A concave/convex configuration of the bone surfaces is more reassuring as it is easier to set the arthrodesis position, is more stable, and produces minimal first ray shortening.

18.1.1.5 Positioning of MTP1 Arthrodesis

The phalanx is placed against the M1 head by applying pressure in the desired position. This position is maintained by inserting an oblique K-wire through the metatarsophalangeal joint from proximal to distal and inside to out. The positioning is checked clinically and radiologically:

- *Horizontal plane:* First ray aligned in slight valgus, ideally 16–18°; good metatarsophalangeal contact; no subluxation; big toe parallel to second toe in a natural position. Less lateral release will allow reduction of phalanx valgus to correct the metatarsus varus through a lever effect.
- *Sagittal plane:* The position of the first phalanx is verified relative to the ground, which is mimicked by placing a radiopaque plate under the sole of the foot. In the ideal case, the P1 axis will have 15° dorsal flexion relative to the M1 axis. This is the angle between the plantar side of P1 and the dorsal side of M1, not the angle between the dorsal sides of P1 and M1.
- *Coronal plane:* The nail of the big toe is positioned parallel to the nail of the second toe and the MTP1 joint locked with a second K-wire inserted distal to proximal from P1 of the big toe into M1 and from medial to lateral.

18.1.1.6 Arthrodesis Fixation

The arthrodesis is secured first with K-wires. One 26-mm screw is inserted retrograde from medial to lateral and inferior to superior, from the medial proximal edge of P1, through the M1 diaphysis, across the arthrodesis site, and sometimes going into the lateral cortex.

After verifying the screw's position on fluoroscopy, an MTP1 arthrodesis plate is set into position (Figs. 18.3 and 18.4). Four self-locking screws are inserted in the plate, which is the stiffest commercially available fixation system. The two temporary K-wires are removed. Primary stability in flexion-extension is verified and then the incision closed without drainage.

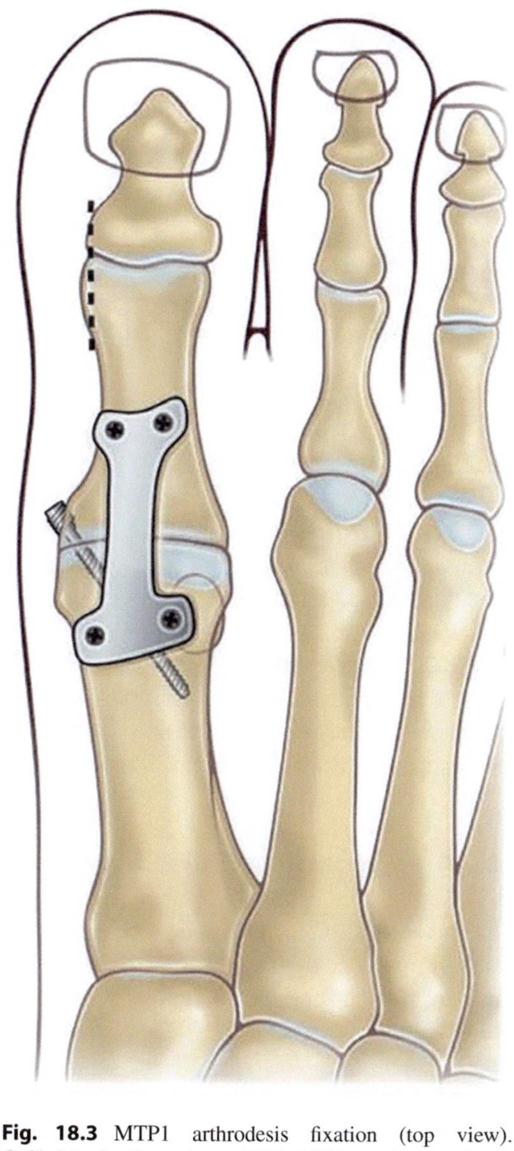

Fig. 18.3 MTP1 arthrodesis fixation (top view).

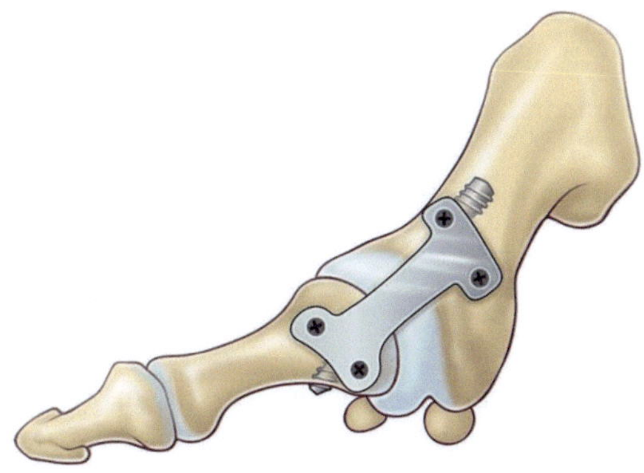

Fig. 18.4 MTP1 arthrodesis fixation (side view).

18.1.2 Postoperative Course

The procedure is usually performed on an outpatient basis. The moderately compressing dressing is left in place for about 15 days and then replaced with a simpler dressing during the first postoperative follow-up visit. Immediate weight-bearing is requested on a postoperative shoe with full, flat rigid sole but protected by crutches or a walker for the first 15 days. Prophylactic antiplatelet therapy is prescribed for 15 days given the protected weight-bearing during this period.

The first radiological and clinical progress checks are done around day 45; if the arthrodesis has fused on radiographs, the patient can start wearing standard shoes and gradually resume heel-toe gait. Other radiological and clinical follow-ups are scheduled at 3 and 6 months postoperative.

The plate may be removed if necessary, generally at 9 months postoperative.

18.1.3 Indications and Results

The indications for open MTP1 fusion are basically the same as for percutaneous MTP1 fusion.

The major advantages of this technique are as follows:

- Small amount of bone stock sacrificed (index minus +++).
- Feasible in patients with severe osteoporosis.
- MTP1 dorsiflexion automatically set at 15° by the plate, which eliminates the high rate of malunion after screw-only fixation.
- Less secondary displacement than after screw-only fixation.
- Fewer cases of nonunion (most recent study reported a 98% MTP1 fusion rate with plate).

The choice of techniques is based on the surgeon's preferences and training. Since a high fusion rate and minimal first ray shortening are very important to us, we use this open technique with locking plate and plantar neutralization screw.

18.1.4 Conclusion

Open MTP1 fusion is a simple procedure that yields results comparable to fusion performed with other techniques. Using a locking plate has reduced the nonunion rate by an appreciable amount, along with the rate of P1 elevatus.

Positioning of the arthrodesis is the key step of this procedure, no matter which technique is used.

The indications for open MTP1 fusion are broad; however, the only indications that absolutely require open surgery are large bone defects requiring bone grafting or severe osteoporosis.

18.2 MTP1 Joint Replacement

18.2.1 Definition

MTP1 joint replacement is the other surgical alternative for end-stage arthritis of the MTP joint in the big toe. Its indications are very limited: MTP1 osteoarthritis centered on both AP and lateral views.

There are two types of arthroplasty procedures:

- Total implant that replaces both articular surfaces.
- Hemiarthroplasty implant that replaces only one side of the joint, typically the phalangeal one.

Unfortunately, these implants often fail, like in the ankle. Using these implants is tricky and surgical revision is even more difficult because it requires bone grafting of the resulting defect (Fig. 18.5).

While this surgery may be attractive, it is anecdotal and should not be used on a regular basis in a forefoot surgery practice.

18.2.2 Indication

Hallux rigidus with arthritis but without elevation or deviation.

18.2.3 Surgical Technique

18.2.3.1 Surgical Approach

A standard medial approach is used, although a dorsal one can be used.

18.2.3.2 Implantation

The technique used depends on the type of implant and instrumentation and must follow the manufacturer's recommendations.

18.2.4 Postoperative Course

The rehabilitation protocol can be more or less aggressive, depending on the type of implant. Weight-bearing is typically allowed immediately.

18.2.5 Outcomes

Very often, the outcomes are disappointing despite the data provided by manufacturers. The

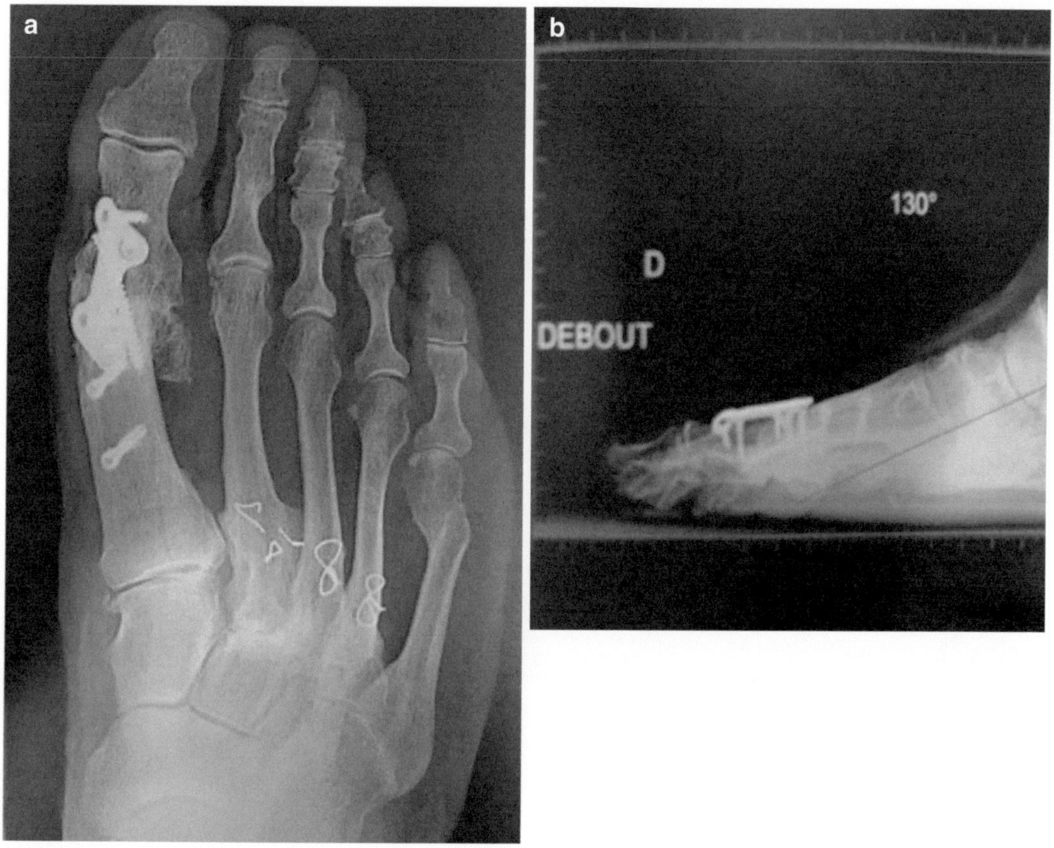

Fig. 18.5 Revision after failed MTP1 joint replacement. Dorsoplantar view (**a**). Mediolateral view (**b**).

immediate risk is persistent pain, which may require early revision for MTP1 fusion that is equally tricky and challenging.

18.2.6 Complications

The infection risk is often higher than in other forefoot surgeries, likely due to the early joint motion, exposure time, and implant volume. The main complications are prolonged inflammation and edema, which contribute to pain and stiffness leading to revision surgery for the failed arthroplasty.

As mentioned previously, surgical revision is tricky because of the resulting bone defect and inflammation which increase the risk of poor healing, discharge, and thereby infection. Repeat surgical procedures always contribute to significant viability problems and subsequent first ray shortening.

18.2.7 Conclusion

In our practice, this type of procedure is banned because of the very high complication rate and poor outcomes when compared to the reliable outcomes of MTP1 arthrodesis, which we believe is the benchmark procedure for advanced first ray osteoarthritis.

The unpredictable results after failed arthroplasty also contribute to our preference to perform first-line arthrodesis in patients with advanced MTP1 osteoarthritis. However, it is not out of the question that in a few years, reliable implants will be introduced that preserve the bone stock and supplant MTP1 arthrodesis.

Percutaneous Fusion of the First Metatarsophalangeal Joint

19

Thomas Bauer and Christophe Cermolacce

19.1 Surgical Technique

19.1.1 Instrumentation

The instrumentation needed for percutaneous MTP1 fusion is the same one used for all percutaneous forefoot surgical procedures. It includes a large conical burr, a Beaver® blade, elevators, rasps, low speed drill with torque limiter, and a fluoroscopy system. Cannulated 3.0-mm compression screws are used with the technique described here, but other percutaneous fixation devices can be used.

19.1.2 Patient Positioning

The patient is positioned supine, with their foot hanging off the end of the table to allow AP and lateral fluoroscopy images to be made. The procedure is typically performed with regional anesthesia; a tourniquet can be used depending on the surgeon's preferences.

T. Bauer (✉)
Orthopedic Department, Ambroise Paré University Hospital, Boulogne-Billancourt, France
e-mail: thomas.bauer@aphp.fr

C. Cermolacce
Institut de Chirurgie Orthopédique et Sportive, Marseille, France

19.1.3 Portals

Percutaneous MTP1 fusion is performed with one main portal and two accessory portals, which can be combined depending on the case (Fig. 19.1).

The main portal is on the medial side at the MTP1 joint and is used to prepare the bone surfaces. Two accessory portals can be useful in some cases: one proximal medial and plantar portal at the head of the first metatarsal (M1) (same portal as for percutaneous hallux valgus exostectomy); one distal lateral and dorsal portal at the base of the proximal phalanx (P1).

The proximal medial accessory portal at the M1 head is used to remove dorsal and medial osteophytes; the distal lateral accessory portal is used to remove dorsal and lateral osteophytes and to release the lateral MTP1 joint capsule and ligaments if necessary. As one becomes more experienced, the procedure can be done using only the main portal; resection of dorsal and medial osteophytes can be carried out through this portal. The accessory dorsolateral portal is only used to resect rare large and painful lateral osteophytes that cannot be completely removed easily through the main portal. Lateral ligament release at the MTP1 joint is rarely done anymore, even in cases of severe deformity.

C. Cazeau, Y. Stiglitz (eds.), *Percutaneous and Minimally Invasive Foot Surgery*,
https://doi.org/10.1007/978-3-030-98791-6_19

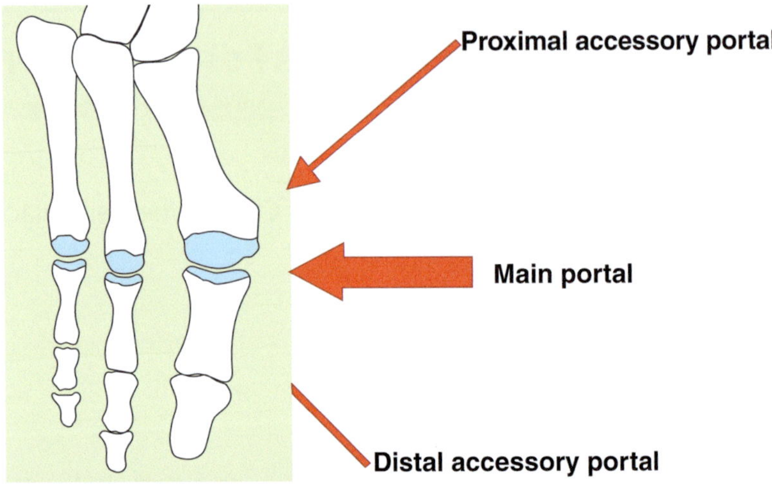

Fig. 19.1 Portals for percutaneous MTP1 fusion. © Thomas Bauer 2015. All Rights Reserved

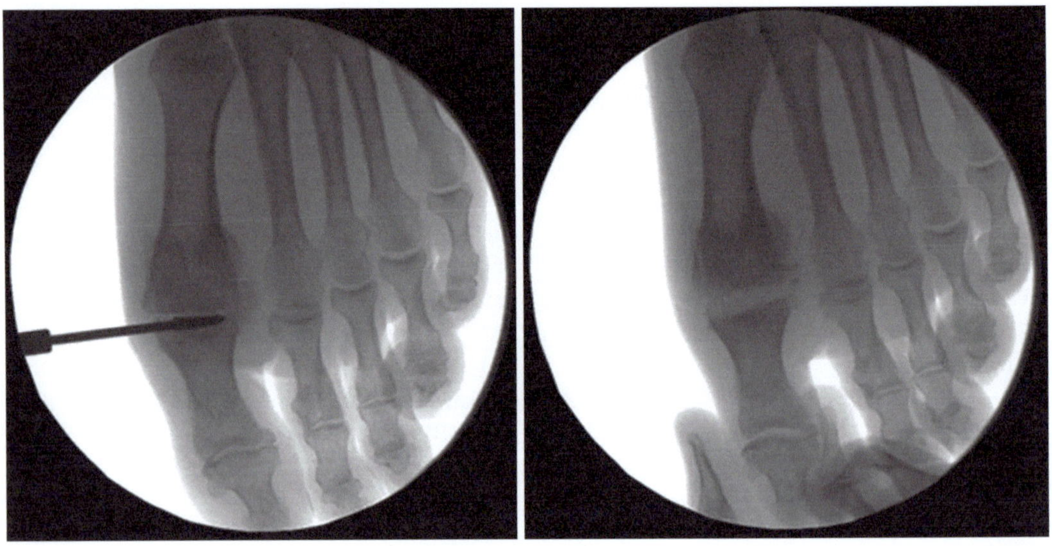

Fig. 19.2 Preparing the bone surfaces at the MTP1 joint. © Thomas Bauer 2015. All Rights Reserved

19.1.4 Preparing the Bone Surfaces

Bone surface preparation begins by removing metatarsal and/or phalangeal osteophytes with a conical burr. This resection is nearly always performed through the main portal (Fig. 19.2). Bone debris is carefully removed, and the resection site is irrigated with copious normal saline. The extent of osteophyte removal must be verified under fluoroscopic control and must be adapted to patient's symptoms. Excessive resection resulting in a bone defect must be avoided since this can compromise the primary stability of the arthrodesis.

Preparing the MTP1 joint is the most important step of this procedure. The conical burr is placed in the MTP1 joint while pulling traction on the hallux. Cartilage resection and bone surface preparation are performed with the burr. Fluoroscopy should be used in a surgeon's early cases to assess the quantity and quality of the bone resection. In this technique, the fusion site is prepared by cutting two flat and parallel surfaces on AP and lateral views. This is the most difficult step of this procedure; the main risk is asymmetrical resection.

The surgeon must be aware of the possibility of the following:

- Excessive metatarsal bone resection: The bone at the P1 base is denser than the bone at the M1 head; thus, the burr will tend to spontaneously remove the weaker bone at the M1 head. If too much bone is removed from the M1 head, this will result in M1 shortening, loss of primary stability, and metatarsus elevatus positioning of the arthrodesis with an increased risk of transfer metatarsalgia due to incorrect first ray loading. Hence, it is important to control the burr and press more on P1 than on the M1 head, while monitoring the position of the burr and the progress of the resection on fluoroscopy.
- Excessive dorsal resection: Since the plantar side of the MTP1 joint is harder to reach than the dorsal side, the burr will tend to spontaneously remove bone on the dorsal side of the joint. The risk is ending up with an asymmetrical V-shaped resection due to excessive dorsal resection, with loss of primary stability and the arthrodesis being positioned in excessive P1 dorsal flexion. Bone preparation must be performed while applying traction on the hallux to open the MTP1 joint; this makes it easier to access the plantar side, monitor the bone resection, and make parallel cuts on lateral fluoroscopy views.
- Osteoporotic bone, especially in patients with inflammatory arthritis and severe hallux valgus. There is a risk of removing too much bone on both sides, which compromises the primary stability and makes the fixation more complex.
- Insufficient resection: This will be evident when a portion of the MTP1 joint is still present when one tries to compress the arthrodesis site. In this case, the bone resection must be redone on the side that still has cartilage, until two flat subchondral bone surfaces are obtained.

After bone resection is completed, the bone debris is removed with rasps, and the arthrodesis site is irrigated with copious normal saline to prevent chronic inflammation.

19.1.5 Positioning of MTP1 Arthrodesis

The phalanx is placed against the M1 head by applying pressure on it; this position is maintained with an oblique K-wire through the phalanx and metatarsal. Positioning of the arthrodesis is assessed two ways:

- Visual inspection: straight alignment of first ray or slight valgus, length of first ray, first phalanx parallel to ground (evaluated by placing a metal plate under the sole of the foot), and neutral position in coronal plane (no medial/lateral rotation of hallux).
- Radiographic controls: straight metatarsophalangeal alignment or slight valgus on AP view (Fig. 19.3); first phalanx parallel to ground in lateral view (Fig. 19.4); good metatarsophalangeal bone contact, no subluxation.

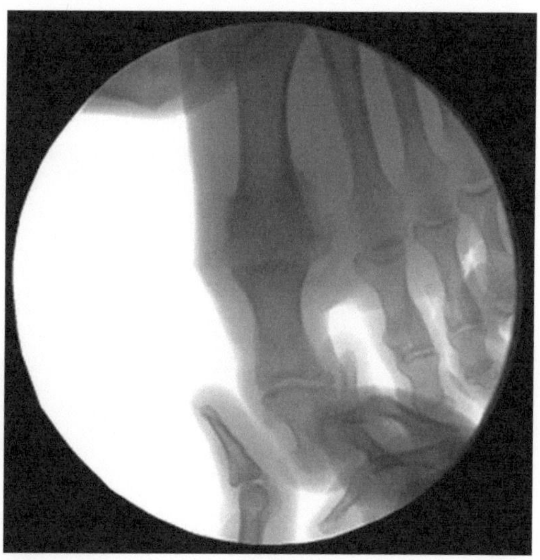

Fig. 19.3 Positioning of arthrodesis on AP view.

A surgeon must be aware of the following traps and pitfalls:

- The most common positioning error is placing the MTP1 joint in excessive dorsal flexion. This misconception has persisted because some surgeons feel that women who wear heals need more dorsiflexion. In the correct position, the dorsal side of P1 is parallel to the ground; this provides good pulpal contact when walking with flat-soled shoes and with heels (6–7 cm, or more) if the interphalangeal joint is flexible in dorsal flexion.
- Plantar subluxation, which is common in hallux rigidus cases, most be avoided to ensure the best possible first ray function and to facilitate fixation.
- Lateral subluxation is the main risk during arthrodesis of severe hallux valgus cases. Reduction can be difficult in such cases because of lateral contracture. Additional bone resection will help to improve MTP1 contact more than lateral arthrolysis will; the latter often has disappointing results because it makes the MTP1 instability worse and further complicates arthrodesis positioning.

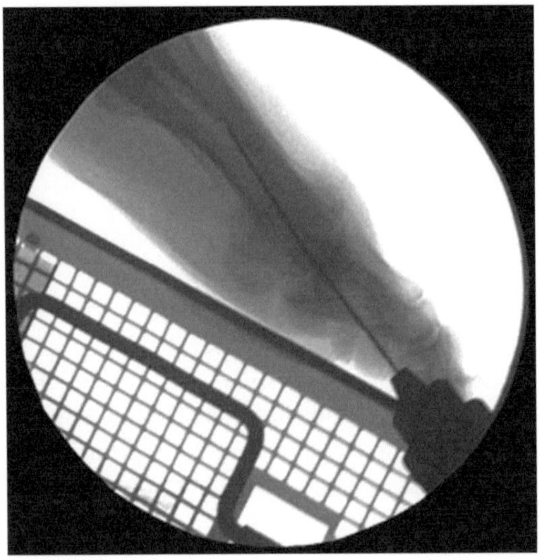

Fig. 19.4 Positioning of arthrodesis on lateral view. © Thomas Bauer 2015. All Rights Reserved

19.1.6 Fixation of the Arthrodesis

The MTP1 arthrodesis is fixed with two cannulated compression screws (Fig. 19.5). The first K-wire is oblique from P1 to M1 from medial-distal to lateral-proximal. The second K-wire goes from M1 to P1 and crosses the first K-wire at the M1 head, not at the previous joint line. The two cannulated screws are inserted, and compression is achieved by tightening each screw alternately.

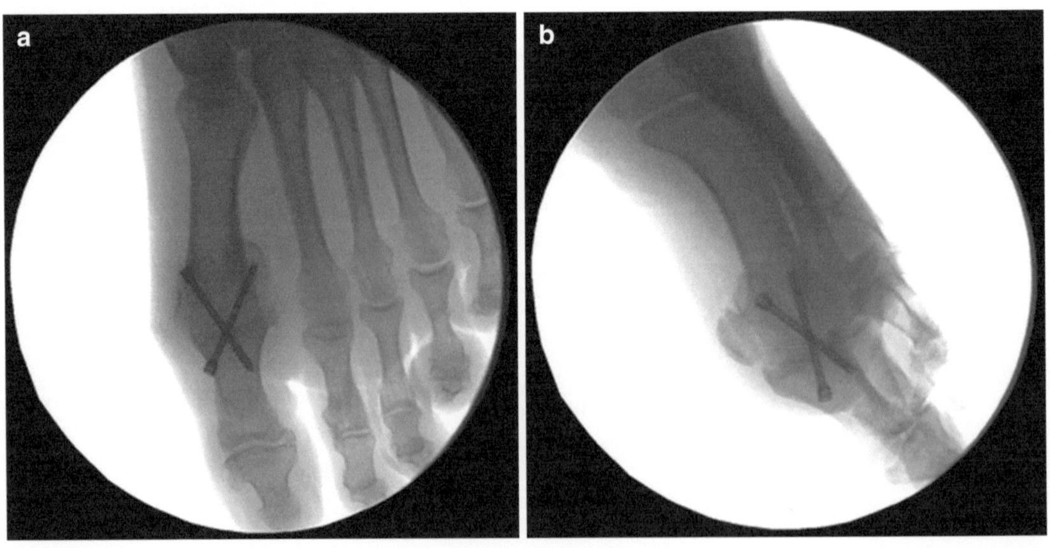

Fig. 19.5 Fixation of arthrodesis with two cannulated compression screws. AP view (**a**) and lateral view (**b**). © Thomas Bauer 2015. All Rights Reserved

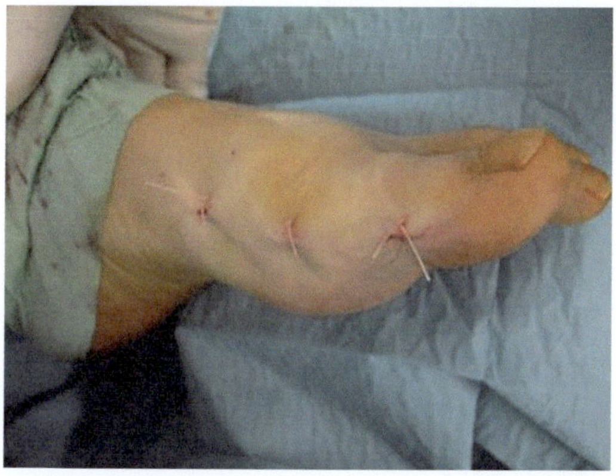

Fig. 19.6 Postoperative appearance.

Primary stability is verified in flexion and extension, and then the portals are closed (Fig. 19.6).

19.2 Postoperative Care

This procedure is performed on an outpatient basis. The initial moderately compressive dressing is left in place for 10 days, and then a simple dressing is applied and changed twice per week until the incision has healed. Immediate full weight-bearing is allowed with a postoperative shoe having a full, flat, and rigid insole. Antithrombotic therapy is not typically done except in patients with known risk factors. The first radiographic check is done on day 10, when the first dressing is changed. The second radiographic and clinical evaluation is done at 1 month postoperative. Patients can start wearing normal shoes after 1 month postoperative, depending on the results of the radiographic and clinical examination.

19.3 Indications and Results

The indications for percutaneous MTP1 fusion are basically the same as for open MTP1 fusion. The best and fastest functional results are obtained in cases of advanced metatarsophalangeal osteoarthritis, which is painful and associated with hallux rigidus and compensatory hypermobility of the interphalangeal joint. Without preoperative interphalangeal hypermobility, return to normal walking and wearing shoes can take longer due to the progressive adaptation of the interphalangeal joint. The main contraindication for percutaneous MTP1 fusion is the presence of extensive bone loss with first ray shortening requiring a bone graft.

19.4 Discussion

Percutaneous MTP1 fusion is a simple and quick procedure that can achieve functional results comparable to those obtained with open MTP1 fusion with a patient satisfaction rate above 90% [1–6].

During open MTP1 fusion procedures, bone preparation requires a large approach, which brings with it a risk of postoperative pain and wound-healing difficulties [1, 7]. One of the benefits of percutaneous MTP1 fusion is less immediate postoperative morbidity (minimal pain, wound healing problems are rare) with the possibility of performing this procedure in an outpatient setting with immediate full weight-bearing in a postoperative shoe.

Bone preparation is a crucial step of this procedure and requires experience in percutaneous forefoot surgery. However, the learning curve is shorter than for percutaneous first metatarsal osteotomy for correcting hallux valgus. The primary risks are first ray shortening and nonunion due to insufficient construct stability.

A concave/convex configuration of the bone surfaces is more reassuring as it is easier to set the arthrodesis position; it is more stable and there is minimal first ray shortening [2, 8]. However, this method of bone preparation is difficult to perform percutaneously.

Arthrodesis positioning is the other crucial step of the procedure. It is not sufficient to only consider the varus/valgus alignment, dorsal/plantar flexion, and medial/lateral rotation. Metatarsus varus, metatarsal cascade, hindfoot shape (valgus flatfoot, pes cavus), clinical symptoms (lateral metatarsalgia, lesser toes deformities), and shoe preferences (flat or high heel shoes) must also be taken into account [1, 7, 9–11]. Setting the arthrodesis position is simple with a percutaneous technique; it can be evaluated at any time clinically and with fluoroscopy. A metal board can be used to mimic ground contact, which makes it possible to correctly position the hallux in the sagittal plane, independent of the shape of the hindfoot or midfoot [1, 7].

The use of crossed cannulated screws for percutaneous MTP1 arthrodesis is a very simple technique. At any point in the procedure, the quality of the contact and positioning of the arthrodesis can be verified, which allows accurate screw positioning under fluoroscopy guidance. However, crossed screws are not the most stable configuration; thus, it is important to verify the screw location to achieve the best possible compression and avoid crossing the screws at the joint line, which will cause excessive stress [1].

19.5 Conclusion

Percutaneous MTP1 fusion is a simple procedure that provides comparable results to fusion performed with open techniques. The postoperative course is simplified with immediate full weight-bearing on rigid flat shoes and quick return to normal walking. Bone preparation is critical and requires experience in percutaneous forefoot surgery. Positioning and fixation of the arthrodesis with this percutaneous procedure are simple and can be verified clinically and radiologically. The indications for percutaneous MTP1 fusion are broad with the only contraindications being severe bone loss or osteoporosis.

Editors' Point of View

Compensatory osteotomies of the first ray must be highly accurate to correct the mechanical factors that hinder MTP1 function. For this reason, MIS (not percutaneous) techniques appear to be essential. Percutaneous MTP1 fusion can be done elegantly with minimal scars; however, the fixation methods are not as reliable as those used during MIS, and immediate full weight-bearing is not always possible. Surgeons must prioritize what is most important: immediate function or small scars?

References

1. Womack JW, Ishikawa SN. First metatarsophalangeal arthrodesis. Foot Ankle Clin. 2009;14:43–50.
2. Goucher NR, Coughlin MJ. Hallux metatarsophalangeal joint arthrodesis using dome-shaped reamers and dorsal plate fixation: a prospective study. Foot Ankle Int. 2006;27:869–76.
3. Coughlin MJ, Shurnas PS. Hallux rigidus: grading and long-term results of operative treatment. J Bone Joint Surg Am. 2003;85:2072–88.
4. Flavin R, Stephens MM. Arthrodesis of the first metatarsophalangeal joint using a dorsal titanium contoured plate. Foot Ankle Int. 2004;25(11): 783–7.
5. Brodsky JW, Passmore RN, Pollo FE, et al. Functional outcome of arthrodesis of the first metatarsophalangeal joint using parallel screw fixation. Foot Ankle Int. 2005;26:140–6.
6. Yee G, Lau J. Current concepts review: hallux rigidus. Foot Ankle Int. 2008;29:637–6.
7. Kelikian AS. Technical considerations in hallux metatarsophalangeal arthrodesis. Foot Ankle Clin. 2005;10:167–90.
8. Curtis MJ, Myerson M, Jinnah RH, et al. Arthrodesis of the first metatarsophalangeal joint: a biomechanical study of internal fixation techniques. Foot Ankle Int. 1993;14:395–9.
9. Conti SF, Dhawan S. Arthrodesis of the first metatarsophalangeal and interphalangeal joints of the foot. Foot Ankle Clin. 1996;1:33–53.
10. Harper MC. Positioning of the hallux for first metatarsophalangeal joint arthrodesis. Foot Ankle Int. 1997;18:827.
11. Alexander IJ. Hallux metatarsophalangeal joint arthrodesis. In: Kitaoka HB, editor. Masters techniques in foot and ankle surgery. 2nd ed. Philadelphia: Lippincott Williams and Wilkins; 2002. p. 45–60.

Percutaneous Osteotomy of the Hallux Proximal Phalanx

20

Cyrille Cazeau and Ali Ghorbani

20.1 Introduction

This osteotomy was first described by Akin in 1925 for the treatment of hallux valgus with or without exostectomy. It was then brought into the modern era by Lavigne in 1978 and is now done with and without other soft tissue procedures like McBride's. And finally, even in the hands of master surgeon L.S Barouk, the scarf osteotomy was only combined with varus shifting of the hallux in an exceedingly small number of cases. This osteotomy has progressively become common place. However, it is truly a supplemental procedure and is never done in isolation to correct a deformity. It cannot make up for an insufficient first metatarsal (M1) osteotomy. On the other hand, if the osteotomy is excessive, it can worsen the hallux metatarsophalangeal joint (MP1) incongruency due to impingement in shoes. Its esthetics are undeniable, which is typically the only thing that matters to many patients.

C. Cazeau (✉)
Clinique Victor Hugo, Paris, France

A. Ghorbani
Clinique Médipôle Garonne, Toulouse, France

20.2 Techniques

Osteotomy of the proximal phalanx is one component of the treatment strategy for hallux valgus or hallux rigidus and is only performed after lateral MP1 arthrolysis and M1 osteotomy.

20.2.1 Standard Surgical Techniques

20.2.1.1 Approach

A dorsomedial approach is made at the P1 base (Fig. 20.1) medial to the extensor hallucis longus. The skin incision is made with a Beaver blade until contact is made with the periosteum, and then an elevator is used to carry out subperiosteal detachment of the entire medial side of P1.

20.2.1.2 Closing Wedge Osteotomy of P1

A straight burr (Shannon 12 × 2 mm) is inserted perpendicular to the P1 axis. The osteotomy is started on the medial side of P1, and then the burr is rotated, using the skin incision as the pivot point, and angled to continue the osteotomy on the plantar and dorsal cortex. The end of the burr is stopped 1–2 mm from the lateral cortex to preserve a lateral cortical hinge (Figs. 20.2, 20.3, and 20.4).

P1 varus is induced by making a forceful varus movement of the hallux while holding it between the thumb and index finger, while the burr contin-

C. Cazeau, Y. Stiglitz (eds.), *Percutaneous and Minimally Invasive Foot Surgery*,
https://doi.org/10.1007/978-3-030-98791-6_20

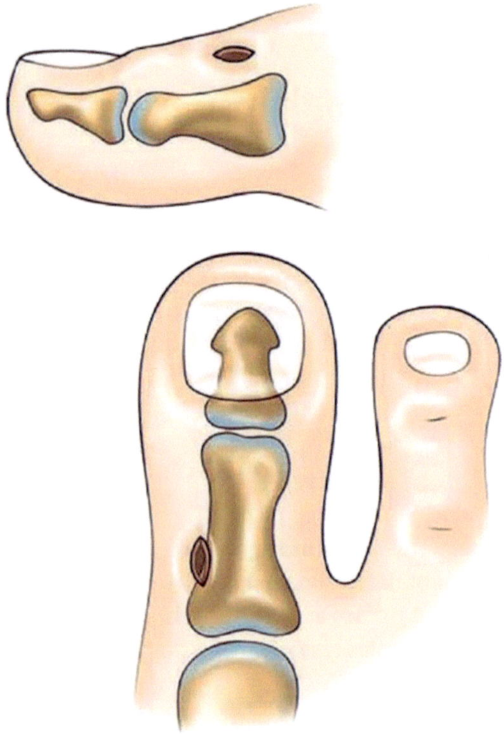

Fig. 20.1 Dorsomedial approach to P1 base.

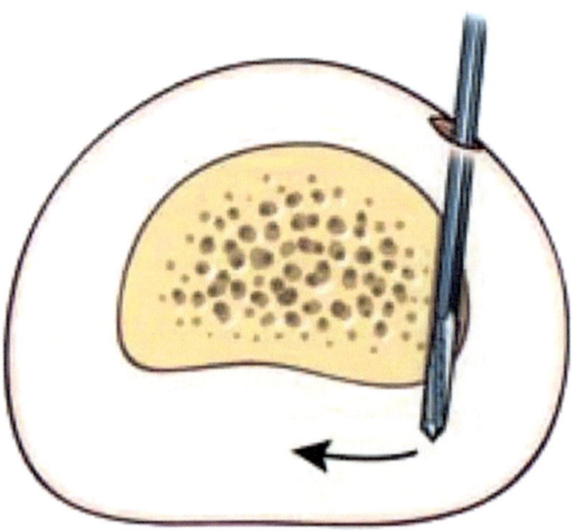

Fig. 20.2 Osteotomy begins with medial cortex.

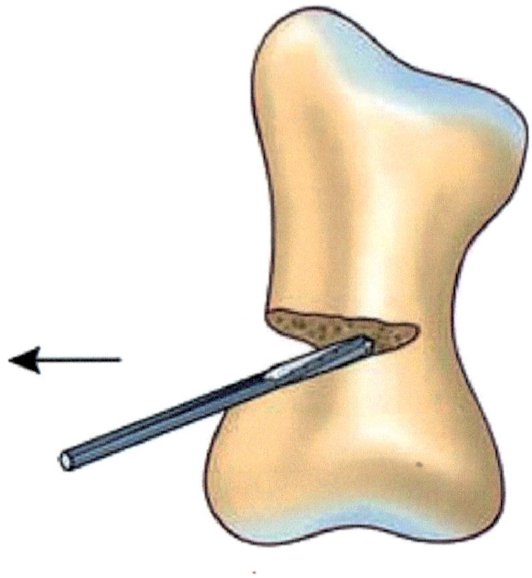

Fig. 20.3 Burr progresses from medial to dorsal and preserves the lateral cortical hinge.

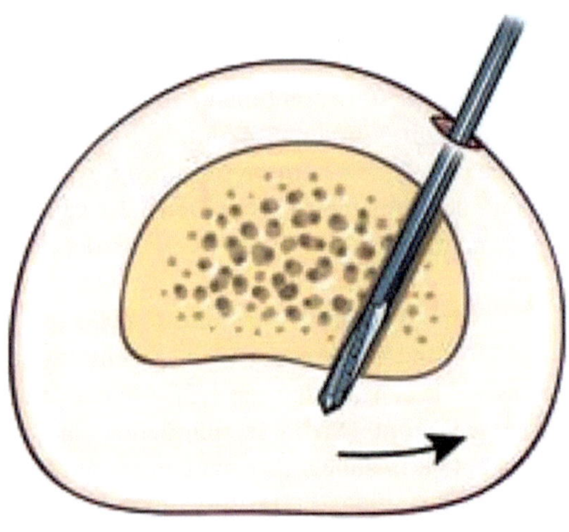

Fig. 20.4 Osteotomy ends back on the medial cortex with more bone resection if needed.

ues to resect the medial four-fifths of P1. This defines the medial wedge needed to achieve the desired correction. Closure and compression of the osteotomy are accomplished by a forceful varus movement. Fluoroscopy is used to check the correction achieved and the stability of the osteotomy when the varus loads are removed.

If there is an indication for dorsal flexion osteotomy, 1–2 mm of the plantar cortex is preserved to act as a plantar hinge. Resection of the dorsal third is continued by performing a forced dorsiflexion movement to produce a wedge with dorsal base.

20.2.2 Technical Variation

A Beaver blade is inserted on the medial side until it contacts bone, halfway between the dorsal and plantar aspects. A working chamber is made using the Beaver blade while ensuring the cutting side of the blade always points toward the bone, i.e., downward when the blade is dorsal and upward when it is plantar. Dissection is performed with an elevator.

Next, a Ø3.1 wedge burr is introduced into the proximal metaphysis area, on the dorsal aspect. Through a continuous plantar translation movement—without going back-and-forth—a compete dorsal, medial, and plantar osteotomy is performed in the medial half of the phalanx. The burr is then inserted horizontally until it makes contact with the intramedullary face of the lateral cortex. This intramedullary route is used to cut away the remaining dorsal and plantar sides of the phalanx until only the lateral cortex remains, which will serve as the hinge (Fig. 20.5).

A forceful varus movement is made, and then by performing the push test (plantar support under M1 head), the phalanx is realigned thanks to the plasticity of the lateral cortical hinge in metaphyseal bone. If resistance is felt, the remaining lateral cortex will need to be thinned out more and the maneuver repeated. The indirect criteria of success are listed in the *Sensing Without Seeing* box.

Fixation is done using a compression screw with differential threads (Fig. 20.6). It is introduced through the distal part of the mini-chevron approach. The entry point is on the medial edge of the phalanx, more on the plantar aspect and angled forward, outward, and upward (Fig. 20.7). A 20-mm length is always enough to place the

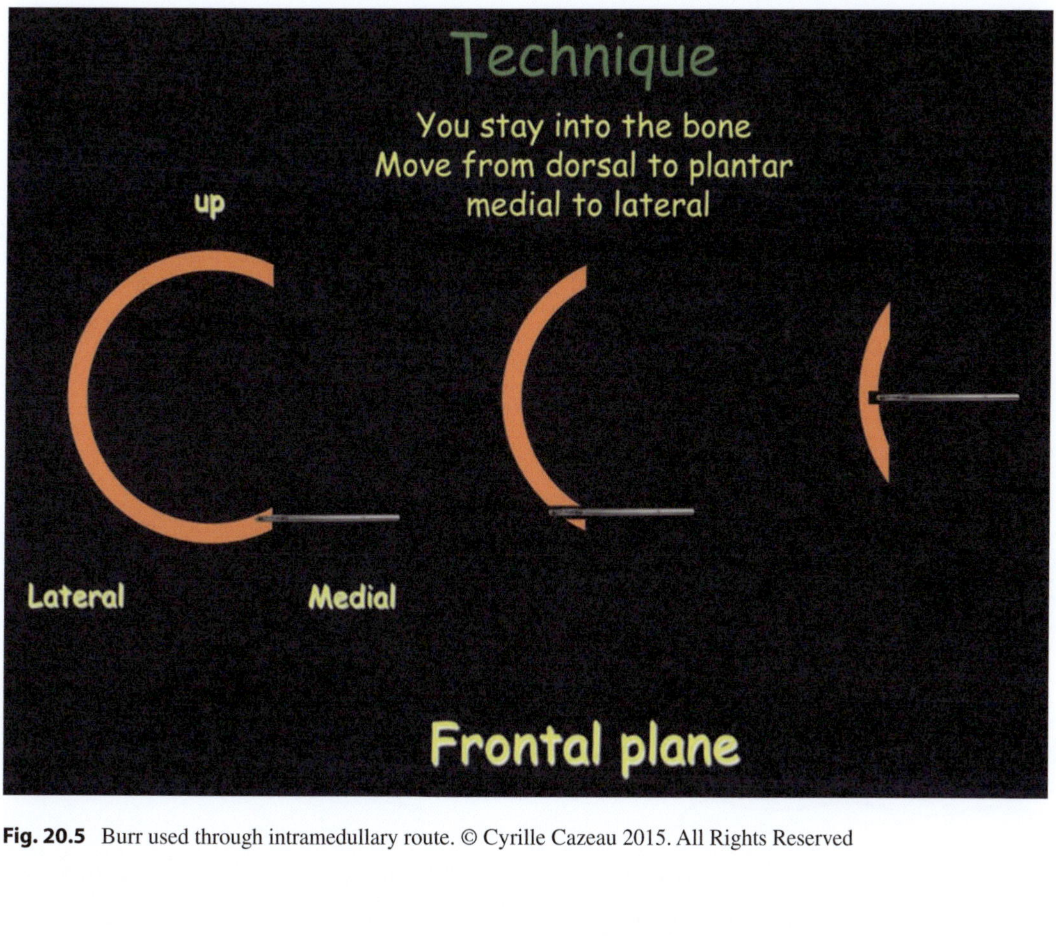

Fig. 20.5 Burr used through intramedullary route. © Cyrille Cazeau 2015. All Rights Reserved

two threads on either side of the osteotomy (Fig. 20.8) and to minimize impingement in the case of false dorsal or plantar passage. The advantage of this technique is that it is easy to carry out, safe because the burr is used inside the medullary canal, and effective at inducing varus because of its 3.1 mm diameter and proximal location. Its metaphyseal location ensures good union and guarantees the plasticity of the hinge. Preserving this lateral hinge (Fig. 20.9), in combination with the screw on the medial side, ensures excellent stability and allows immediate mobilization of the MP1 joint. The postoperative dressing no longer has a support function. The various steps of the procedure are summarized in Fig. 20.10.

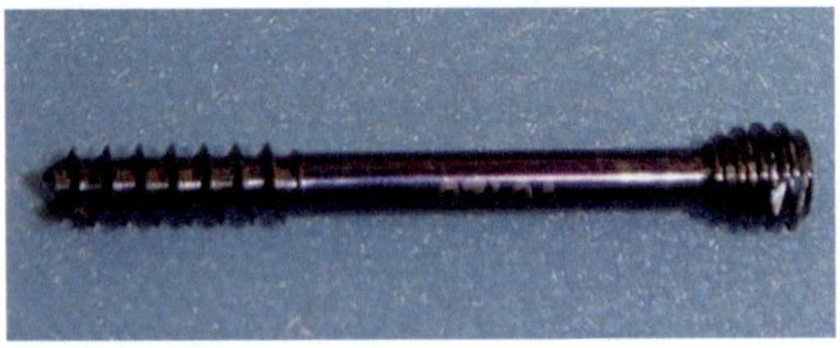

Fig. 20.6 Dual thread compression screw.

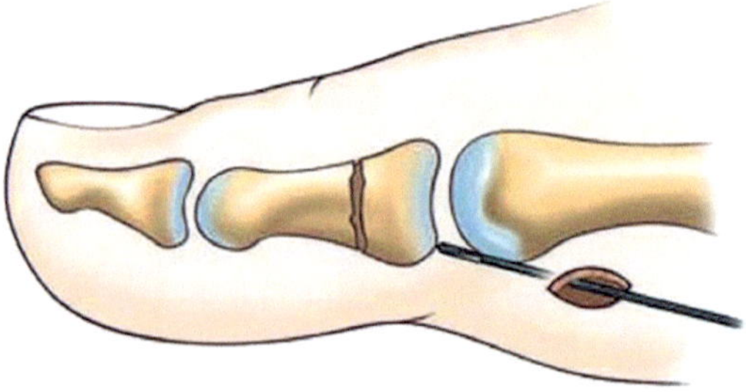

Fig. 20.7 Entry point.

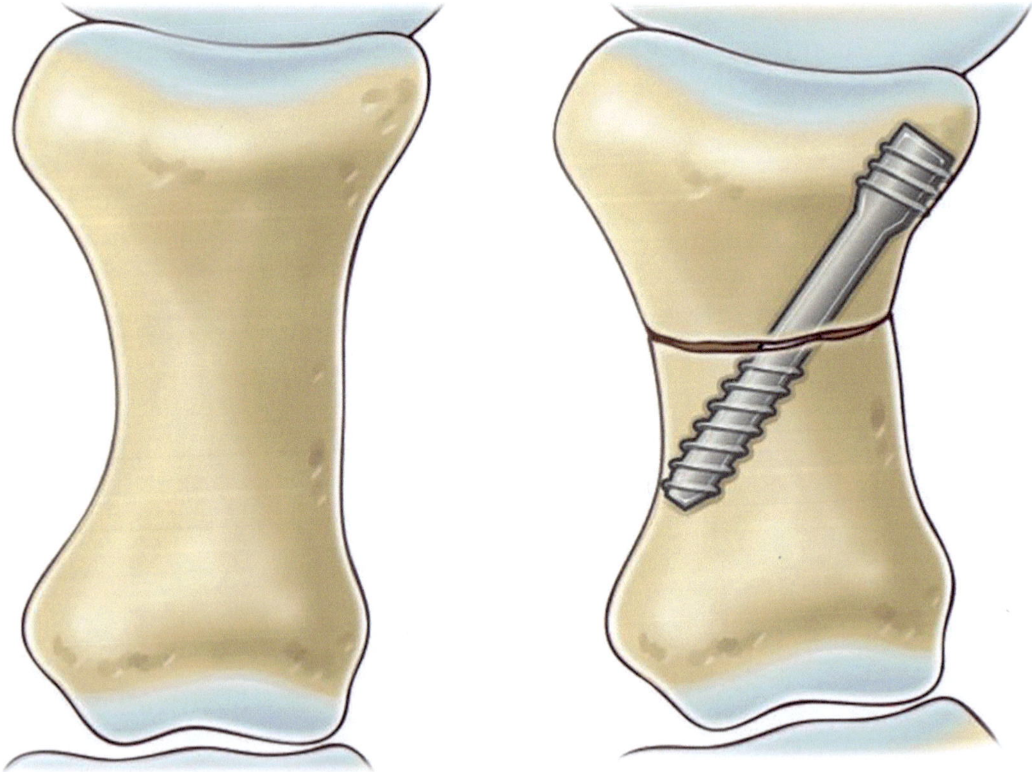

Fig. 20.8 A 20-mm screw is used to compress the osteotomy site.

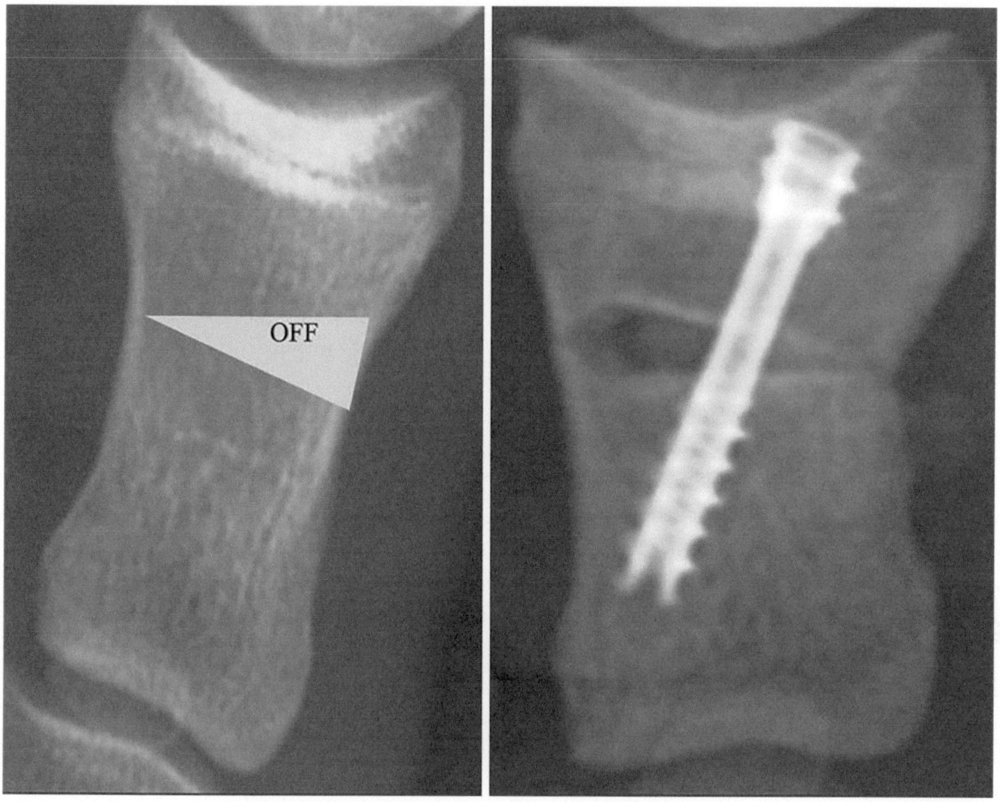

Fig. 20.9 Preserving the lateral hinge. © Cyrille Cazeau 2015. All Rights Reserved

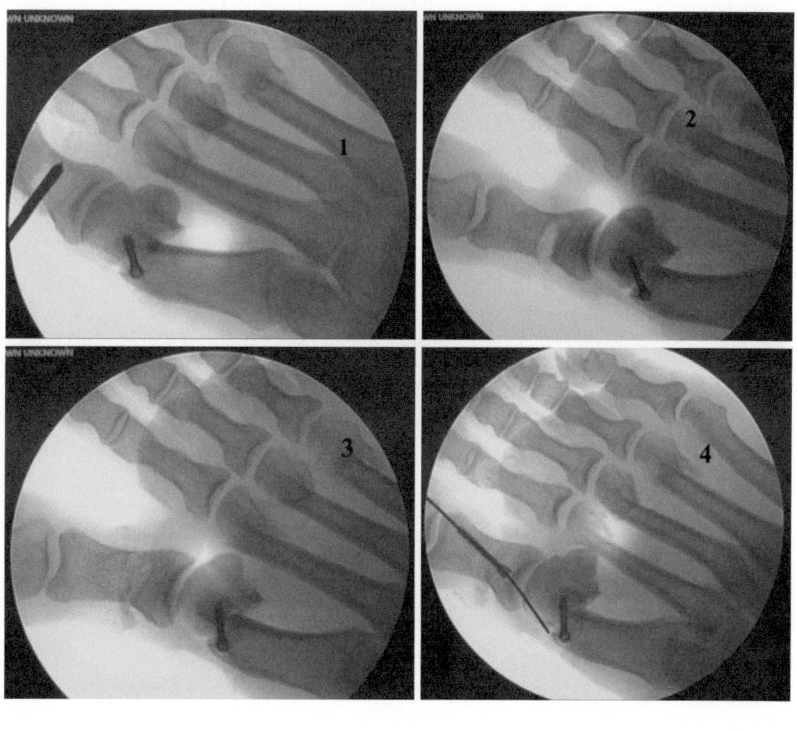

Fig. 20.10 Summary of the procedure: (1) Medial osteotomy with 3-mm diameter burr, (2) Burr removal and lateral hinge check, (3) Medial closing to induce varus; the lateral hinge's plasticity provides stability, (4) Screw fixation. © Cyrille Cazeau 2015. All Rights Reserved

20.3 General Mechanical Advantage

Overall, this osteotomy contributes to the correction in all three anatomical planes and helps to correct the first ray's alignment initiated by the M1 osteotomy. It also helps to reduce bowing of the long tendons, thereby helping to restore joint congruency. Improving all of these parameters helps to increase stability and reduce the mechanical loads that are present.

20.4 Osteotomy by Location

The proximal, diaphyseal, and distal locations of this osteotomy have different indications and goals (Fig. 20.11).

20.4.1 Proximal Osteotomy

This osteotomy is performed proximally in the cancellous bone. Its advantages are as follows:

- Large varus produced due to the significant moment arm.
- Ease of preserving a lateral bone hinge due to plasticity of the metaphyseal bone.
- Medialization of the FLD and EDL tendons, with reduction of the bowing.
- Possibility of dorsal flexion in cases of hallux rigidus, by keeping a plantar hinge, which improves the push-off phase.
- Stable, easy, and reproducible procedure with predictable union.

20.4.2 Diaphyseal Osteotomy

A diaphyseal osteotomy has a higher risk of nonunion or delayed union. To reduce this risk, one will try to perform a monocortical osteotomy. However, some cases may be better addressed with a bicortical osteotomy.

20.4.2.1 Shortening

Hallux rigidus or Egyptian foot are treated with a variable osteotomy depending on which burr is

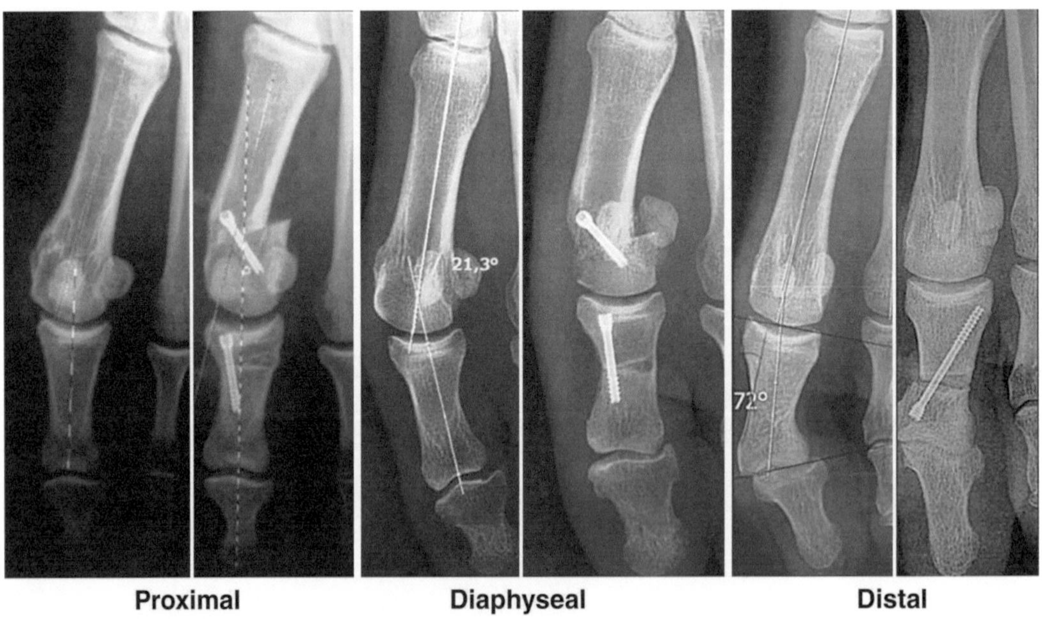

Fig. 20.11 Proximal, diaphyseal, and distal osteotomies have different abilities to induce varus.

chosen (3.1- or 4.1-mm wedge burr). It reduces the risk of recurrence as it eliminates rubbing in shoes and tension exerted by the FDL and EDL tendons. The diaphyseal axis needs to be carefully controlled when the phalanx is shortened significantly to avoid inducing varus.

20.4.2.2 Derotation

Additional supination is possible if the osteotomy done at M1 was not sufficient. This shifts the pressure from the medial side of the hallux to its plantar surface. The push-off phase becomes easier. However, this osteotomy is unstable and delayed union often happens.

20.4.3 Distal Osteotomy

The indication for distal osteotomy is interphalangeal valgus, also called distal epiphyseal cross. The more the osteotomy is placed at the apex of the deformity, the more effective it is geometrically. But it is technically more difficult to carry out, especially the fixation step; interphalangeal joint stiffness is common.

20.5 Complications

20.5.1 Transection of FDL and EDL Tendons

This is a rare complication given that the working space is developed early on. The vibration-induced movements and soft nature of these tissues means that they do not react to the burr's action. Nevertheless, one must make sure not to press the FDL and EDL tendons against the bone with the hand that is not holding the burr.

20.5.2 Nonunion

Nonunion can occur in the diaphyseal location. It is more apparent on radiographs than clinically and worries the radiologist more than the surgeon. Delayed union does not prevent the possibility of immediate weight bearing and moving the toes.

20.5.3 Skin Burns

This is a common complication early in the learning curve related to the burr's position and to not having used the pivot point correctly.

20.5.4 Rupture of Lateral Cortical Hinge

This occurs in an estimated 5% of cases, either deliberately or due to a technical error such as excessive osteotomy, osteoporosis, or diaphyseal osteotomy with insufficient elasticity or made too distally. In these cases, closing is more difficult because the cortical bone in this area already has little capacity for plastic deformation and is fragile, thus increasing the risk of the hinge breaking. The possibilities of correction are more limited. Breaking of the lateral cortical hinge may lead to secondary displacement.

20.5.5 Secondary Displacement

This mainly occurs into dorsal flexion and varus (Fig. 20.12). The risk factors for secondary displacement are rupture of the hinge, diaphyseal location, no fixation, and osteoporosis.

20.5.6 Screw Protrusion

This mainly occurs in the plantar zone. A plantar start is essential with the K-wire angled upward, forward, and outward. Using a larger-diameter K-wire is recommended before inserting the more flexible K-wire that will be used to guide the screw insertion.

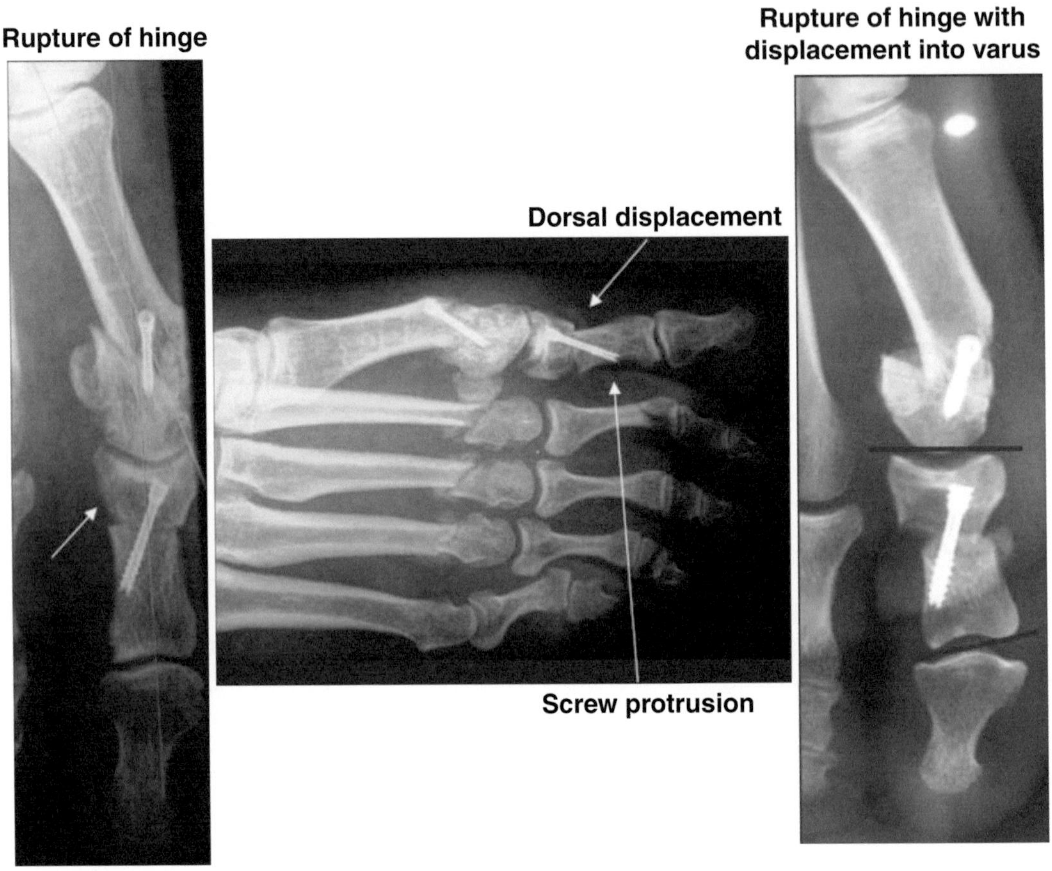

Fig. 20.12 Secondary displacement due to rupture of hinge.

20.5.7 Overabundant Bone Callus

Healing of the percutaneous P1 osteotomy sometimes occurs with the development of a large bone callus, which causes edema and prolonged discomfort in the hallux area. This is more frequent in the diaphysis.

20.6 Dressings and Postoperative Care

If no fixation devices are used, the correction is maintained by the dressings. For varus-inducing procedures, this dressing applies a varus load on the phalanx to hold the osteotomy closed. It is essential to verify the bone correction on fluoroscopy after the dressing has been applied (see chapter 38 on dressings for more details). For dorsal flexion osteotomy cases, the dressing is less important because the osteotomy is held closed mainly by the immediate weight-bearing.

Immediate full weight-bearing is allowed with a postoperative shoe having a flat or curved rigid insole. Radiological and clinical follow-up visits are scheduled on day 10 and day 21 if no fixation was used, day 21 after screw fixation, and then at day 45. The goal is to check that no secondary displacement has occurred and to look for signs of bone union.

20.7 Results

Percutaneous closing wedge and shortening osteotomy of P1 in the context of hallux treatment produces an average varus of 7° (−5° to 20)

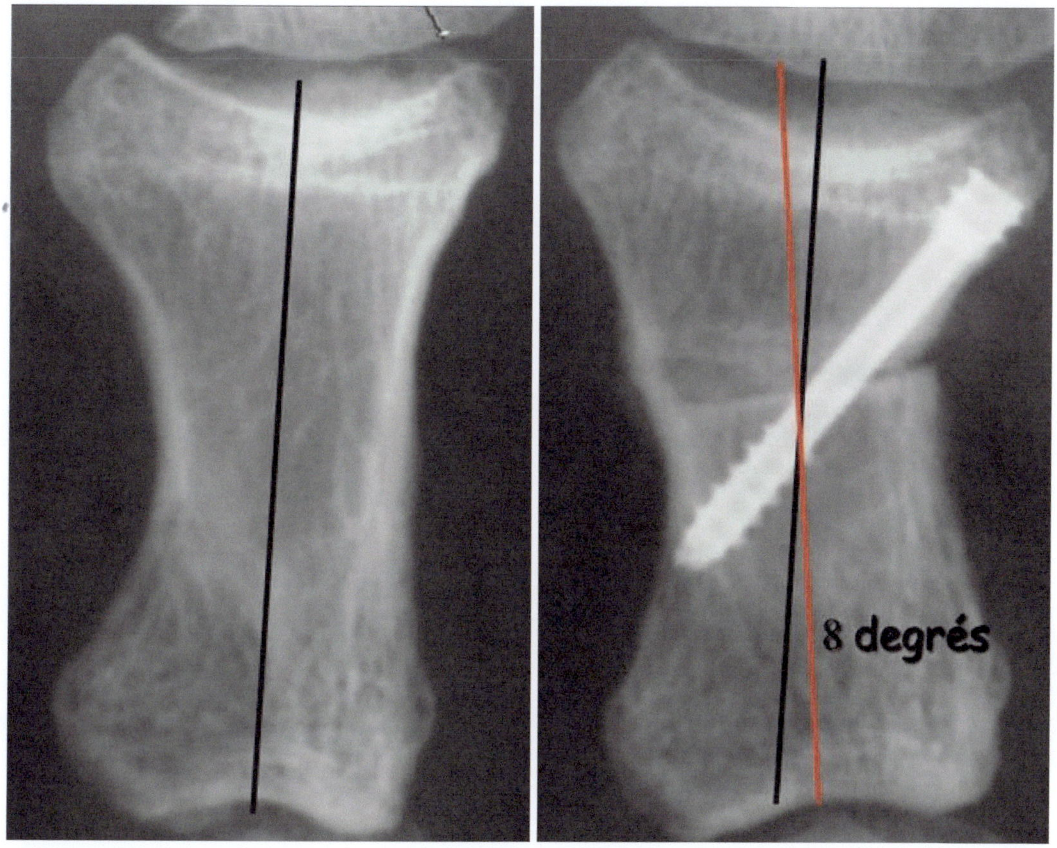

Fig. 20.13 Closing wedge and shortening osteotomy result in 8° varus.

(Fig. 20.13) and average shortening of 3 mm (maximum = 6 mm) at P1. No cases of nonunion have been reported.

Sensing Without Seeing

- Feeling that P1 changes shape during the forced varus movement. This may not occur if the hinge is still too thick (repeated burring will fatigue it) or the osteotomy was done too distally or in the diaphysis, which will often result in it breaking.
- Lack of cracking is evidence that the hinge is preserved.
- Persistence of correction without holding it during the push test, with direct visual confirmation that M1/P1 is straight.
- Discharge from bone marrow during the forced varus movement is evidence that high intramedullary pressure was induced during the maneuver.
- The elasticity of an 0.8-mm or 0.9-mm K-wire often leads to a false passage. This can be prevented by first inserting a stiffer 1.5-mm K-wire, which exits the phalanx laterally at its most distal portion, then replacing it with the flexible K-wire that will serve as a guide wire.
- Inserting the screw at slow drill speeds makes it easier to feel the resistance when the larger diameter thread is seated inside the bone, thereby confirming that it is positioned correctly.

Editors' Point of View

Percutaneous osteotomy of the hallux proximal phalanx produces the same corrections as open procedures with excellent stability provided by the lateral bone hinge and compression screw fixation.

Simultaneous Proximal and Distal Surgery of the First Ray: The Mechanical Principle of "Decoupling"

21

Yves Stiglitz and Cyrille Cazeau

21.1 Introduction

One of the options in the treatment of forefoot deformities has been described a long time ago by Lapidus with the tarsometatarsal (TMT) fusion of the first ray and a 1–2 intermetatarsal fusion. It was his way of treating hallux valgus at a time when few solutions were available and percutaneous surgery was not even an idea.

Nowadays surgical teams are in the trend to reduce the aggressivity of their numerous procedures defined in the meantime.

Proposing a percutaneous technique for TMT1 fusion has become possible, but it's accompanied with technical pitfalls and limitations of indications. This led us to define the new mechanical concept of "decoupling" in the simultaneous proximal and distal surgery of the first ray.

21.2 Pitfalls and Limitations of TMT1 Fusion

TMT1 fusion, also named modified-Lapidus fusion, is not as simple as a single joint fusion. In most cases the first ray deformity is complex, and surgery aims to have the disappearance of the "bunion" and the restauration of the biomechanics of the forefoot. Therefore a preoperative 3D planning is defined to address a first ray 3D reconstruction.

Many surgeons fear this procedure because it requires the completion of requisites related to both the first ray's correction and the fusion.

21.2.1 First Ray's Correction Requisites

Three main steps are under specific watch in the correction of a hallux valgus with a TMT1 fusion.

Lateral MTP1 joint release is considered mandatory by some authors in order to be able to mobilize the metatarsal and achieve the fusion in good position in the next steps. When performed in an open procedure, a separate lateral approach may be needed. If done percutaneously the perception of the sesamoïdometatarsal ligament's cutting is poor, which doesn't guarantee its complete section.

One of the main complications after TMT1 fusion is the positioning of the metatarsal in a sagittal plane. A metatarsal head elevation may happen in the case of an unprecise position when fixing the arthrodesis and/or when returning to weight-bearing where the forces are applied under the head.

Another usual complication is the excess of metatarsal shortening. Preparing the bone surfaces implies removing two layers of cartilage (on the metatarsal base and on the cuneiform)

Y. Stiglitz (✉) · C. Cazeau
Clinique Victor Hugo, Paris, France

C. Cazeau, Y. Stiglitz (eds.), *Percutaneous and Minimally Invasive Foot Surgery*,
https://doi.org/10.1007/978-3-030-98791-6_21

and two layers of subchondral bones (one on each side). Shortening reaches often 4 mm and sometimes more. In the case of a preoperative relative metatarsal length excess, shortening could be a part of the preop planning. However, in the case of a preoperative already short metatarsal, adding any amount of shortening is a concern, and some would consider it a contraindication in this procedure.

21.2.2 Fusion Requisites

The achievement of a fusion in orthopedics obeys to the same fundamentals for any joint.

Adjusting the bone surfaces to maximize their reciprocal contact is a key point. The TMT1 joint suffers from a highly variable anatomy in its geometry. Therefore, a precise preoperative planning is necessary, and the risk of shortening is high because of the significant amount of bone resection required.

When the surfaces are in a sufficient contact the fusion is enhanced by providing compression. The question of the hardware mount's mechanical strength is central because after any modern forefoot procedure compression, and resistance to immediate full weight-bearing is needed. Open procedures offer a wider choice for hardware selection (including plates) and positioning (medial, dorsal, plantar), whereas percutaneous surgeries are limited to the use of compressive screws (even if their design may slightly vary).

21.2.3 Contradictions of the Requisites

Whether needed by fusion or by first ray's correction, the requisites may be in conflict with each other. Removing an important amount of bone may be needed for a better fusion and correction but puts at risk of excessive shortening and elevating. Improving the hardware strength with a larger approach and bulkier plate is more aggressive but delays faster recovery. An extensive lateral MTP1 joint release is necessary to help mobilize the metatarsal thus correct the deformity but provides the fusion with more risk of secondary displacement.

Forefoot deformities correction and fusion appear to be opposites; however, they are to be achieved in the same procedure. This is the reason why we define here the new concept of "decoupling."

21.3 Mechanical Concept of "Decoupling"

Following several objectives is difficult and in several aspects contradictory for one reason: surgery is carried out in a single procedure in a single site.

The concept of decoupling consists of achieving exactly the same objectives, but with a procedure split in two sites in order to remove the contradictions.

There is no other way than to fuse proximally the TMT1 joint. Therefore, all the non-conflictual objectives are treated in the modified Lapidus procedure: cartilage resection, bone preparation, surfaces adjustment, compression, and if possible part of metatarsus varus correction. All these steps are easily achievable if they are considered as providing no distal consequences (e.g., shortening).

A distal metatarsal procedure is unavoidable to perform a lateral MTP1 release and one of the most often used to treat forefoot deformity (e.g., with a chevron osteotomy). It is then logical to do distally what's necessary and adjust the remaining correction after the fusion is complete (Fig. 21.1): lateral MTP1 release; metatarsus varus correction, for example, with a chevron; adjust metatarsal length; and even lengthen if the fusion produced too much shortening, lower the head to avoid or correct elevation.

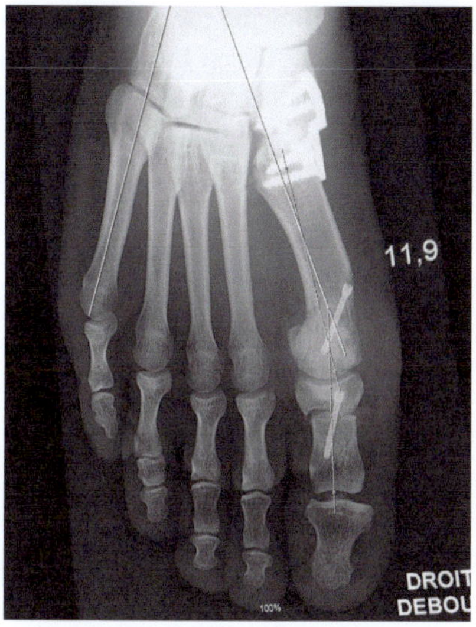

Fig. 21.1 MIS proximal and distal corrections for first ray reconstruction. Lapidus is achieved here with a plate which provides with a good contact and compression in the fusion site. The metatarsal angle is corrected, partially thanks to the Lapidus and partially thanks to the distal chevron. Shortening is prevented thanks to distal adjustment. © Yves Stiglitz 2015. All Rights Reserved

21.4 Application Thanks to MIS and PC

The concept of decoupling as defined above is a split of a highly difficult single-site procedure in two-site usual procedures. It implies a multiplication of the surgical aggressivity, approaches, and potential complications, which is barely admissible when considering standard open procedures.

Since the spreading of MIS (Fig. 21.2) and PC (Fig. 21.3) procedure, a two-site procedure has become much more acceptable. Not only are the wounds limited but the postoperative course has been improved for each separate procedure and adds another benefit to the decoupling.

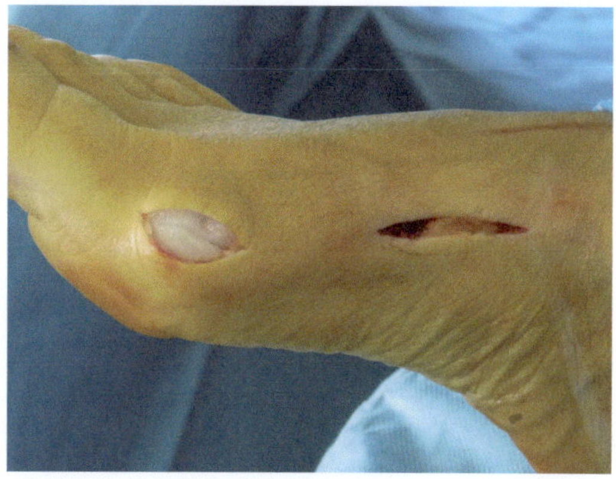

Fig. 21.2 Proximal and distal MIS approaches for simultaneous Lapidus and chevron. © Yves Stiglitz 2015. All Rights Reserved

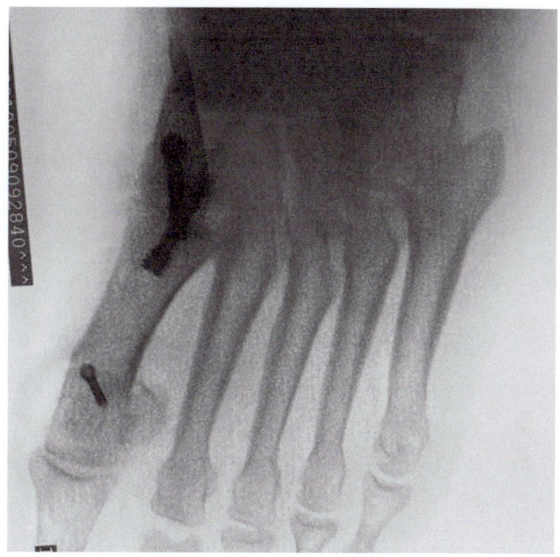

Fig. 21.3 Peroperative view of a percutaneous Lapidus and MIS chevron. Metatarsus varus reduction is appropriate and achieved both proximally and distally. Chevron adjustment prevents from excessive shortening. © Yves Stiglitz 2015. All Rights Reserved

21.5 Conclusion

Decoupling the correction of a first ray deformity consists in splitting a procedure and thus simplifying the surgery. It increases the chances of success on each site allowing the other site to adjust to the weaknesses induced by the first steps. It became possible thanks to MIS and PC surgery, which is part of the concept.

Role of the Lapidus Procedure for Treating Hallux Valgus

22

Patrice Determe

22.1 General Principles

Surgical treatment of hallux valgus aims to restore a patient's function and anatomy as close to normal as possible. The specifications of this surgery consist of recentering the joint, restoring good mechanics at the metatarsophalangeal and metatarsoseasmoid joints, reloading the first ray, redistributing the loads—especially the anterior ones—and rebalancing the soft tissue to ensure the correction lasts.

In the best-case scenario, this correction will achieve these specifications while providing the patient with the simplest and fastest functional recovery possible. Currently, the most widely used surgical techniques involve distal osteotomy of the first metatarsal (M1). These techniques simultaneously provide good-quality correction, good hold over time, and relatively quick functional recovery. But one wonders why we would perform a procedure that deforms a normal bone but does not impact the tarsometatarsal joint involved in the metatarsus varus, which is inexorably linked with hallux valgus.

Unfortunately, in such situations, these techniques are not enough to meet the objectives that were set out. In particular, there is considerable cuneometatarsal instability in these deformities.

In fact, in every case of hallux valgus, there is dual motion combining hallux valgus and metatarsus varus. The presence of metatarsus varus itself implies that the biomechanics of the cuneometatarsal joint are altered. In most cases, this likely developed because as the deformity worsened, the joint adapted to the new loads placed on it and remained stable. In certain cases, cuneometatarsal instability may be observed clinically. It manifests itself by hypermobility, altered distribution of the anterior loads, and a vicious circle where the hallux valgus becomes worse due to transverse pressure of the proximal phalanx (P1) base on the mobile M1 head.

Stabilizing the medial cuneometatarsal joint is one option for correcting and stabilizing the first ray in three-dimensions (Fig. 22.1). If one is unable to perform a completely stable capsule and ligament repair, tarsometatarsal arthrodesis can be proposed.

The intention of this article is not to specify the indications for the original Lapidus procedure (with additional arthrodesis of second ray) and the modified Lapidus described here, but instead to describe in detail the technical features that are essential to a successful tarsometatarsal arthrodesis.

P. Determe (✉)
Clinique Médipôle Garonne, Toulouse, France

C. Cazeau, Y. Stiglitz (eds.), *Percutaneous and Minimally Invasive Foot Surgery*,
https://doi.org/10.1007/978-3-030-98791-6_22

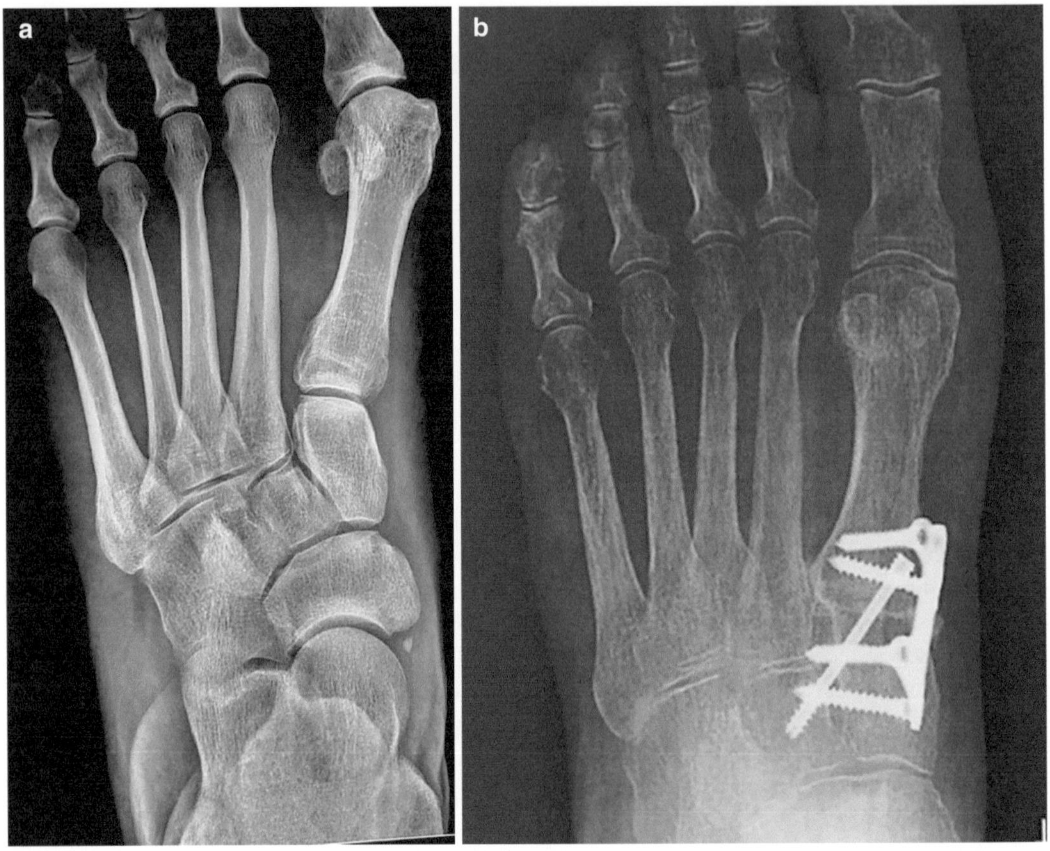

Fig. 22.1 (**a**) Preoperative appearance (**b**) Postoperative appearance after Lapidus.

22.2 Clinical Findings

It is often difficult to define boundaries beyond which one surgical technique should be used and another eliminated. The surgeon's skill and experience come into play when making these difficult choices. Setting an indication for a Lapidus procedure is a decision with serious consequences that is based on a range of arguments. The required postoperative immobilization and its social and professional impact must be evaluated and balanced with the risk of a poor outcome or recurrence from a different procedure that is easier for the patient to deal with.

The clinical findings form the basis of the surgical indication. It consists of direct and indirect signs. The benefit of imaging is relative: small deformities may be accompanied by incomplete weight bearing on the first ray, while major angular deviations may be completely stable. This poor reliability was confirmed in a 2014 anatomy study.

22.2.1 Direct Signs

The direct signs consist mainly of elements involved in the first ray's stability. This stability is evaluated in non-load-bearing conditions during clinical examination of the foot but also during weight-bearing.

- Vertical instability (Fig. 22.2): This is the best-know element and the easiest to evaluate. This examination is done without loading. The examiner stands at the patient's foot. The lateral metatarsals are held in the palm of one hand, while the M1 head is held between the thumb and index finger of the other hand and then mobilized vertically. One can then see first ray elevation.

- Horizontal instability (Fig. 22.3): This is a lesser-known element; it is evaluated by holding the lateral metatarsals in one hand while using the other hand to place axial pressure on the big toe. Reduction through transverse loading of the M1 head contributes to evaluating the instability. This examination is done without weight-bearing, like the vertical instability test.
- Overall instability: Asking the patient to alternately load and unload the foot can be very informative. When instability is present, the patient will feel the foot spreading out during loading. During weight-bearing, it is easy to see that the M1–M5 opening angle increases, even without quantifying it.

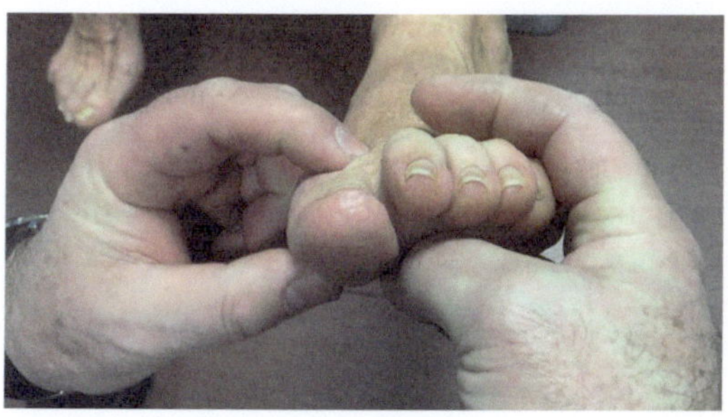

Fig. 22.2 Assessment of vertical stability. © Patrice Determe 2015. All Rights Reserved

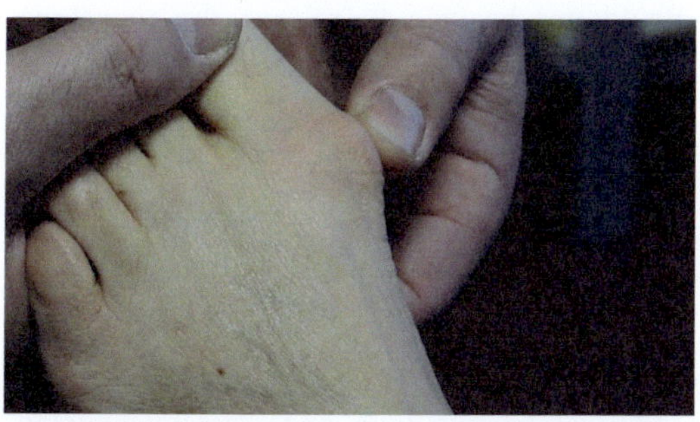

Fig. 22.3 Assessment of horizontal stability. © Patrice Determe 2015. All Rights Reserved

- Pain: While not disease-specific, pain or even thickening over the first cuneometatarsal joint is a sign of chronic damage in this joint.

22.2.2 Indirect Signs

The indirect signs consist of all the clinical evidence of insufficient loading of the first ray during weight-bearing. The main one is metatarsalgia. This overloading occurs in the context of cavus forefoot.

First off, the presence of mechanical pain with hyperkeratosis but without round forefoot is a sign of first ray instability (Fig. 22.4). This is a distinct possibility when it affects the second and third metatarsals, especially when pes cavus is not present.

If the lesser rays are overloaded, it may be due to cuneometatarsal instability; however, a diagnosis of posterior chain contracture is more likely (medial gastrocnemius stronger than lateral one). The latter possibility must be evaluated specifically.

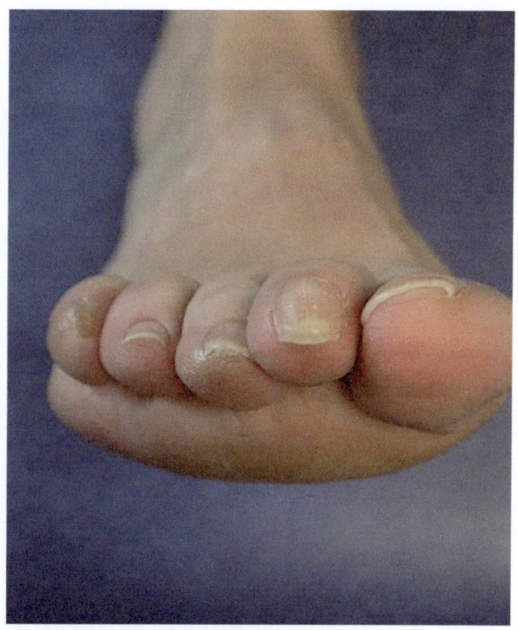

Fig. 22.4 Hyperkeratosis/round forefoot. © Patrice Determe 2015. All Rights Reserved

Another clue is that the bunion is more dorsal than usual. This specific finding is due to a dorsomedial impingement because the metatarsal head elevates during load; this is an indirect sign of instability.

On a different note, one must look for pes planovalgus. Collapse of the talus head into the open space between the navicular and the sustentaculum.

Tali in fact triggers rotational adaptation of the entire medial column and compensatory supination of the forefoot, which destabilizes the first cuneometatarsal joint. Ignoring the pes planovalgus during surgical hallux valgus treatment increases the risk of recurrence.

22.3 General Criteria

While the hallux valgus being treated surgically may occur in the context of cuneometatarsal instability, this does not mean the only option is tarsometatarsal arthrodesis. The treatment choice must be made in a broader context in which several parameters are considered. Along with the clinical examination, one must take into consideration the patient's profession, family situation, psychological context, and whether the deformity is unilateral or bilateral. Some patients prefer to take the (measured) risk of recurrence or inadequate correction rather than to undergo a procedure with serious functional repercussions. In fact, while stabilization techniques that use a plantar plate appear to allow immediate weight-bearing, the postoperative restrictions are more extensive than for a distal osteotomy, and it is difficult to entertain the possibility of bilateral correction.

22.4 Surgical Technique

22.4.1 Hospitalization

This surgery, like any foot surgery, can be done as an outpatient procedure. The prescriptions are given beforehand, and the patient can be discharged from the facility after standing up and undergoing lymphatic drainage, 2–3 h after exiting the operating suite.

22.4.2 Anesthesia

As with any forefoot surgery, the Lapidus procedure (or modified Lapidus) is now performed with regional anesthesia. This is carried out in the pre-anesthesia room. For this procedure, the saphenous nerve innervating the surgical incision area must be anesthetized, along with the sciatic nerve or its terminal branches innervating all the foot bones. Ultrasound is used to identify the nerves in question, which improves the reliability of this nerve block and makes it possible do very distal anesthesia that preserves the foot's motor control. Long-lasting local anesthesia (naropeine or levobupivacaine) is used to help with postoperative analgesia. Dexamethasone, which is used as an adjuvant for local anesthetics (intravenous or perineural), helps to extend their action beyond the first 24 h. Hence, the postoperative pain can be controlled fully by the paracematol-NSAID combination.

22.4.3 Patient Positioning

The patient is supine with his foot at the end of the table. A tourniquet is placed immediately above the malleoli. While this distal tourniquet position is well tolerated, one must be aware of a *tourniquet effect* upon inflation that induces claw toe deformity and alters the foot's appearance during simulated loading conditions. These temporary deformities are likely due to a tenodesis effect associated with tightening. One should not hesitate to release the tourniquet intraoperatively to avoid correcting a nonexisting claw toe deformity.

22.4.4 Surgical Procedure

22.4.4.1 Incisions

Our preferred strategy is to combine cuneometatarsal stabilization with wide metatarsophalangeal joint arthrolysis. Consequently, two incisions are needed (Fig. 22.5). The first, 15-mm-long incision is made at the junction of the plantar skin and dorsal skin over the M1 head; the second is more posterior and centered over the medial side

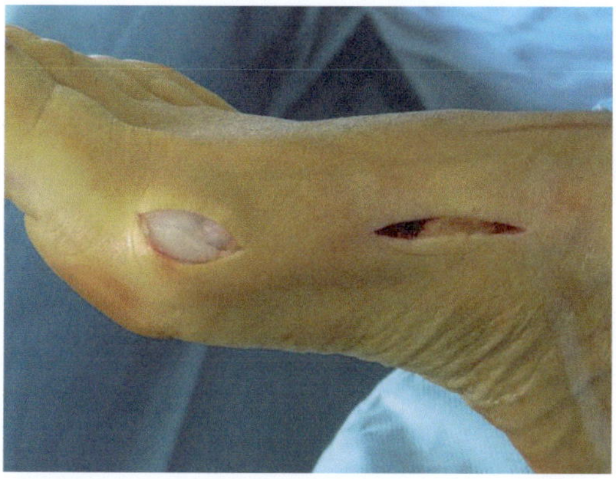

Fig. 22.5 Incisions. © Patrice Determe 2015. All Rights Reserved

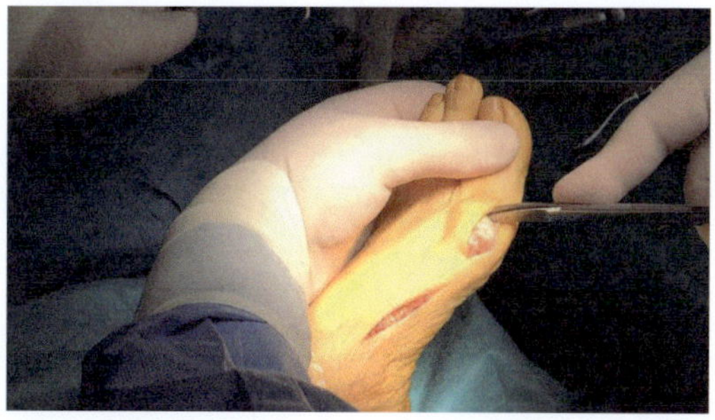

Fig. 22.6 Arthrolysis. © Patrice Determe 2015. All Rights Reserved

of the first cuneometatarsal joint. This second incision is slightly longer (30–40 mm). While using a plantar plate results in better stability, the drawback is that a larger approach is needed.

22.4.4.2 Metatarsophalangeal Arthrolysis

The standard arthrolysis approach is used. If needed, a skin and joint capsule wedge can be removed to improve visibility. The medial meniscus-like structure can be excised as needed. Next, arthrolysis is performed with the aim of moving the head, so it can be repositioned on the sesamoid band. This is especially useful in more severe cases because the sesamoid is sequestered in the first intermetatarsal space. In this scenario, the physical presence of the lateral sesamoid can prevent good reduction of the metatarsal. Thus, is it important to be able to move the joint freely by cutting the lateral metatarsal sesamoid ligament. This wide release can be done with scissors by passing inside the joint between the M1 head and the P1 base (Fig. 22.6).

22.4.4.3 Cuneometatarsal Approach

This approach is not particularly difficult (Fig. 22.7); however, one must be aware of the superficial venous network and especially a vertical vein that needs to be coagulated or ligated. The joint can then be entered. The expansions of the distal attachment of the tibialis anterior tendon must be reflected proximally. This exposes the cuneometatarsal joint, which appears damaged and has capsule dehiscence that can let inflammatory synovial fluid leak out.

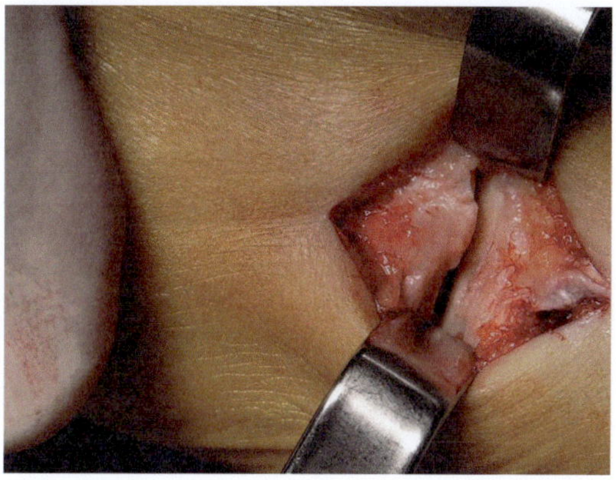

Fig. 22.7 Medial exposure of cuneometatarsal joint. © Patrice Determe 2015. All Rights Reserved

The dorsal and plantar aspects of the joint are then released to allow its mobilization. The plantar release is more difficult because of the insertion of the peroneus longus fibers, which reinforce the capsule at the lateral-plantar corner. An osteotome can be used to detach these fibers and allow the M1 base to be mobilized fully. If needed, a rongeur can be used to cut away bone at this corner.

22.4.4.4 Joint Preparation

- Metatarsal side: Once released, the joint can be mobilized. The M1 base is dislocated medially (Fig. 22.8). This procedure provides an excellent view of the cartilage, which will be removed sparingly and evenly over its entire surface. This resection is performed manually, typically with rongeur. Remember that the

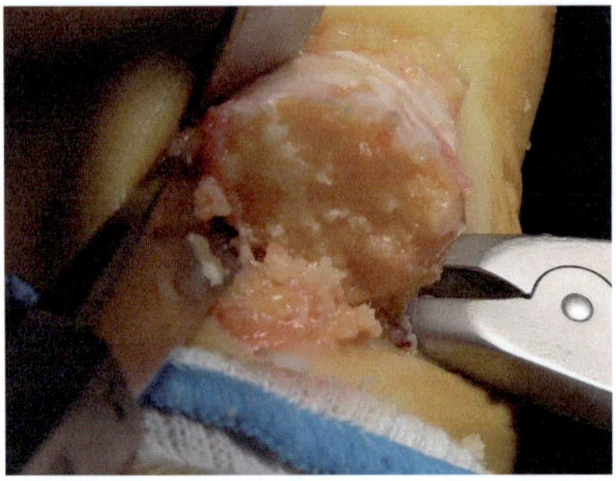

Fig. 22.8 Preparing the metatarsal base.

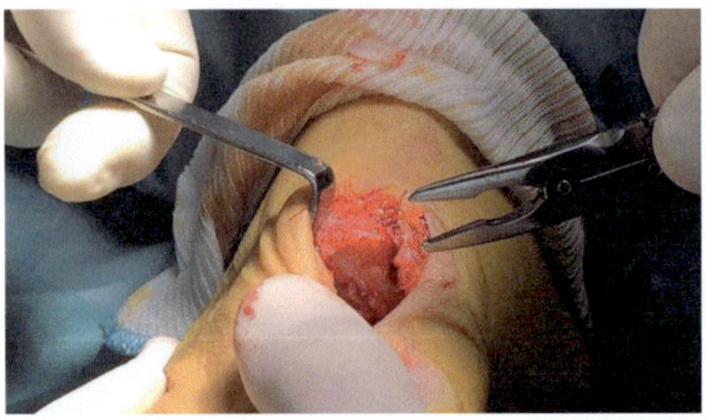

Fig. 22.9 Preparing the cuneiform base.

goal is stabilization and repositioning, not anatomical correction. Thus, there is no reason to cut away the lateral corner to induce valgus in the metatarsal. Holes can be made in the subchondral bone if necessary.
- Cuneiform side: The same process is used with a rongeur, with the same goal of removing a minimal amount of cartilage and trying not to remove more bone laterally. In order to ensure the exposure needed for good bone preparation, the metatarsal base can be tipped downward and held in this position by a Hohmann retractor (Fig. 22.9).

22.4.4.5 Reduction and Temporary Fixation

Once the joint has been prepared, the most difficult step—and the one that requires the nimblest of fingers—is the reduction step. The metatarsal must be positioned correctly in all three anatomical planes while simultaneously applying compression on the cuneometatarsal joint (Fig. 22.10). One trick is to hold the big toe firmly in one hand and to use it to position the metatarsal by applying axial pressure. This accomplishes two goals:

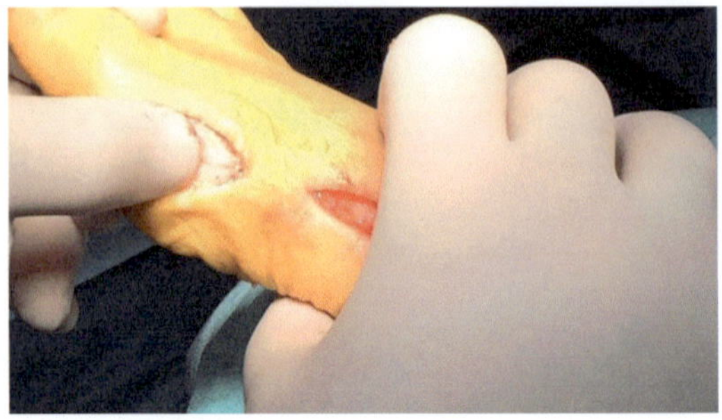

Fig. 22.10 Reduction maneuver.

- Compresses the arthrodesis site
- Stabilizes the metatarsal head in the chosen position to allow temporary fixation.

This temporary fixation is done with a 1.5-mm K-wire inserted transversely between the M1 and M2 heads (Fig. 22.11).

Now, the angle correction, toe position, and metatarsal head height can be checked. It is important to restore the arch without overloading the joint due to excessive lowering. Contact at the arthrodesis site and the overall position of the metatarsal are confirmed. All these checks are done with simulated loading.

22.4.4.6 Fixation

The arthrodesis will be fixed using the surgeon's preferred method. We prefer to start by inserting a 3-mm compression screw, positioned in a retrograde manner between the first metatarsal and the second cuneiform (Fig. 22.12). This screw stabilizes the correction and ensures the arthrodesis site is compressed. It is wise at this stage to apply simulated loading to confirm the desired correction is maintained.

The next step is to position the locking plate (Fig. 22.13) in a neutral position on either side of the joint line. In our experience, the plate ends up medial, although several authors position it dor-

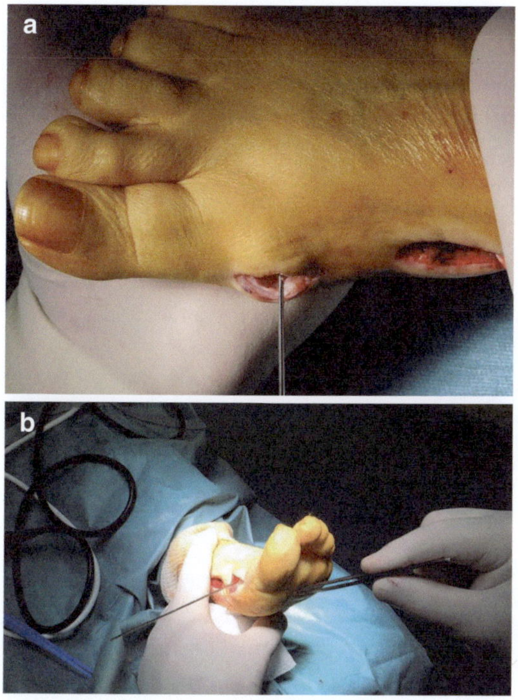

Fig. 22.11 Temporary fixation with M1 to M2 K-wire (**a**) Verification that anterior arch is restored (**b**).

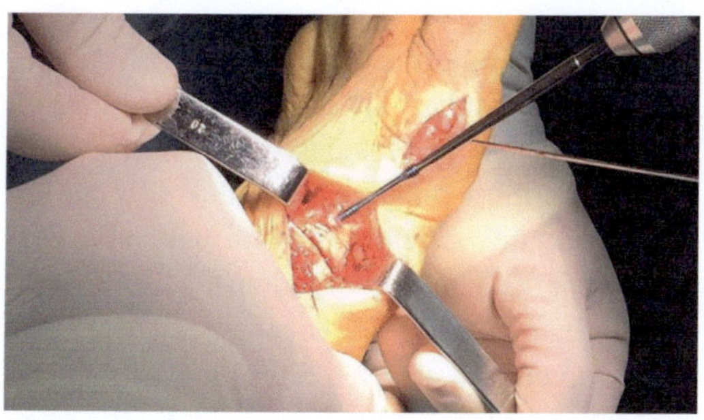

Fig. 22.12 Insertion of oblique screw through M1/C2.

sally, which may require shifting the incision upward. However, this position may reduce tolerance and compromise stability. Several recent studies have featured plantar plates, which are harder to set in place, but cause less discomfort and are more stable biomechanically.

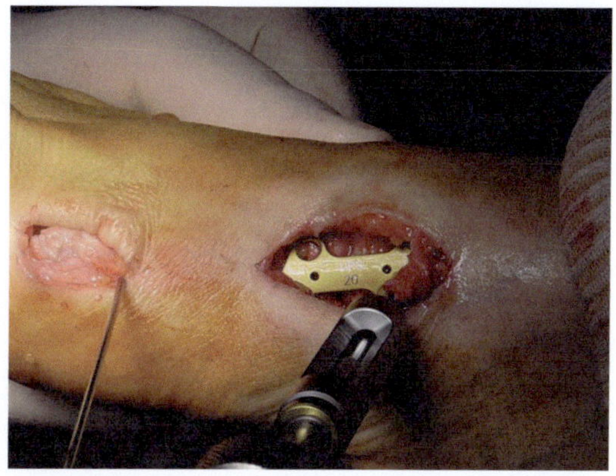

Fig. 22.13 Fixation of locking plate.

22.4.5 Additional Procedures

22.4.5.1 Distal Osteotomy

It is sometimes difficult or even impossible to correct the deformity fully, especially in a surgeon's early cases. In this scenario, it may be useful to add a distal osteotomy. This osteotomy (most often a modified chevron) aims to put the finishing touches on the correction, either by translating the head or by de-rotating it, especially in severe congenital cases. The surgical approach is the same one used for the arthrolysis; standard screw fixation is used.

22.4.5.2 Akin Osteotomy

Correcting the hallux valgus and stabilizing the first cuneometatarsal joint does not depend on if a crossover toe deformity is present. If this is the case—and mainly to limit the recurrence risk by refocusing the work of the musculotendinous structures—an Akin phalangeal osteotomy can be performed. The main goal is to induce varus at the distal end of P1, although this osteotomy can also be used to make up for insufficient axial correction by modifying the toe's pronation/supination. The fixation methods are based on the surgeon's preferences, but typically involves axial screw fixation.

22.4.5.3 Lengthening of Extensor Mechanism

In instances of severe deformity, there is often a certain amount of extensor mechanism contracture, which pulls the toe into valgus and extension. This tension actively contributes to making the deformity worse. No matter which surgical technique is used, if this excess tension is not addressed, these lateral and dorsal forces can prevent the deformity from being corrected. Moreover, they contribute to imbalances that greatly increase the risk of recurrence.

When a Lapidus procedure is done, the low fixation position on the metatarsal generates a tenodesis effect that increases tension on the extensors. Adding a tendon-lengthening procedure to the bone correction may be useful, if only to prevent stiffening in plantar flexion of the first metatarsophalangeal joint.

22.4.5.4 Second Toe Shortening

While the goal is to trim away the least amount of cartilage, this procedure is innately shortening.

If the patient has a Greek foot shape, this shortening may cause discomfort and specifically irritate the second toe when wearing shoes. If justified by the foot's preoperative shape, one can propose a simultaneous toe-shortening procedure. When claw toe is not present, this shortening is done within P1, either percutaneously or open, using an implantable material such as TOEGRIP® 0°. When claw toe deformity is present, one can use the claw's flattening to achieve as much of the shortening as possible.

22.4.6 Checks, Closure, and Dressings

As with every forefoot surgery, it is important to regularly perform simulated loading to ensure the toes, and especially the first ray, are in the correct position. Taking regular intraoperative fluoroscopy views is also essential, especially in a surgeon's early cases.

Closure is done in the standard manner, in several layers with a running intradermal absorbable suture. A drain is not necessary.

The dressing applied in the operating room can be left in place for 1–2 weeks. If needed, it will subsequently be replaced by a nurse with a simple dressing.

22.5 Postoperative Course

The seriousness of the postoperative course is one of the main reasons the indications for this surgical technique are limited.

Since the tarsometatarsal arthrodesis in the vertical plane is subjected to shear forces during weight-bearing, it is especially vulnerable to loading. Thus, it is advisable to prohibit weight-bearing during the first weeks, at least until bone union is achieved. The recent use of low-profile locking plates means that we can consider allowing loading, especially since these plates are positioned on the plantar side. But the return to weight-bearing is a surgical decision; the unloading period can range from 0–6 weeks depending on the surgeon's preferences. During the unloading period, antithrombotic prophylaxis should be prescribed and the ankle immobilized at 90° most of the time to prevent stiffening in Equinus.

It is obvious that this unloading period has a high social and professional cost; even though around the third month postoperative, there are practically no differences with patients who underwent distal osteotomy. Conversely, bilateral surgery cannot be proposed; one should wait at least 3 months between performing surgery on the first and second foot. This is likely the most onerous scenario.

During the postoperative phase, like in every forefoot surgery, steps must be taken to control edema. The forefoot must be elevated, and the foot iced regularly. Rehabilitation must be gentle and not cause trauma. While we do not recommend toe mobilization, it important for the patient to undergo daily lymphatic drainage massage.

Lastly, adjuvant treatments can be implemented, depending on the surgeon's preferences (homeopathy, vitamin C, etc.).

22.6 Conclusion

While the Lapidus procedure has been extensively documented in the literature and it is frequently used in several countries to the point that it makes up 30% of hallux valgus surgery procedures, it remains a fringe procedure in France. Several surgeons prefer to push the boundaries of the indications for distal osteotomy or to perform metatarsophalangeal arthrodesis instead of giving the first cuneometatarsal joint the stability it is missing.

This is without doubt a difficult procedure, with a restrictive postoperative course, but it is essential to master it as should be proposed in very specific clinical situations.

Thus, beyond pes planovalgus, one must look for and evaluate cuneometatarsal instability, either by observing abnormal mobility or by finding indirect signs such as overloading of the lateral rays due to an inadequate first ray.

Other than the fact that a surgery targeted at the first cuneometatarsal joint is best suited to get at the source of the deformity, it allows a surgeon to treat several ailments through a single procedure, and in particular, to avoid doing lateral ray osteotomies that are often not well tolerated by patients.

Editors' Point of View

This excellent technique is most widely used in German- and English-speaking countries. It can be done either with MIS or percutaneously. The direction of forces, related to the location of the C1/M1 joint at the top of the longitudinal arch, provides a geometric fit between bones upon weight-bearing, which can be immediate.

Appendix (Dr. Cyrille Cazeau)

The intention of this chapter is not to describe the technique and indications for the original Lapidus procedure (Fig. 22.14), which supplements the

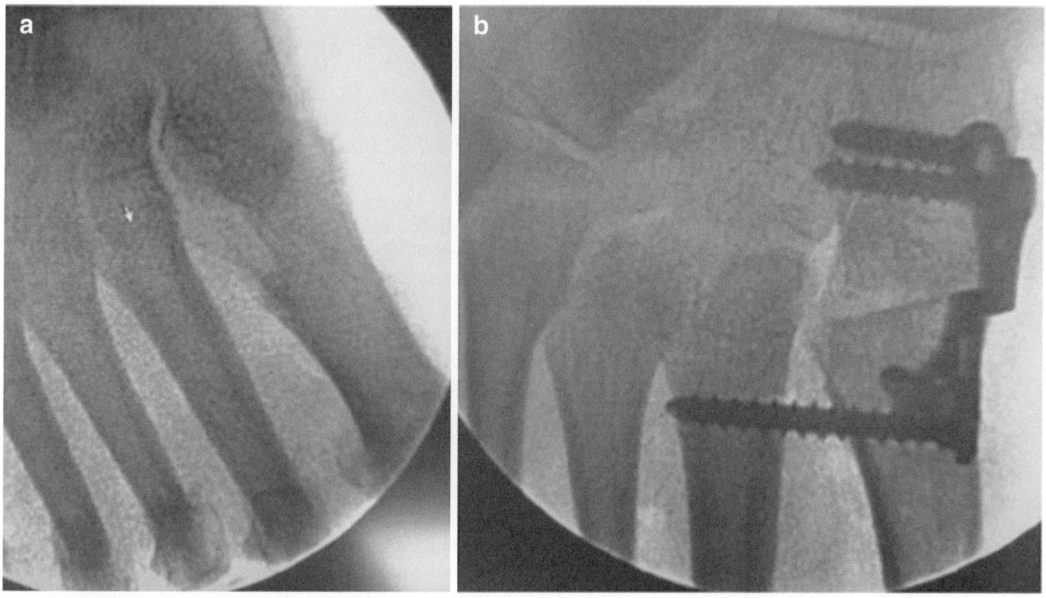

Fig. 22.14 Original Lapidus: arthrodesis of C1/M1 and R1/R2 (M1/M2, C1/C2, M1/C2) (**a**, **b**).

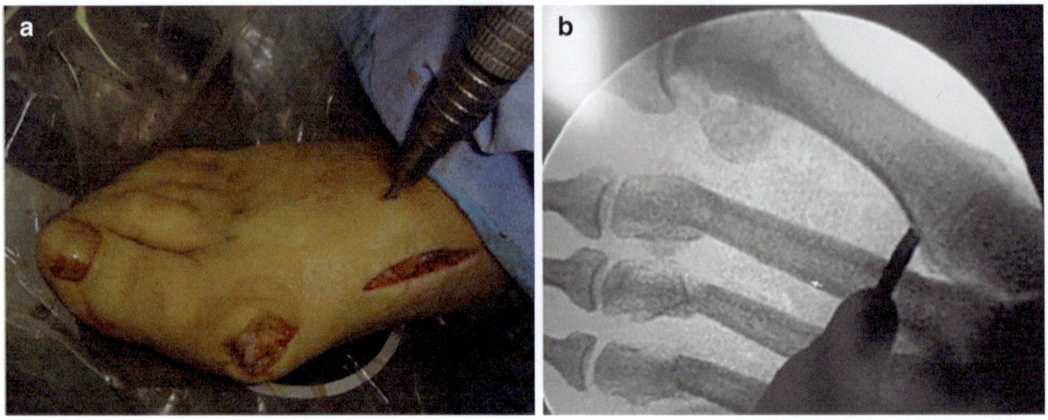

Fig. 22.15 Percutaneous decortication of M1/M2. Intraoperative (**a**) and fluoroscopy (**b**) views.

first tarsometatarsal arthrodesis with fixation of the first and second ray. The decortication between M1 and M2, C1 and C2, and M1 and C2 can be performed percutaneously, thus supplementing the technique described in this chapter (Fig. 22.15).

Suggested Reading

Angthong C, Kanitnate S, Angthong W. Hallux valgus correction using a mini TighTrope device: a report of the short-term outcomes in 3 feet. J Med Assoc Thail. 2011;94(Suppl 7):S66–72.

Avino A, et al. The effect of the Lapidus arthrodesis on the medial longitudinal arch: a radiographic review. J Foot Ankle Surg. 2008;47(6):510–4.

Bacardi BE, Boysen TJ. Considerations for the Lapidus operation. J Foot Surg. 1986;25(2):133–8.

Baravarian B, Ben-Ad R. Contemporary approaches and advancements to the Lapidus procedure. Clin Podiatr Med Surg. 2014;31(2):299–308.

Baravarian B, Briskin GB, Burns P. Lapidus bunionectomy: arthrodesis of the first metatarsocuneiform joint. Clin Podiatr Med Surg. 2004;21(1):97–111. vi

Basile P, Cook EA, Cook JJ. Immediate weight bearing following modified Lapidus arthrodesis. J Foot Ankle Surg. 2010;49(5):459–64.

Bednarz PA, Manoli A 2nd. Modified Lapidus procedure for the treatment of hypermobile hallux valgus. Foot Ankle Int. 2000;21(10):816–21.

Bierman RA, Christensen JC, Johnson CH. Biomechanics of the first ray. Part III. Consequences of Lapidus arthrodesis on peroneus longus function: a three-dimensional kinematic analysis in a cadaver model. J Foot Ankle Surg. 2001;40(3):125–31.

Blitz NM. The versatility of the Lapidus arthrodesis. Clin Podiatr Med Surg. 2009;26(3):427–41. Table of Contents

Blitz NM. Early weightbearing of the Lapidus bunionectomy: is it feasible? Clin Podiatr Med Surg. 2012;29(3):367–81.

Blitz NM, et al. Early weight bearing after modified Lapidus arthrodesis: a multicenter review of 80 cases. J Foot Ankle Surg. 2010;49(4):357–62.

Butson AR. A modification of the Lapidus operation for hallux valgus. J Bone Joint Surg (Br). 1980;62(3):350–2.

Catanzariti AR, et al. The modified Lapidus arthrodesis: a retrospective analysis. J Foot Ankle Surg. 1999;38(5):322–32.

Chang TJ, Ruch JA. Lapidus arthrodesis. A different perspective. J Am Podiatr Med Assoc. 1994;84(6):281–8.

Clark HR, Veith RG, Hansen ST Jr. Adolescent bunions treated by the modified Lapidus procedure. Bull Hosp Jt Dis Orthop Inst. 1987;47(2):109–22.

Coetzee JC, et al. The Lapidus procedure as salvage after failed surgical treatment of hallux valgus: a prospective cohort study. J Bone Joint Surg Am. 2003;85-A(1):60–5.

Coetzee JC, et al. The Lapidus procedure as salvage after failed surgical treatment of hallux valgus. Surgical technique. J Bone Joint Surg Am. 2004;86-A(Suppl 1):30–6.

Coetzee JC, Wickum D. The Lapidus procedure: a prospective cohort outcome study. Foot Ankle Int. 2004;25(8):526–31.

Cottom JM. Fixation of the Lapidus arthrodesis with a plantar interfragmentary screw and medial low profile locking plate. J Foot Ankle Surg. 2012;51(4):517–22.

Cottom JM, Rigby RB. Biomechanical comparison of a locking plate with intraplate compression screw versus locking plate with plantar interfragmentary screw for Lapidus arthrodesis: a cadaveric study. J Foot Ankle Surg. 2013;52(3):339–42.

Cottom JM, Vora AM. Fixation of Lapidus arthrodesis with a plantar interfragmentary screw and medial locking plate: a report of 88 cases. J Foot Ankle Surg. 2013;52(4):465–9.

Dayton P, et al. Relationship of frontal plane rotation of first metatarsal to proximal articular set angle and hallux alignment in patients undergoing tarsometatarsal arthrodesis for hallux abducto valgus: a case series and critical review of the literature. J Foot Ankle Surg. 2013;52(3):348–54.

Dayton P, Kauwe M, Feilmeier M. Is our current paradigm for evaluation and management of the bunion deformity flawed? A discussion of procedure philosophy relative to anatomy. J Foot Ankle Surg. 2015;54(1):102–11.

Dayton P, et al. Observed changes in first metatarsal and medial cuneiform positions after first metatarsophalangeal joint arthrodesis. J Foot Ankle Surg. 2014;53(1):32–5.

Desmet M, et al. I.V. and perineural dexamethasone are equivalent in increasing the analgesic duration of a single-shot interscalene block with ropivacaine for shoulder surgery: a prospective, randomized, placebo-controlled study. Br J Anaesth. 2013;111(3):445–52.

Didomenico LA, et al. Correction of frontal plane rotation of sesamoid apparatus during the Lapidus procedure: a novel approach. J Foot Ankle Surg. 2014;53(2):248–51.

Dietze A, et al. First ray instability in hallux valgus deformity: a radiokinematic and pedobarographic analysis. Foot Ankle Int. 2013;34(1):124–30.

Doty JF, Coughlin MJ. Hallux valgus and hypermobility of the first ray: facts and fiction. Int Orthop. 2013;37(9):1655–60.

Doty JF, et al. First metatarsocuneiform joint mobility: radiographic, anatomic, and clinical characteristics of the articular surface. Foot Ankle Int. 2014;35(5):504–11.

Ellington JK, et al. The use of the Lapidus procedure for recurrent hallux valgus. Foot Ankle Int. 2011;32(7):674–80.

Espinosa N, Wirth SH. Tarsometatarsal arthrodesis for management of unstable first ray and failed bunion surgery. Foot Ankle Clin. 2011;16(1):21–34.

Faber FW, et al. Mobility of the first tarsometatarsal joint in hallux valgus patients: a radiographic analysis. Foot Ankle Int. 2001a;22(12):965–9.

Faber FW, Mulder PG, Verhaar JA. Role of first ray hypermobility in the outcome of the Hohmann and the Lapidus procedure. A prospective, randomized trial involving one hundred and one feet. J Bone Joint Surg Am. 2004;86-A(3):486–95.

Faber FW, van Kampen PM, Bloembergen MW. Long-term results of the Hohmann and Lapidus procedure for the correction of hallux valgus: a prospective, randomised trial with eight to 11-year follow-up involving 101 feet. Bone Joint J. 2013;95-B(9):1222–6.

Faber FW, et al. Quantification of first tarsometatarsal joint stiffness in hallux valgus patients. Clin Biomech. 2001b;16(8):714–6.

Fleming JJ, et al. Intraoperative evaluation of medial intercuneiform instability after Lapidus arthrodesis: intercuneiform hook test. J Foot Ankle Surg. 2015;54(3):464–72.

Fleming L, et al. Results of modified Lapidus arthrodesis procedure using medial eminence as an interpositional autograft. J Foot Ankle Surg. 2011;50(3):272–5.

Frankel JP, Larsen DC. The misuse of the Lapidus procedure: re-evaluation of the preoperative criteria. J Foot Ankle Surg. 1996;35(4):355–61. discussion 371–2

Galli MM, et al. Enhanced Lapidus arthrodesis: crossed screw technique with middle cuneiform fixation further reduces sagittal mobility. J Foot Ankle Surg. 2015;54(3):437–40.

Galli MM, Protzman NM, Brigido SA. Arthrodiastasis of the lateral column with medial fusion: a retrospective examination of medial double and Lapidus arthrodeses. J Foot Ankle Surg. 2015;54(3):412–6.

Grace D, et al. Modified Lapidus arthrodesis for adolescent hallux abducto valgus. J Foot Ankle Surg. 1999;38(1):8–13.

Gutteck N, et al. Comparative study of Lapidus bunionectomy using different osteosynthesis methods. Foot Ankle Surg. 2013;19(4):218–21.

Haas Z, et al. Maintenance of correction of first metatarsal closing base wedge osteotomies versus modified Lapidus arthrodesis for moderate to severe hallux valgus deformity. J Foot Ankle Surg. 2007;46(5):358–65.

Habbu R, et al. Operative correction of arch collapse with forefoot deformity: a retrospective analysis of outcomes. Foot Ankle Int. 2011;32(8):764–73.

Hamilton GA, et al. Revision Lapidus arthrodesis: rate of union in 17 cases. J Foot Ankle Surg. 2007;46(6):447–50.

Hansen ST Jr. Hallux valgus surgery. Morton and Lapidus were right! Clin Podiatr Med Surg. 1996;13(3):347–54.

Hernandez A, Hernandez PA, Hernandez WA. Lapidus: when and why? Clin Podiatr Med Surg. 1989;6(1):197–208.

Hofbauer MH, Grossman JP. The Lapidus procedure. Clin Podiatr Med Surg. 1996;13(3):485–96.

Johnson KA, Kile TA. Hallux valgus due to cuneiform-metatarsal instability. J South Orthop Assoc. 1994;3(4):273–82.

Kazzaz S, Singh D. Postoperative cast necessity after a Lapidus arthrodesis. Foot Ankle Int. 2009;30(8):746–51.

King CM, Hamilton GA, Ford LA. Effects of the Lapidus arthrodesis and chevron bunionectomy on plantar forefoot pressures. J Foot Ankle Surg. 2014;53(4):415–9.

King CM, et al. Modified Lapidus arthrodesis with crossed screw fixation: early weightbearing in 136 patients. J Foot Ankle Surg. 2015;54(1):69–75.

Klaue K. Hallux valgus and hypermobility of the first ray-causal treatment using Tarso-metatarsal reorientation arthrodesis. Ther Umsch. 1991;48(12):817–23.

Klaue K, Hansen ST, Masquelet AC. Clinical, quantitative assessment of first tarsometatarsal mobility in the sagittal plane and its relation to hallux valgus deformity. Foot Ankle Int. 1994;15(1):9–13.

Klos K, et al. Stability of medial locking plate and compression screw versus two crossed screws for Lapidus arthrodesis. Foot Ankle Int. 2010;31(2):158–63.
Klos K, Simons P. Lapidus arthrodesis plus osteochondral autograft transplantation in the management of hallux rigidus with an elevated first ray. Foot Ankle Spec. 2014;7(2):135–9.
Klos K, et al. Plantar versus dorsomedial locked plating for Lapidus arthrodesis: a biomechanical comparison. Foot Ankle Int. 2011;32(11):1081–5.
Klos K, et al. Modified Lapidus arthrodesis with plantar plate and compression screw for treatment of hallux valgus with hypermobility of the first ray: a preliminary report. Foot Ankle Surg. 2013;19(4):239–44.
Kopp FJ, et al. The modified Lapidus procedure for hallux valgus: a clinical and radiographic analysis. Foot Ankle Int. 2005;26(11):913–7.
Lagaay PM, et al. Rates of revision surgery using Chevron-Austin osteotomy, Lapidus arthrodesis, and closing base wedge osteotomy for correction of hallux valgus deformity. J Foot Ankle Surg. 2008;47(4):267–72.
Lamm BM, Wynes J. Immediate weightbearing after Lapidus arthrodesis with external fixation. J Foot Ankle Surg. 2014;53(5):577–83.
Lapidus PW. The author's bunion operation from 1931 to 1959. Clin Orthop. 1960;16:119–35.
Lopez AM, et al. Ultrasound-guided ankle block for forefoot surgery: the contribution of the saphenous nerve. Reg Anesth Pain Med. 2012;37(5):554–7.
Lui TH. Symptomatic first metatarsocuneiform nonunion revised by arthroscopic Lapidus arthrodesis. J Foot Ankle Surg. 2012;51(5):656–9.
Lui TH, et al. Arthroscopy-assisted correction of hallux valgus deformity. Arthroscopy. 2008;24(8):875–80.
Lui TH, Chan KB, Ng S. Arthroscopic Lapidus arthrodesis. Arthroscopy. 2005;21(12):1516.
Magin MN. Full weight-bearing after Lapidus arthrodesis in hallux valgus deformity using the IVP plate fixation (V-TEK((R)) system). Oper Orthop Traumatol. 2014;26(2):184–95.
Mallette JP, Glenn CL, Glod DJ. The incidence of nonunion after Lapidus arthrodesis using staple fixation. J Foot Ankle Surg. 2014;53(3):303–6.
Mcinnes BD, Bouche RT. Critical evaluation of the modified Lapidus procedure. J Foot Ankle Surg. 2001;40(2):71–90.
Menke CR, McGlamry MC, Camasta CA. Lapidus arthrodesis with a single lag screw and a locking H-plate. J Foot Ankle Surg. 2011;50(4):377–82.
Michels F, et al. The arthroscopic Lapidus procedure. Foot Ankle Surg. 2011;17(1):25–8.
Mote GA, Yarmel D, Treaster A. First metatarsal-cuneiform arthrodesis for the treatment of first ray pathology: a technical guide. J Foot Ankle Surg. 2009;48(5):593–601.
Myerson MS, Badekas A. Hypermobility of the first ray. Foot Ankle Clin. 2000;5(3):469–84.
Neylon TA, Johnson BA, Laroche RA. Use of the Lapidus bunionectomy in first ray insufficiency. Clin Podiatr Med Surg. 2001;18(2):365–75.
Patel S, et al. Modified lapidus arthrodesis: rate of nonunion in 227 cases. J Foot Ankle Surg. 2004;43(1):37–42.
Paulick TA, et al. A retrospective study of two Lapidus groups, each with a different method of rail application. J Foot Ankle Surg. 2015;54(3):323–5.
Pinney SJ, Song KR, Chou LB. Surgical treatment of severe hallux valgus: the state of practice among academic foot and ankle surgeons. Foot Ankle Int. 2006;27(12):1024–9.
Popelka S, et al. Hypermobility of the first metatarsal bone in patients with rheumatoid arthritis treated by Lapidus procedure. BMC Musculoskelet Disord. 2012;13:148.
Popelka S, et al. Our results of the Lapidus procedure in patients with hallux valgus deformity. Acta Chir Orthop Traumatol Cechoslov. 2008a;75(4):271–6.
Popelka S, et al. Lapidus procedure in patients with rheumatoid arthritis-short-term results. Z Orthop Unfall. 2008b;146(1):80–5.
Redborg KE, et al. Ultrasound improves the success rate of a tibial nerve block at the ankle. Reg Anesth Pain Med. 2009;34(3):256–60.
Rink-Brune O. Lapidus arthrodesis for management of hallux valgus–a retrospective review of 106 cases. J Foot Ankle Surg. 2004;43(5):290–5.
Sangeorzan BJ, Hansen ST Jr. Modified Lapidus procedure for hallux valgus. Foot Ankle. 1989;9(6):262–6.
Saxena A, Nguyen A, Nelsen E. Lapidus bunionectomy: early evaluation of crossed lag screws versus locking plate with plantar lag screw. J Foot Ankle Surg. 2009;48(2):170–9.
Schmid T, Krause F. The modified Lapidus fusion. Foot Ankle Clin. 2014;19(2):223–33.
Shi K, et al. Surgical treatment of hallux valgus deformity in rheumatoid arthritis: clinical and radiographic evaluation of modified Lapidus technique. J Foot Ankle Surg. 2000;39(6):376–82.
Shinabarger AB, et al. Isolated first metatarsocuneiform joint fusion for correction of metatarsus primus varus deformity and literature review. J Foot Ankle Surg. 2014;53(5):624–7.
Simons P, et al. First Tarsometatarsal arthrodesis: an anatomic evaluation of dorsomedial versus plantar plating. J Foot Ankle Surg. 2015;54(5):787–92.
Sorensen MD, Hyer CF, Berlet GC. Results of Lapidus arthrodesis and locked plating with early weight bearing. Foot Ankle Spec. 2009;2(5):227–33.
Taylor NG, Metcalfe SA. A review of surgical outcomes of the Lapidus procedure for treatment of hallux abductovalgus and degenerative joint disease of the first MCJ. Foot (Edinb). 2008;18(4):206–10.
Thompson IM, Bohay DR, Anderson JG. Fusion rate of first tarsometatarsal arthrodesis in the modified Lapidus procedure and flatfoot reconstruction. Foot Ankle Int. 2005;26(9):698–703.
Treadwell JR. Rail external fixation for stabilization of closing base wedge osteotomies and Lapidus procedures: a retrospective analysis of sixteen cases. J Foot Ankle Surg. 2005;44(6):429–36.

Trnka HJ, Hofstatter S. The modified Lapidus arthrodesis. Orthopade. 2005;34(8):735–41.
Vieira PA, et al. Dexamethasone with bupivacaine increases duration of analgesia in ultrasound-guided interscalene brachial plexus blockade. Eur J Anaesthesiol. 2010;27(3):285–8.
Wang JC, Riley BM. A new fixation technique for the Lapidus bunionectomy. J Am Podiatr Med Assoc. 2005;95(4):405–9.
Willegger M, et al. Correction power and complications of first tarsometatarsal joint arthrodesis for hallux valgus deformity. Int Orthop. 2015;39(3):467–76.
Wu DY. Salvaging of a failed Lapidus procedure by the soft tissue osteodesis procedure: a six-year follow-up case report. Foot (Edinb). 2015;
Young NJ, Zelen CM. New techniques and alternative fixation for the Lapidus arthrodesis. Clin Podiatr Med Surg. 2013;30(3):423–34.

23 Percutaneous Arthrodesis of the First Tarsometatarsal Joint

Julien Laborde and Joël Vernois

23.1 Introduction

In patients with substantial first ray deformity and large metatarsus varus, a more proximal procedure may be necessary at the first metatarsal (M1). Tarsometatarsal arthrodesis or the Lapidus procedure is an excellent corrective procedure in patients who have a hypermobile first tarsometatarsal joint or who have poor quality bone (>60 years of age) that may compromise the fixation of a basal osteotomy.

Tarsometatarsal arthrodesis provides at least 10° correction of the M1–M2 angle. As with a basal osteotomy, there is a risk of increasing the lateral orientation angle of the distal M1 articular surface (DMAA). This procedure may need to be supplemented with M1 distal osteotomy. Note that the shortening inherent to this technique is balanced by M1 lowering during the arthrodesis, or even the distal osteotomy, since realignment of the first ray contributes to reloading.

23.2 Surgical Technique

23.2.1 Lateral Release

The first step is lateral release of the first metatarsophalangeal joint. Given the large deformity, this release must be extensive. It is done using a Beaver blade under fluoroscopy control and often involves all the lateral layers.

23.2.2 Arthrodesis Groundwork

For the results to be reproducible, the bone cuts must follow a guide. This is accomplished by inserting two 1.2-mm diameter K-wires vertically in the dorsoplantar direction under fluoroscopy control (Fig. 23.1).

The first K-wire goes into the first cuneiform and must be set parallel to and 2 mm behind the joint line to capture all the cartilage and end up in the cancellous bone. The second K-wire (also dorsoplantar) goes into the M1 base and will define the plantar corner to be removed by the bone cut (Fig. 23.2) and will induce M1 lowering.

J. Laborde (✉)
Clinique de l'Union, Saint-Jean, France

J. Vernois
Sussex Orthopaedic NHS Treatment Centre,
Haywards Heath, UK

C. Cazeau, Y. Stiglitz (eds.), *Percutaneous and Minimally Invasive Foot Surgery*,
https://doi.org/10.1007/978-3-030-98791-6_23

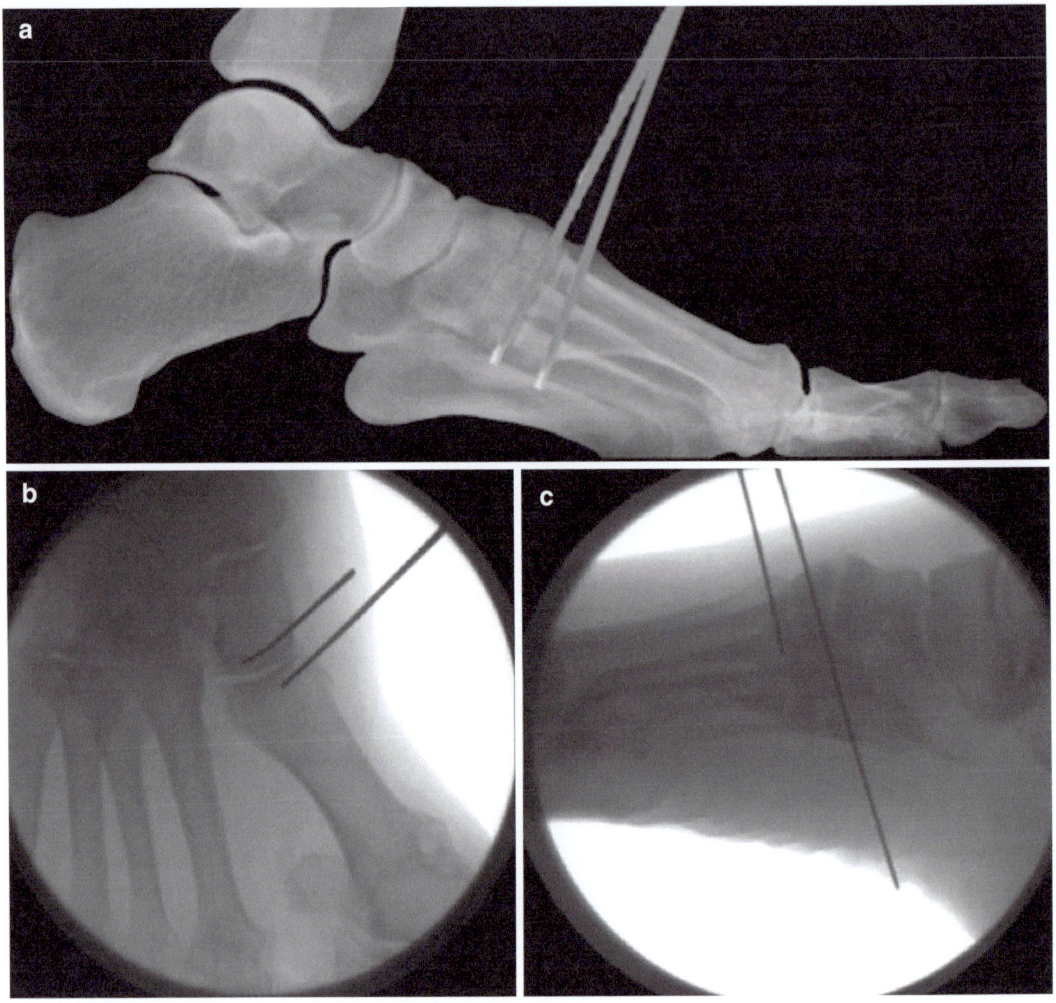

Fig. 23.1 Two K-wires inserted vertically and medially to act as a cutting guide. Conceptual view (**a**) AP fluoroscopy view (**b**) Mediolateral fluoroscopy view (**c**). © Julien Laborde 2015. All Rights Reserved

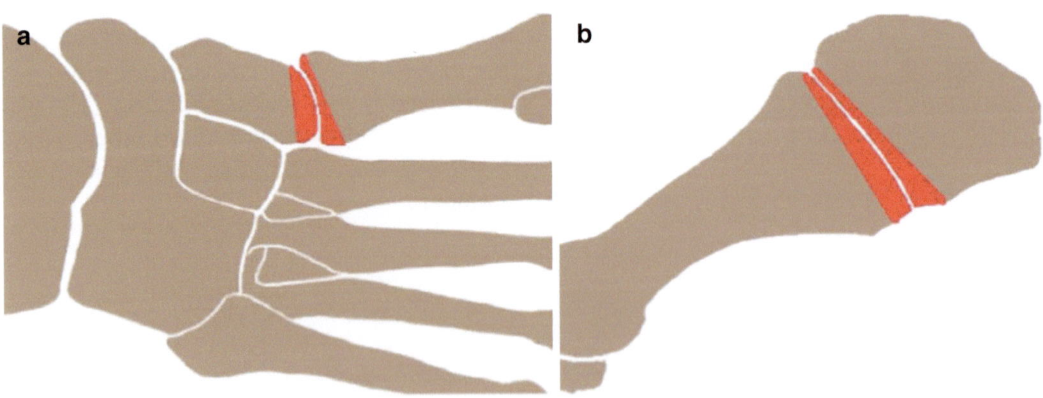

Fig. 23.2 Bone wedges to be removed during arthrodesis seen in the frontal (**a**) and sagittal planes (**b**). © Julien Laborde 2015. All Rights Reserved

23.2.3 Bone Cuts

The bone cuts are done using a 3 × 20-mm burr. The first cut is made in the medial cuneiform (Fig. 23.3a). A slit is made medially in the skin over the joint and then the burr inserted. It is placed perpendicular to the second metatarsal (M2). The cut starts at the K-wire, and then progresses in an apical-caudal windshield wiper movement, while staying perpendicular to M2. This is a true bone cut, not a bone grinding maneuver; thus, it does not generate bone dust. Halsted mosquito clamps are used to extract the resulting bone fragments (Fig. 23.3b).

The next cut is at the M1 base. The M1–M2 angle is closed manually to achieve the desired correction in the frontal plane (Fig. 23.4a), and then the cut is made. A K-wire can be inserted through M1/M2 to hold the correction temporarily.

The metatarsal cut is made according to the same principle, while staying perpendicular to M2. Again, Halsted mosquito clamps are used to extract the bone fragments (Fig. 23.4b–d).

23.2.4 Arthrodesis Fixation (Modified Lapidus)

Fixation is done by crossing two anteroposterior, compressive, 4-mm diameter screws. The first screw is inserted distal to proximal and dorsal to plantar. It is aimed at the inferomedial corner of the first cuneiform, which is the most solid part of this bone (Fig. 23.5).

23.2.5 Additional Fixation (Original Lapidus)

Once the arthrodesis has been performed, the M1/M2 mobility is tested by pressing on the first intermetatarsal space. If any mobility remains, additional fixation by C1–C2 arthrodesis must be performed (Fig. 23.7).

The 3 × 20-mm burr is inserted under fluoroscopy guidance between the first and second cuneiform and between M1 and M2 to decorticate their articular surfaces (Fig. 23.8). Next, M1 and M2 are joined by a 4-mm-diameter

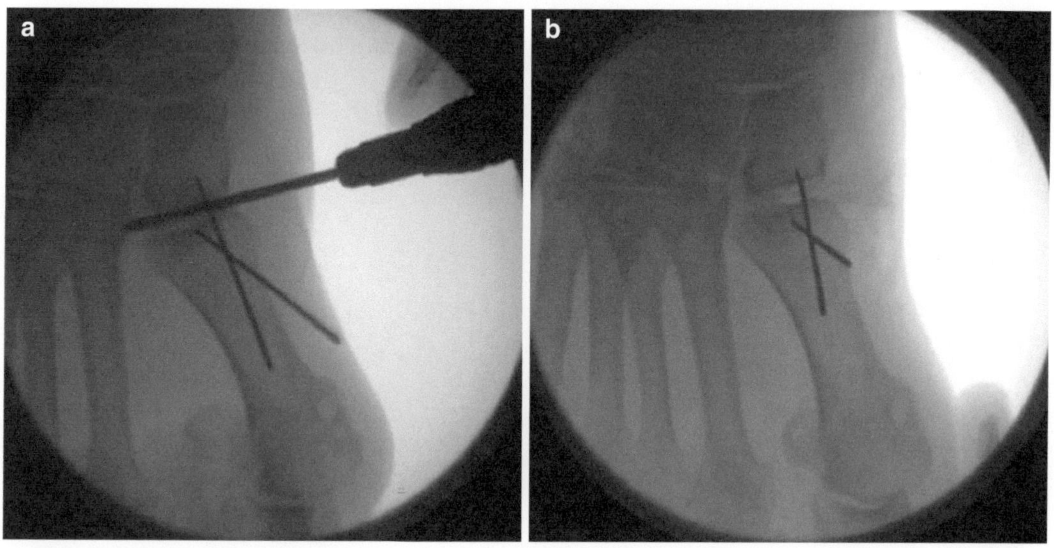

Fig. 23.3 First cut made with burr in medial cuneiform (**a**). Cut surface is perpendicular to M2 (**b**).

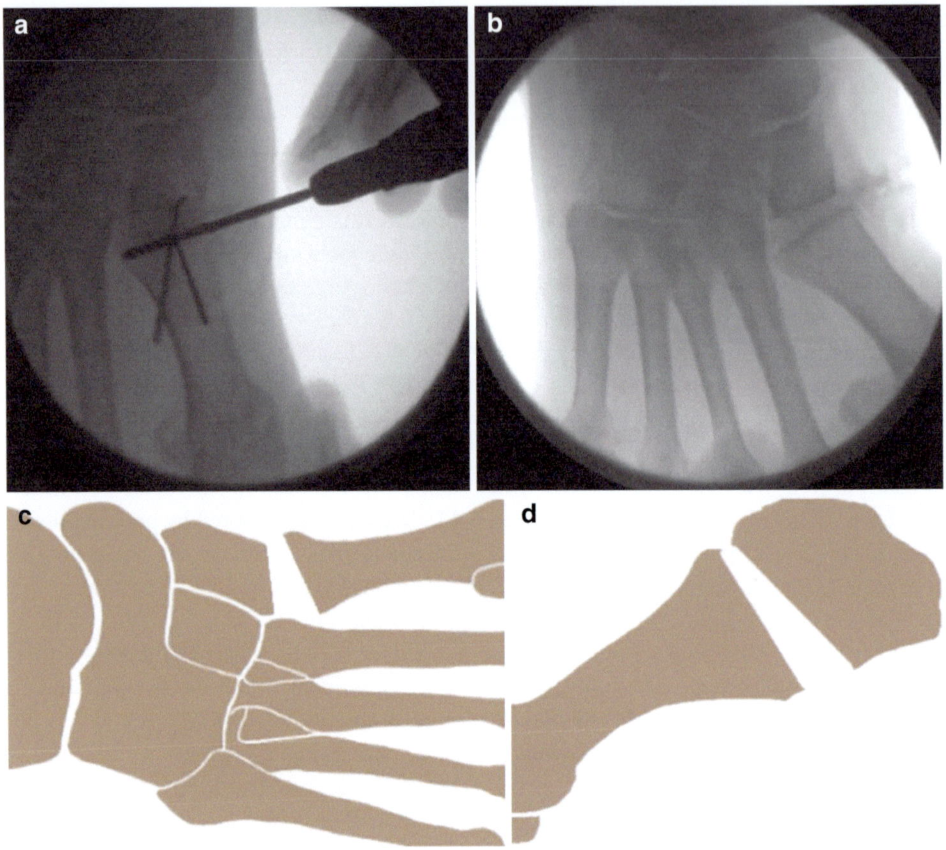

Fig. 23.4 The M1–M2 angle is closed manually to achieve the desired correction the frontal plane (**a**). Lateral closing wedge osteotomy on an AP fluoroscopy view (**b**). Bone wedges removed during arthrodesis seen in frontal (**c**) and sagittal planes (**d**). © Julien Laborde 2015. All Rights Reserved

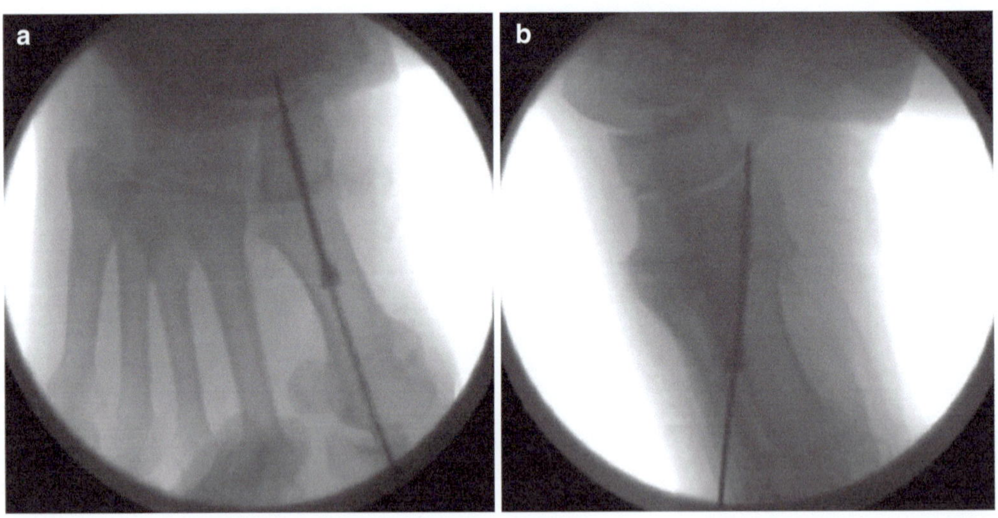

Fig. 23.5 First screw inserted distal to proximal (**a**), while aiming for the inferomedial corner of the first cuneiform (**b**) The second screw goes proximal to distal and dorsal to plantar and is lateral to the first screw. It must cross the plantar cortex of M1 and the first cuneiform to achieve solid hold (Fig. 23.6). © Julien Laborde 2015. All Rights Reserved

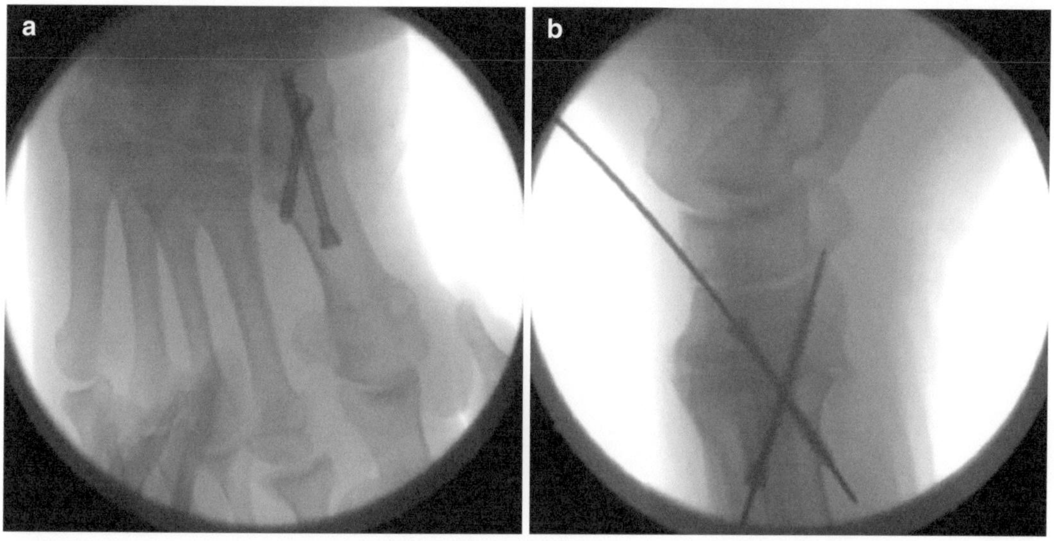

Fig. 23.6 Second screw inserted proximal to distal (**a**). Good hold achieved when screw crosses M1 plantar cortex and first cuneiform (**b**).

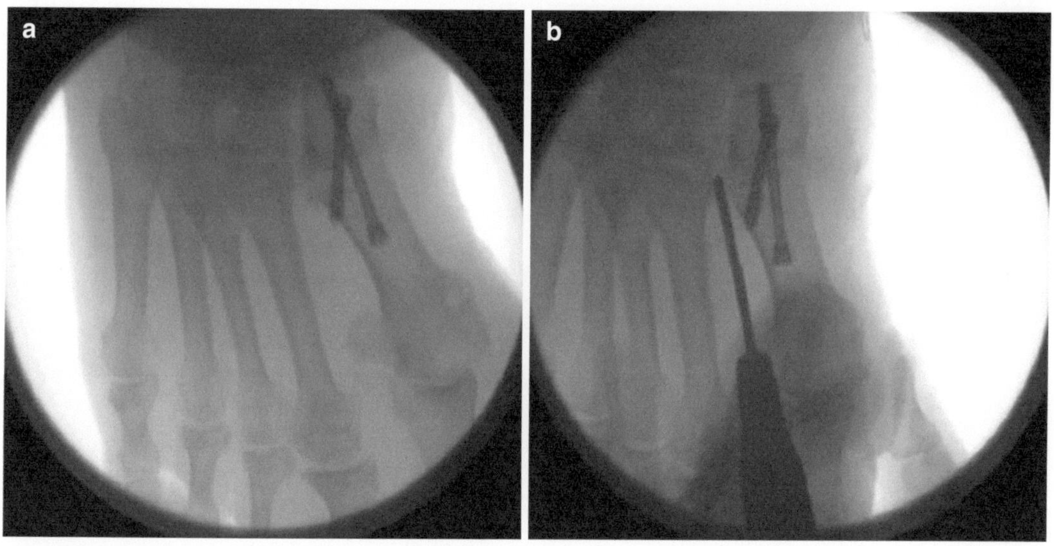

Fig. 23.7 Fluoroscopy (**a**) used to check the burr's position in the first intermetatarsal space (**b**).

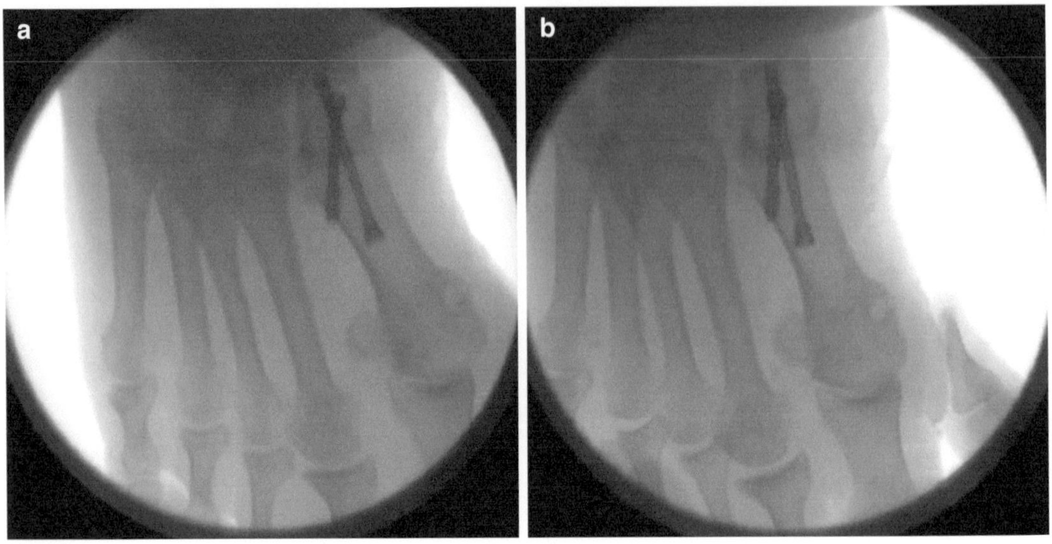

Fig. 23.8 Fluoroscopy (**a**) used to monitor the burr's progress during decortication of the surfaces between the first and second cuneiform and between M1 and M2 (**b**).

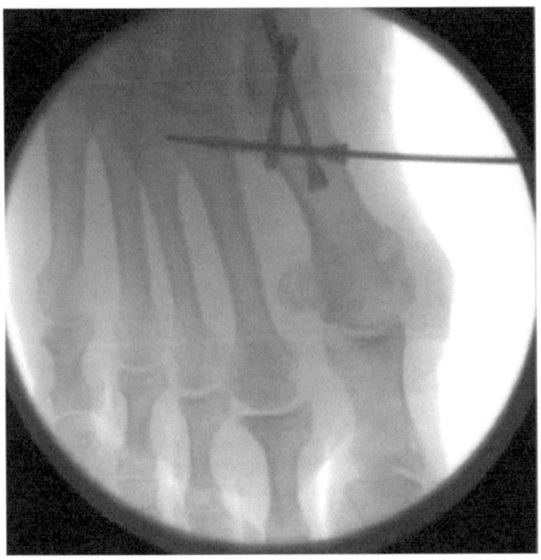

Fig. 23.9 A 4-mm-diameter compressive screw is used to join M1 and M2.

compressive screw, placed horizontally at the proximal third of M1, and perpendicular to M2 (Fig. 23.9).

Note The screw only needs to enter the medial cortex of M2. The screw head must not penetrate any deeper than the medial cortex of M1; if the screw goes through M1, the correction will be lost.

Supplementary Procedures

- The procedure is finished in the typical manner.
- An Akin osteotomy can be done at P1; it is secured with a compressive 2.5-mm diameter screw.
- Lavage with copious saline is required.
- The skin incision does not need to be closed, thus allowing any hematoma to drain.
- A corrective dressing is left in place for the first 15 days.
- The patient wears a heel contact shoe for 6 weeks to allow full healing of the arthrodesis site and to limit its loading.

24 Minimally Invasive and Percutaneous Arthrodesis of the Hallux Interphalangeal Joint

Christophe Piat and Cyrille Cazeau

24.1 Introduction

Arthrodesis of the hallux interphalangeal joint (IPJ) is indicated in patients with degenerative or inflammatory cartilage damage, and in those with painful, irreversible static or dynamic deformities of this joint. While some of these cases are congenital, the vast majority are acquired over time.

24.2 Indications

IPJ arthrodesis is performed in patients with joint or ligament lesions and with joint deformity (Fig. 24.1). The origin can be degenerative or arthritic. Rarely primary, it is mainly secondary to open or closed trauma such as a crush injury.

Posttraumatic osteoarthritis is the most common indication. This osteoarthritis develops quickly, in the year following an injury such as intra-articular fracture of the distal phalanx (P2) base or proximal phalanx (P1) head (closed or even open). It can also be secondary to reduced or unreduced dislocation, and to traumatic subluxations, or even hallux IPJ sprains.

Unlike hallux rigidus, primary hallux IPJ arthritis is very rare and may be related to crystal arthropathy.

C. Piat (✉) · C. Cazeau
Clinique Victor Hugo, Paris, France

The arthritis can have a degenerative origin, developing secondary to arthrodesis of the hallux metatarsophalangeal joint, especially if it was done in an incorrect position. In fact, the excess dorsiflexion is countered by IP flexion, which causes dorsal impingement and osteoarthritis in the dorsal, non-loaded part of the joint, with progressive stiffening of the flexion deformity, which is initially reducible, then becomes fixed.

Other than this degenerative origin, cartilage destruction can also be observed in cases of inflammatory arthropathy.

Hallux IPJ arthrodesis is proposed for treating ruptures of the flexor hallucis brevis tendon secondary to trauma, or more often, secondary to foot surgery, such as hallux valgus surgery with lateral sesamoidectomy (Petersen or McBride), which have more extensive lateral release.

Neurological or neuropathic cases are rarer; there are no cartilage or ligament lesions initially. The neuropathy can result in a deficit of the flexor hallucis brevis. It can occur as part of pes cavus, no matter the etiology, and may be accompanied by claw toes, especially of the hallux with an IPJ flexion deformity.

In tendon-related or neurological deformities, the cartilage is initially intact with the deformity still being reducible but then stiffens up over time. Arthritic lesions appear in areas where the cartilage is not loaded in the upper portion of the joint for IP flexion deformity cases. This condi-

C. Cazeau, Y. Stiglitz (eds.), *Percutaneous and Minimally Invasive Foot Surgery*,
https://doi.org/10.1007/978-3-030-98791-6_24

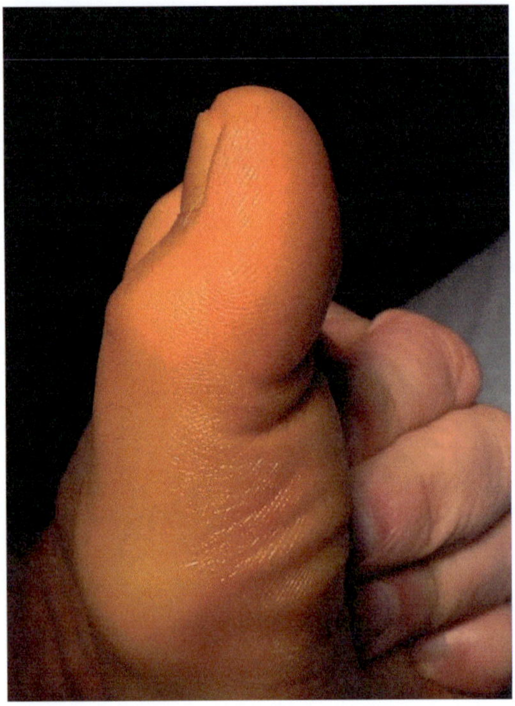

Fig. 24.1 Hallux interphalangeal joint deformity.

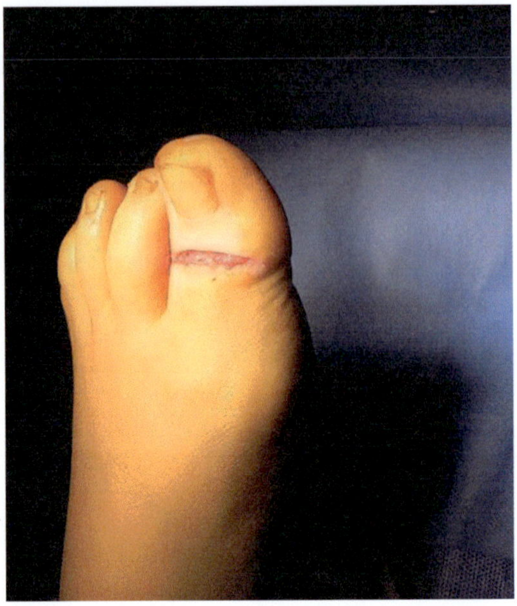

Fig. 24.2 IPJ transverse dorsal approach.

tion then progresses like posttraumatic osteoarthritis, making it nearly impossible to preserve the joint.

24.3 Methods and Technique

24.3.1 Minimally Invasive

The procedure is done under regional anesthesia through a minimally invasive transverse dorsal approach at the base of the joint. The incision goes through the extensor tendon, slightly behind the base of the nail matrix (Fig. 24.2). This approach is straight forward but must be accompanied by elliptical cutaneous resection in flexion deformity cases. This allows the excess dorsal skin and corn that has developed to be excised, initially starting out slowly. In cases of hyperextension, the dorsal approach is trickier. No cutaneous resection should be done. Closure is only feasible by making cuts on either side of the joint of several millimeters, which will reduce the length of the big toe and help to cover the arthrodesis zone while preserving the hyperextension correction with hallux straightening.

The bone cuts for the arthrodesis are made with an oscillating saw, aiming to make them parallel to the final desired position, i.e., taking into account the sagittal or horizontal deformity and any potential translation, along with the posttraumatic or acquired malunion. There is no reason to add a tendon graft. Fixation is performed using a 3.5-mm-diameter Maconor stainless steel screw (Fig. 24.3). Burring is carried out by going back-and-forth on the arthrodesis surface, while making sure to use the medullary canal as a guide and not piercing through the P1 base. Compression is applied manually by maintaining contact between the arthrodesis surfaces during fixation. It can be supplemented by drilling into P2 with a 3.5-mm bit, while P1 is drilled with a 2.7-mm bit or by using cancellous bone screws with distal threads. Verifying the contact and compression between the arthrodesis surfaces is a tricky phase of the procedure because visibility is greatly reduced by the correction of the flexion deformity. Small retractors can facilitate this task. The tendon and

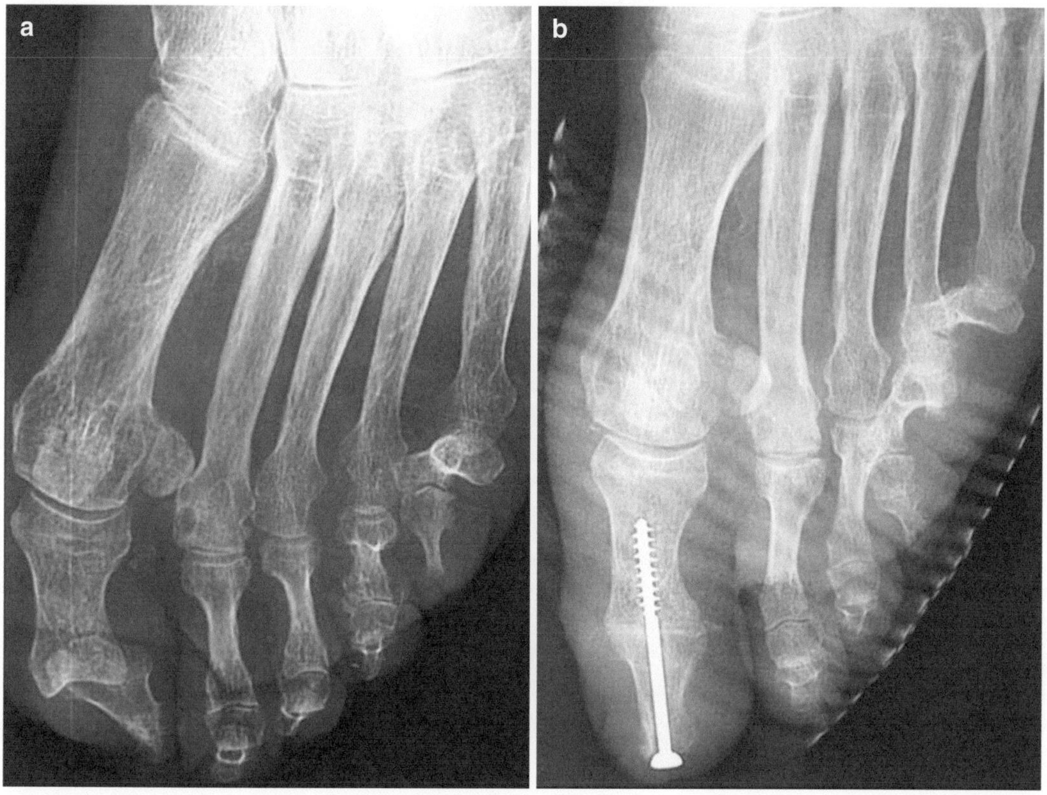

Fig. 24.3 Preoperative view of hallux interphalangeal joint deformity (**a**); postoperative view after axial screw fixation of the arthrodesis (**b**).

skin layers are then closed. The patients can bear weight while using a rigid postoperative shoe for 4 weeks.

24.3.2 Percutaneous

A percutaneous technique can also be used, especially when there are skin lesions on the dorsal side of the IPJ. A medial or lateral approach is used depending on whether the surgeon is right or left-handed and which foot is being operated on. A Beaver blade is used for the arthrotomy (Fig. 24.4a). This is followed by placement of a 3.1-mm-diameter Wedge burr or 12 × 2-mm Shannon burr (Fig. 24.4b), which is used to sparingly remove cartilage until subchondral bone is exposed (Fig. 24.5a). In cases of locked flexion deformity, it is recommended to start by carefully performing a plantar capsulotomy using a Beaver blade, and slight shortening through back-and-forth movements of the burr. A second arthrotomy can be made on the opposite side to make it easier to remove the cartilage debris using a syringe—debris that is known to cause an inflammatory reaction. The various steps are verified with fluoroscopy, especially the bone fixation. Fixation can be done with crossed screws, with a compressive screw having differential pitch threads, or more simply by single or double axial screw fixation, inserted distal to proximal through P2 (Fig. 24.5b).

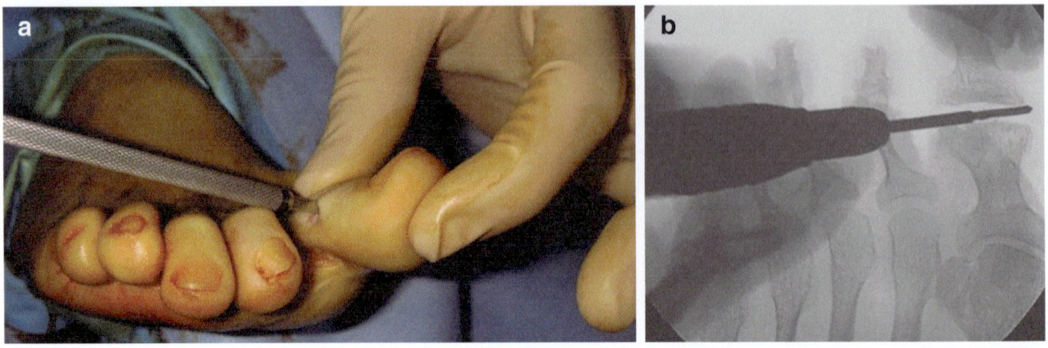

Fig. 24.4 Beaver blade for lateral percutaneous IPJ approach and plantar release (**a**); cartilage and subchondral bone removal with burr under fluoroscopy control (**b**). © Cyrille Cazeau 2015. All Rights Reserved

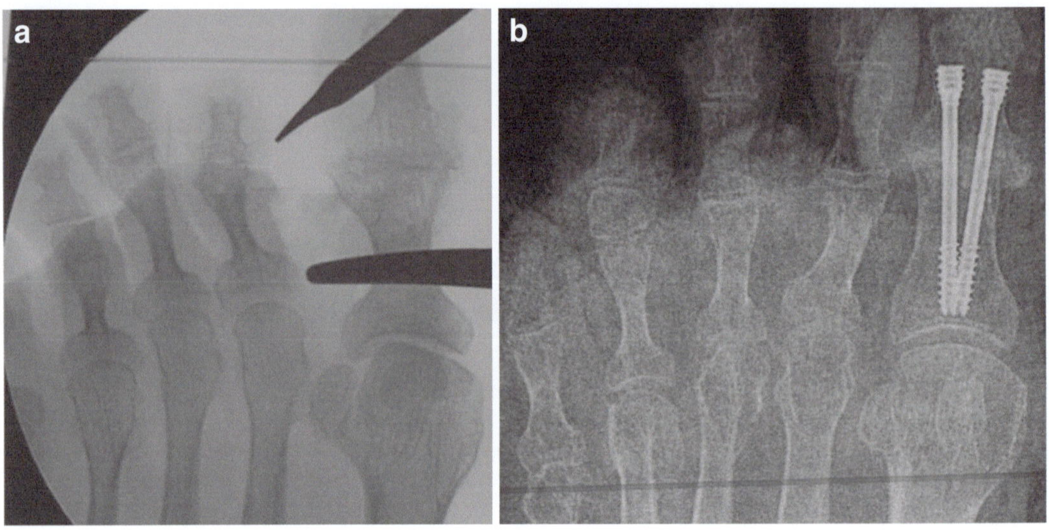

Fig. 24.5 Arthrodesis surfaces approximated (**a**); double axial screw fixation (**b**). © Cyrille Cazeau. All Rights Reserved

24.4 Postoperative Course

Nonunion is the most common complication. It is always attributed to an interfragmentary gap resulting from incorrect cuts or capsule/tendon interposition. Nevertheless, tight fibrous ankylosis is rarely symptomatic. The hardware can be removed in nonunion cases or in young patients. Improvements such as pain relief, better walking distance, possibility of wearing traditional shoes with reduction, or discontinuation of orthotics, along with disappearance of dorsal or pulp calluses, have been reported; however, the acquired dystrophic nail problems are unchanged. Cases attributed to arthritis have better outcomes than those attributed to neurological deficits, except for instances of highly sclerotic posttraumatic osteoarthritis that do not fuse.

24.5 Discussion

Arthrodesis of the hallux IPJ can return this deformed joint to its original (correct) position and recreate new tendon balance, which improves stability and reduces pain. The arthrodesis allows the flexor hallucis longus to lower both P1 and P2 overall. The dorsal transverse approach has no negative effects on the nail matrix and causes technical problems only in patients who have a dorsal flexion deformity, which requires a slightly more extensive bone cut to allow healing. In this scenario, another medial or lateral approach should be considered, which is straightforward when using a percutaneous technique. Axial screw fixation is enough to stabilize the arthrodesis site and to ensure good compression, particularly when the distal reaming has allowed the fixation to be compressive. One or more axial screws are used to place the arthrodesis in a satisfactory position. The location in the P1 and P2 diaphysis help to automatically correct the joint deformity. Conversely, poor contact due to the surfaces not being parallel or soft tissue interposition will lead to the development of an interfragmentary gap that is nearly always synonymous with nonunion. Thus, during the procedure, it is crucial to confirm good contact between the arthrodesis surfaces either visually or by fluoroscopy.

24.6 Conclusion

Hallux IPJ arthrodesis is a reliable procedure that corrects the hallux deformity and is likely to reduce the patients' pain and improve their function and walking ability. A minimally invasive dorsal approach or a medial or lateral percutaneous approach combined with axial screw fixation are critical to the success of this procedure. The limiting factor is the difficulty in making the bone cuts due to the deformity and achieving extended contact between the arthrodesis surfaces without interposition.

Editors' Point of View

IPJ arthrodesis is much easier to do with a percutaneous technique than an open one. Signs of delayed union on radiographs are not a concern, as fusion will occur after the third month.

Suggested Reading

Cracchiolo AC. Arthrodesis of the hallux MTP joint and IP joint. In: Wülker N, Stephens M, Cracchiolo AC, editors. An atlas of foot and ankle surgery. London: Dunitz; 1998. pp. 59–66.

Derner R, Meyer AJ. Hallux interphalangeal joint arthrodesis. J Foot Ankle Surg. 2009;48(3):408–10.

Frankel JP, Turf R, Tirone M. Arthrodesis of the hallux interphalangeal joint using a diagonally placed 2-mm cortical bone screw. J Foot Surg. 1989;28:466–70.

Jahss MH. Disorders of the hallux and the first ray. In: Jahss MH, editor. Disorders of the foot and ankle, medical and surgical management. 2nd ed. Philadelphia: W.B. Saunders Company; 1991. p. 943–1106.

Piat C, Cazeau C, Stiglitz Y. Arthrodèse interphalangienne de hallux. Lille (France): Journées de Printemps de l'AFCP; 2013.

Piat C. Pied creux de l'adulte. In: Cahiers d'enseignement de la SOFCOT 97. Issy-les-Moulineaux: Elsevier Masson; 2008. pp. 97–118.

Steensma MR, Jabara M, Anderson JG, Bohay DR. Flexor hallucis longus tendon transfer for hallux claw toe deformity and vertical instability of the metatarsophalangeal joint. Foot Ankle Int. 2006;27:689–92.

DMMO

25

Jean Yves Coillard

25.1 Introduction

Open metatarsal osteotomy procedures for treating metatarsalgia were first described in the early 1900s by Meisenbach. However, the gold standard technique is the one described by Lowell S. Weil in 1991. Several modifications to his technique have been proposed (e.g., OCRA, shortening chevron) to get around the potential side effects (stiffness, pain).

Minimally invasive metatarsal osteotomy procedures have also been used for a long time but are not well described and have not been properly evaluated. Stephen Isham was the first to advocate the use of this type of osteotomy, which he taught to members of the American Society of Podiatric Surgeons.

Mariano de Prado, an orthopedic surgeon from Spain, was the first European surgeon to adopt Isham's techniques, and he introduced them to Europe.

This is a percutaneous extra-articular distal osteotomy that results in malunion of the metatarsal heads in elevation and shortening. The aim is to reduce forefoot pressure and pain that often occurs in combination with first ray insufficiency. The goal of the percutaneous method is to eliminate the side effects of open osteotomy with fixation:

- Pain and stiffness due to the capsule (intra-articular)
- Dorsal contracture of the soft tissues (extra-articular)
- Insufficient metatarsal head elevation after Weil osteotomy that results in persistent metatarsalgia.

For a long time, this osteotomy was incorrectly called the *percutaneous Weil*. It is now referred to as distal metatarsal minimally invasive osteotomy (DMMO).

25.2 Anatomical Considerations

The lateral metatarsal heads form a harmonious curve known as Lelièvre's parabola. Maestro defined various forefoot types based on precise metatarsal length measurements. Metatarsalgia can in part be explained by these anatomical relationships. This foot disorder can be attributed to the length of one or two metatarsals, or to other associated deformities. Be that as it may, excessive pressure is concentrated under the middle metatarsal heads and manifests itself as isolated pain in the forefoot, then by painful calluses. Later, degenerative anatomical lesions appear in the soft tissues (plantar plate) and bone tissue (fatigue fracture). Because of tendon contractures, claw toe deformity develops, which accen-

J. Y. Coillard (✉)
Clinique du Parc, Lyon, France
e-mail: jean-yves.coillard@cliniqueduparclyon.com

C. Cazeau, Y. Stiglitz (eds.), *Percutaneous and Minimally Invasive Foot Surgery*,
https://doi.org/10.1007/978-3-030-98791-6_25

tuates the joint deformities and results in a rigid deformity. Together this results in a painful, contracted forefoot.

25.3 Objectives and Principles

The aim of these minimally invasive osteotomies is to reduce the excessive plantar pressure and release the dorsal contractures by shortening and elevating the metatarsal heads. The metatarsophalangeal (MTP) joint retracts after the osteotomy due to muscle and tendon activity and the passive plantar pressure that occurs during weight-bearing. This displacement corresponds to shortening in the mechanical axis of the metatarsal. This results in metatarsal malunion but also places the pathological joint into a better position with relaxation of the musculotendinous system and elimination of the excessive plantar pressure.

To accomplish this, one needs to perform an osteotomy of the metatarsal neck (like a fracture) and then allow the patient to gradually resume weight bearing. Through the effects of plantar pressure and musculotendinous traction, the now mobile heads and joints will move into the appropriate functional position to allow the development of a fibrous callus and then a bony one. While the result is bone malunion, this configuration is mechanically better.

This situation resembles the functional treatment of metatarsal head fractures, which leads to very good outcomes: balanced displacement, no stiffness, good quality callus, and no secondary metatarsalgia even though the heads are not in an anatomical position. One likely needs to supplement this osteotomy with procedures on the lateral rays; however, the most important step is to fully and permanently resolve the first ray insufficiency that triggered the metatarsalgia in the first place. Otherwise the procedure will fail, or the deformity will recur.

Strictly speaking, there is no preoperative planning for this osteotomy. This philosophy is completely different than that of fixed osteotomies. Instead, we rely on functional displacement of the metatarsal heads resulting from the reloading and the action of the foot's intrinsic muscles and tendons.

25.4 Conventional DMMO

There are several variations of the basic technique depending on whether the emphasis is on elevating or shortening the lateral rays. We will describe Isham's original technique as taught to us by M. de Prado.

25.4.1 Instrumentation

Minimally invasive surgery of the metatarsals requires the same instrumentation as any other minimally invasive surgery on the foot.

- Beaver® type blade when possible
- Raspatory and elevator
- Rasps (not essential) to create the working space
- Small-powered surgical tool with slow rotation (less than 8000 rpm) and if possible, a torque limiter to avoid burning skin and especially, bone tissue
- Long Shannon 44 burr or a wider burr when shortening is the priority (long M2)
- Low-radiation image intensifier (fluoroscopy) to verify the burr position in early cases and to evaluate the result at the end of the procedure

25.4.2 Surgical Technique

25.4.2.1 Anesthesia

In most cases, regional anesthesia is performed through a popliteal or posterior tibial/peroneal nerve block, supplemented as needed by a calcaneopedal block and anterior coronal block of the midfoot.

25.4.2.2 Patient Setup

No specific setup is needed for this surgical technique; the patient's position is chosen based on the procedure being done on the first ray, typically during the same session. However, one must factor in the possibility of intraoperative radiographs being made. If the first ray will also be operated using a minimally invasive technique, the patient will be positioned as described in the relevant chapter.

25.4.2.3 Approach

The skin incision is made with a Beaver blade in the intercapitometatarsal space, immediately besides the head and parallel to the extensor tendons. The scalpel is angled 45° in the direction of the metatarsal neck. The incision must be large enough to allow burr movements without damaging the skin (3–4 mm). The raspatory or elevator is inserted to create a working space and prevent any contact with the soft tissues; this requires stripping off the lateral edge below the metatarsal head. A fluoroscopy image can be taken at this point to verify the osteotomy level.

25.4.2.4 Osteotomy

Next, the wide or long Shannon 44 burr is inserted into the working space, against the metatarsal cortex (Fig. 25.1). To start the osteotomy, the burr is angled 45° relative to the ground, making a clear-cut cortical groove to prevent incorrect orientation and displacement of the burr. Then, using a rotational movement around the neck, the burr cuts through the entire medial cortex of the metatarsal (for a right foot and right-handed surgeon), then the plantar cortex, lateral cortex, and dorsal cortex. The burr's shaft always remains angled at 45°.

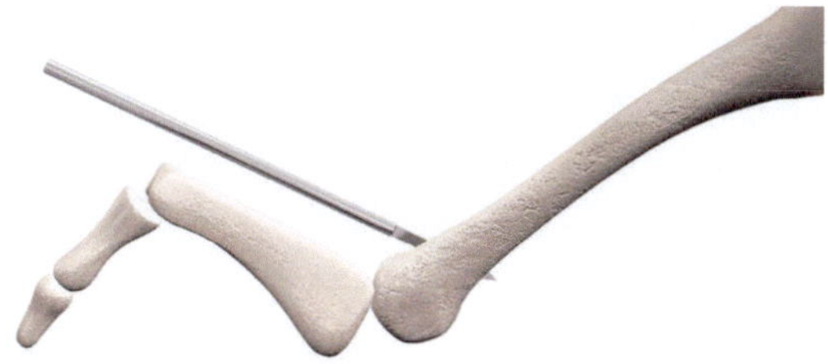

Fig. 25.1 Orientation of burr during conventional DMMO.

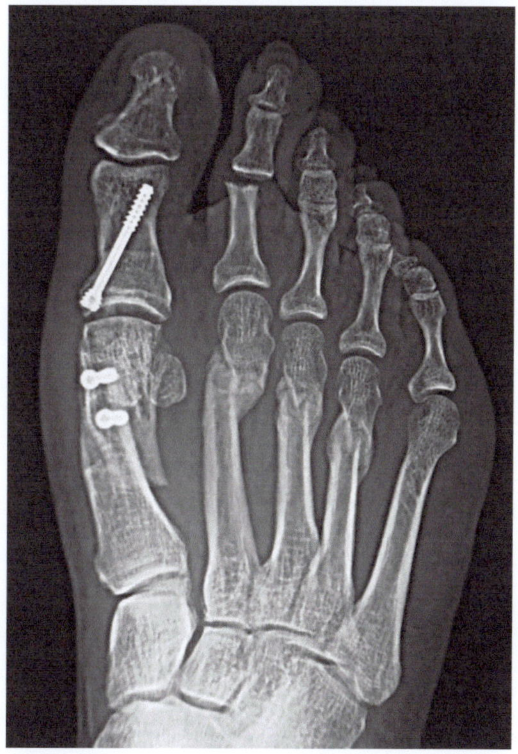

Fig. 25.2 Radiograph of conventional DMMO.

Another option is to shift the burr laterally without rotation around the metatarsal axis, although there is a higher risk of soft tissue damage. At this point, the osteotomy's position can be checked with fluoroscopy and the head's mobility checked clinically.

During the osteotomy, it is important to control the rotation speed. If the skin is burned accidentally, it is crucial to immediately excise the damaged skin and then to suture the healthy edges together.

The number of osteotomy procedures will depend on the degree of plantar hyperkeratosis, although the standard procedure is to perform an osteotomy on the three middle metatarsals. Since the fifth ray is shorter and more mobile, it rarely needs to be shortened. One possibility is combining M3 and M4 DMMO with a moderate M2 osteotomy with fixation.

Once the osteotomy is finished, the metatarsal heads should have equal displacement, with shortening and often slight lateral shift (Figs. 25.2 and 25.3).

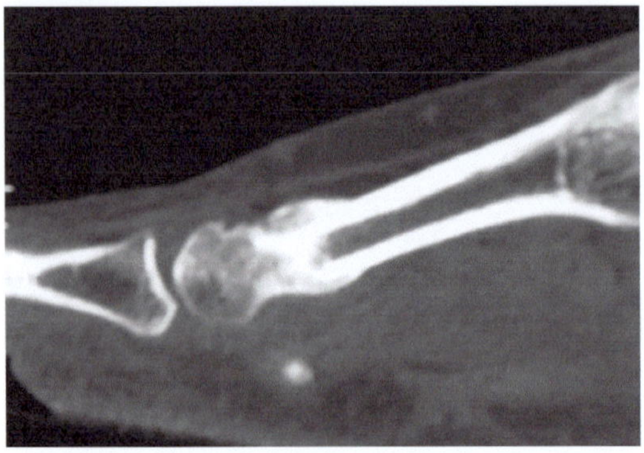

Fig. 25.3 CT scan of conventional DMMO.

25.4.2.5 Closure and Postoperative Course

The skin is closed with sutures, although some surgeons choose not to close it. The dressing must be meticulously assembled, given the absence of fixation. Gauze dressings are used to angle the toes inward toward the hallux, in order to limit excessive lateral displacement of the metatarsals. This helps counter any lateral deviation of the lesser toes induced by first ray instability. Some surgeons insist on placing the MTP joints in plantar flexion right away, to ensure shortening of the heads.

25.5 Oblique DMMO (DOMMO)

This osteotomy variation was developed because insufficient head displacement was observed in some cases. This was like the outcome of certain Weil osteotomy procedures in which the head remained jammed under the metatarsal neck and caused persistent metatarsalgia. This led some surgeons to perform a sagittal and oblique osteotomy cut that will induce mechanically safer shortening in the metatarsal axis by telescoping, while eliminating the risk of leaving the head jammed under the metatarsal neck. Also, by increasing the bone contact area, the already low risk of delayed union is reduced even more. The elevation effect is no longer a hindrance either.

The top to bottom osteotomy described initially was improved by Marius Uscatu, who executed it very precisely from bottom to top. This is the modified technique that we now use.

25.5.1 Osteotomy Technique

The anesthesia, patient positioning, and approach are as described above.

Once the burr has been inserted against the metatarsal neck, the aim is to pass under the neck (Fig. 25.4). After the burr is stabilized in the infe-

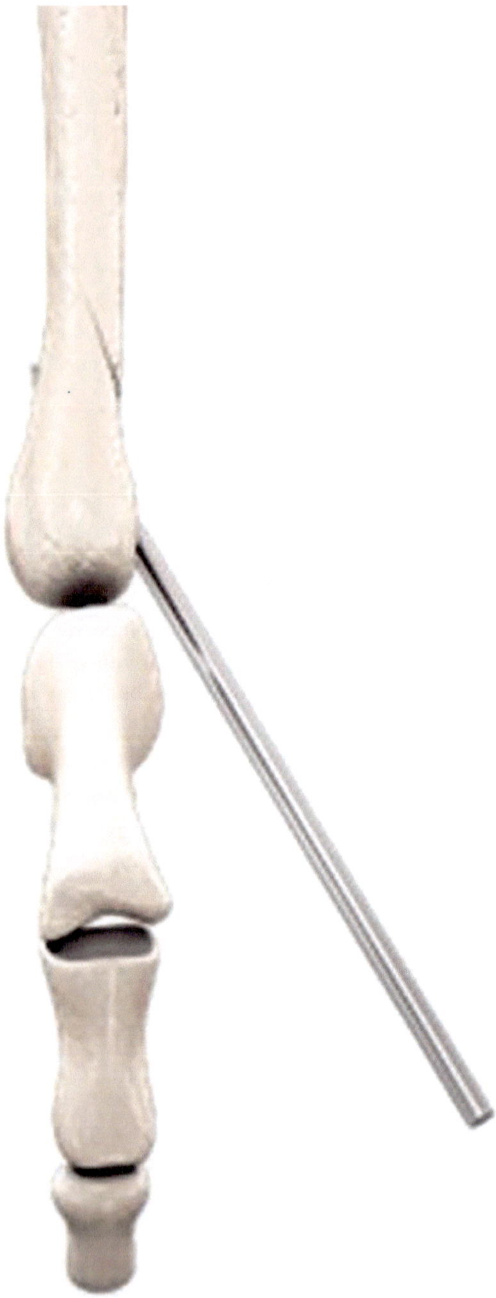

Fig. 25.4 Burr orientation for oblique DMMO.

rior concave surface of the metatarsal neck, the burr is angled relative to the bone axis of the metatarsal. Next, with a steady motion from bottom to top, the metatarsal neck is cut in the sagittal plane. Retrograde pressure on the head provides bone telescoping without resistance. The more oblique the osteotomy, the larger the burr diameter and the greater the shortening. If the osteotomy axis diverges (front to back and inside to outside), the lateral displacement happens easily; conversely, if the axis converges, less displacement will occur.

This osteotomy simplifies metatarsal head shortening and elevation and appears to limit the reduction problems and delayed union. We now use this technique regularly in our practice (Figs. 25.5 and 25.6).

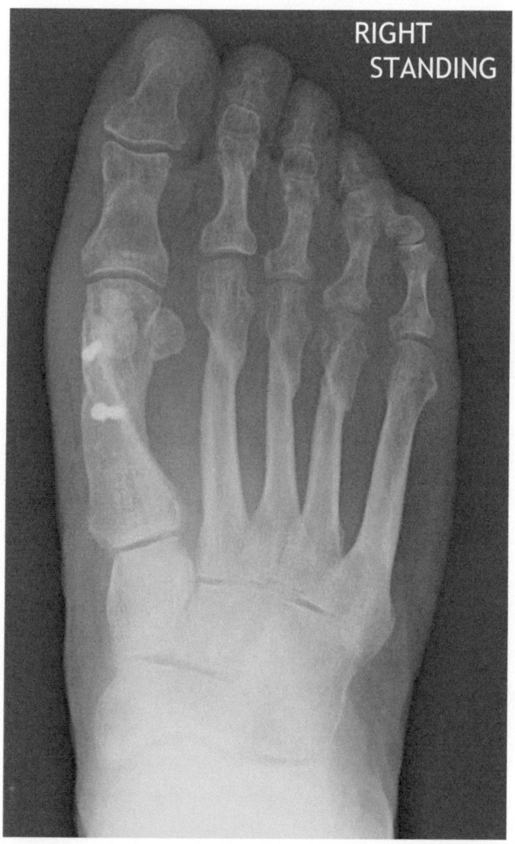

Fig. 25.5 Radiograph of oblique DMMO. © Jean Yves Coillard 2015. All Rights Reserved

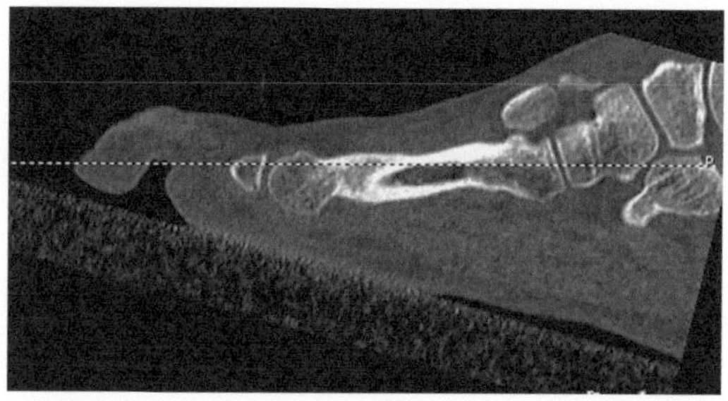

Fig. 25.6 CT scan of oblique DMMO. © Jean Yves Coillard 2015. All Rights Reserved

25.6 Reverse DMMO

The reverse DMMO technique is a modification based on the idea of elevating the metatarsal heads without shortening the metatarsal. This is relevant in some cases of very painful isolated calluses without soft tissue contracture in which we wish we could remove the heads without using an invasive approach. Thus, a different osteotomy plane is needed that provides simple head elevation.

25.6.1 Osteotomy Technique

The surgical approach, or more specifically the entry point, is more proximal and before the metatarsal heads. The burr is vertical but angled slightly downward and forward, contrary to the conventional DMMO, with the tip aimed slightly forward and downward (Fig. 25.7). The burr must be positioned against the neck and the head cut with an oblique transverse stroke. The surgeon must stand at the patient's instep, not in front of the foot. It is recommended to place the index of the opposite hand under the metatarsal head. One palpates under the tip of the burr, and once the head is cut, the index finger is used for reduction.

This osteotomy provides significant head elevation with small displacement in the axis. And since the inter-fragment movement is minimal, it results in simpler postoperative course, less pain,

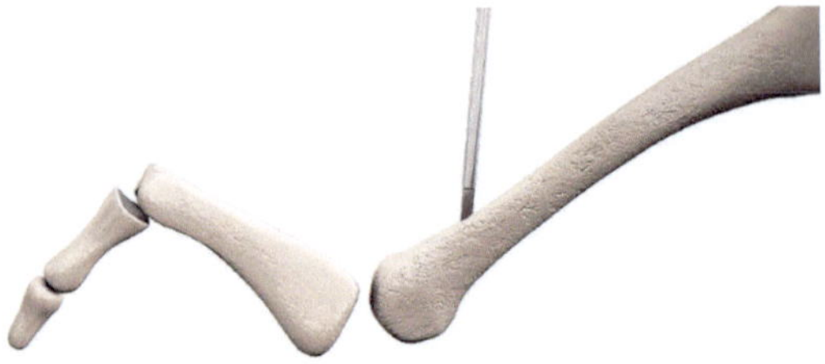

Fig. 25.7 Orientation of burr for reverse DMMO. © Jean Yves Coillard 2015. All Rights Reserved

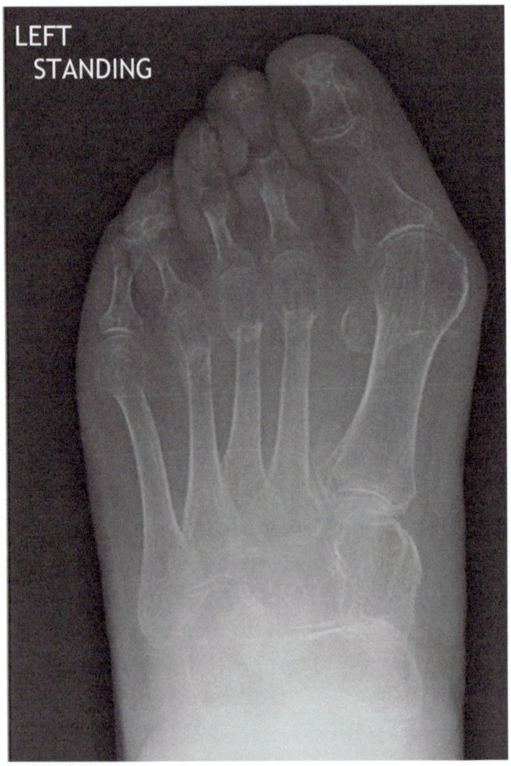

Fig. 25.8 Radiograph of reverse DMMO. © Jean Yves Coillard 2015. All Rights Reserved

and none of the usual edema. However, the head elevation is so substantial that one must perform this osteotomy on the four lateral metatarsals to eliminate the risk of transfer metatarsalgia on M5. This is the mechanical equivalent of metatarsal head resection without being invasive. The absence of shortening means that hallux arthrodesis is no longer necessary to reduce the risks of secondary misalignment of the first toe (Figs. 25.8 and 25.9).

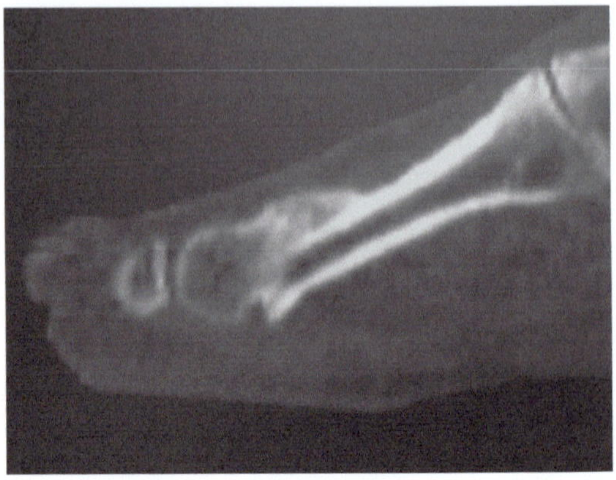

Fig. 25.9 CT scan of reverse DMMO. © Jean Yves Coillard 2015. All Rights Reserved

25.7 Metatarsophalangeal Dislocation

(Cyrille Cazeau)

25.7.1 Introduction

MTP dislocation is usually a contraindication for DMMO. It generally requires so much metatarsal shortening that it is theoretically preferable to perform a Weil osteotomy. But can this be done percutaneously in certain technical conditions? On Fig. 25.10 we can see a case of MTP2 dislocation, which has been reduced following DMMO with a 4.1-mm wedge burr, with 3-month follow-up.

25.7.2 Osteotomy Technique

The following steps are critical to technical success: wide and extensive percutaneous release, DMMO performed with shortening burr (4.1-mm wedge), and additional PIP arthrodesis. A high-quality dressing is essential for a successful outcome.

The first step is a release; it must be thorough, broad, and performed with a Beaver blade. It includes full dorsal capsulotomy, EDL and EDB

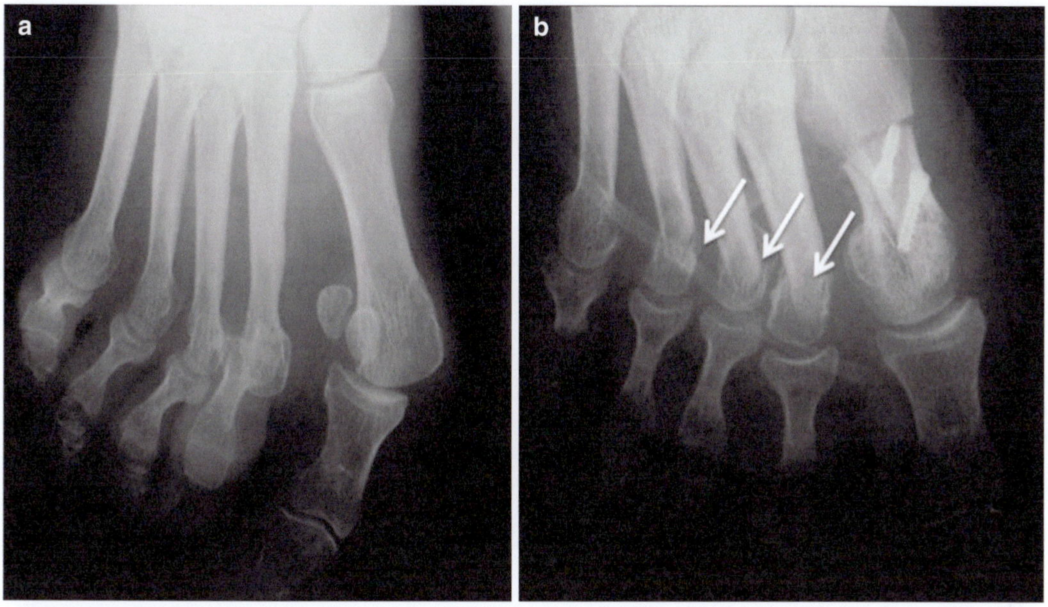

Fig. 25.10 MTP2 dislocation (**a**). Correct osteotomy location, just behind the metatarsal heads (**b**). © Cyrille Cazeau 2015. All Rights Reserved

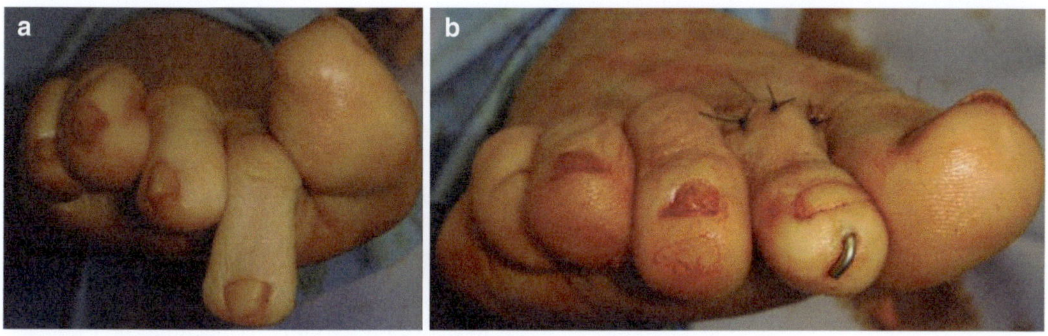

Fig. 25.11 Toe ptosis present after joint release (**a**) which is corrected with PIP arthrodesis (**b**). © Cyrille Cazeau 2015. All Rights Reserved

tenotomy, and transection of the metatarsophalangeal ligaments. The Beaver blade is often inserted horizontally between the plantar face of P1 and the dorsal face of M1 because of the dorsal dislocation; the joint is reduced by applying firm traction on the toe during the release. The result is ptosis of the toe (Fig. 25.11), related to the fact that all the dorsal suspensory elements have been completely transected. If this does not occur, then the release was insufficient and ineffective.

The second step is the DMMO. A normal approach is used. However, it must be located below the metatarsal heads (Fig. 25.10), in a dense cancellous bone. The osteotomy is performed with a 4.1-mm wedge burr; however, it is not straightforward because this type of burr is intended for exostectomy procedures. Like in the standard DMMO, one makes an initial osteotomy track and then always stays within it while making sure not to jam the burr. The burr orientation and trajectory are the same as the standard DMMO.

Given the shortening nature of this osteotomy, potentially accentuated by back-and-forth motions, the procedure must always be done on M2, M3, and M4 (Fig. 25.10). Forced plantar flexion is applied to ensure shortening.

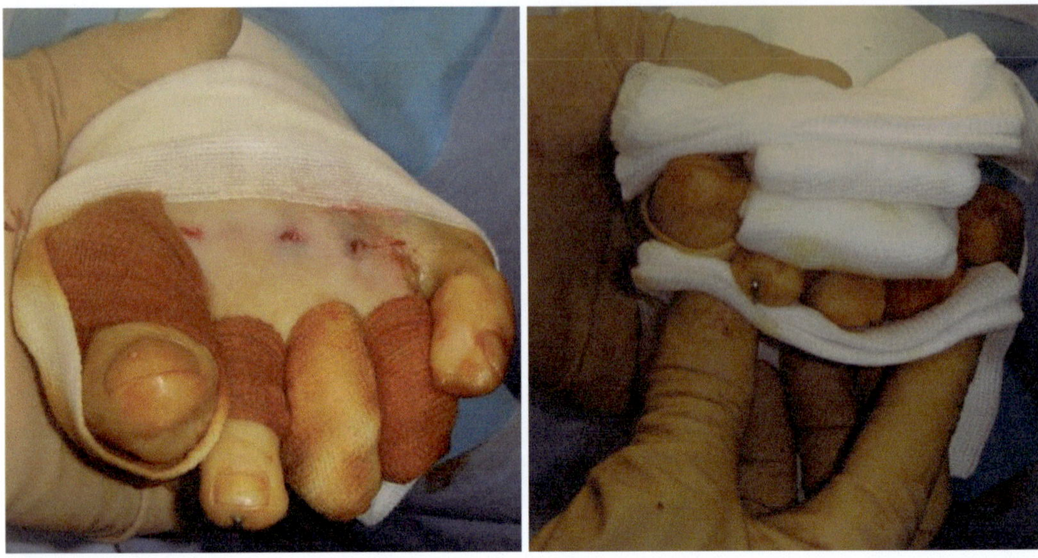

Fig. 25.12 Postoperative dressing.

The third step is correcting the toe ptosis resulting from the extensive release. This correction is achieved through a flat PIP arthrodesis (Fig. 25.11), either percutaneous or minimally invasive. The nearly universal fixed PIP flexion deformity is a reason to implement it.

If residual instability is present, the construct can be stabilized by pushing a K-wire into the M1 head. But this procedure must not be done to achieve reduction, as it will be lost when the K-wire is removed.

The postoperative dressing is essential (Fig. 25.12). Three principles must be followed: MTP joints placed in maximum plantar flexion; plantar translation of the toes by placing two gauze pieces folded into quarters on their dorsal side. This dressing is worn for 3–4 days. Immediate weight-bearing is recommended using a shoe with rockered sole. You can also place a compresse under the metatarsal heads, M2, M3, M4, to obtain their elevation thanks to the full weight bearing.

25.7.3 Conclusion

This is not a standard procedure, done at the start of a surgeon's learning curve. If reduction does not happen easily after the release, it is best to convert to a conventional Weil osteotomy.

25.8 Outcomes

The outcomes have been very encouraging in various published studies: patient satisfaction above 95%, elimination of metatarsalgia by the third month, bone union achieved in 99% of cases within 2 months.

Minor joint stiffness has been reported although it is difficult to measure, evaluate, and compare. There are no reports of the dorsal soft tissue contractures typical of a Weil osteotomy, which are responsible for toe elevatus that limits pulp contact.

25.9 Indications

It is always difficult to define the exact indications for a relatively new surgical technique. This requires the surgeon's discretion. Some favorable scenarios have emerged however, and they are described below.

25.9.1 Mechanical Metatarsalgia in Older Adults

The most obvious indication is that of mechanical and degenerative metatarsalgia in older adults associated with first ray insufficiency and lateral toe deformity. This is called static mechanical metatar-

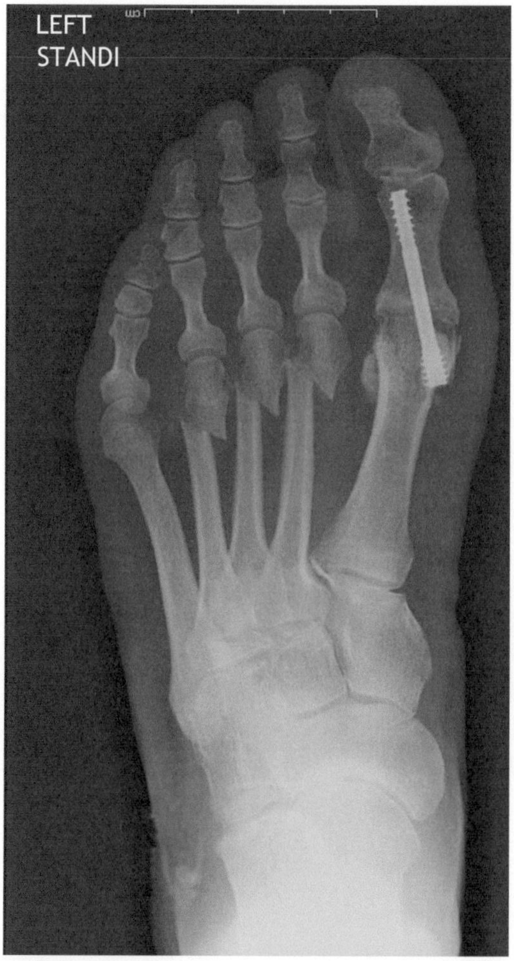

Fig. 25.13 Radiograph of DMMO. © Jean Yves Coillard 2015. All Rights Reserved

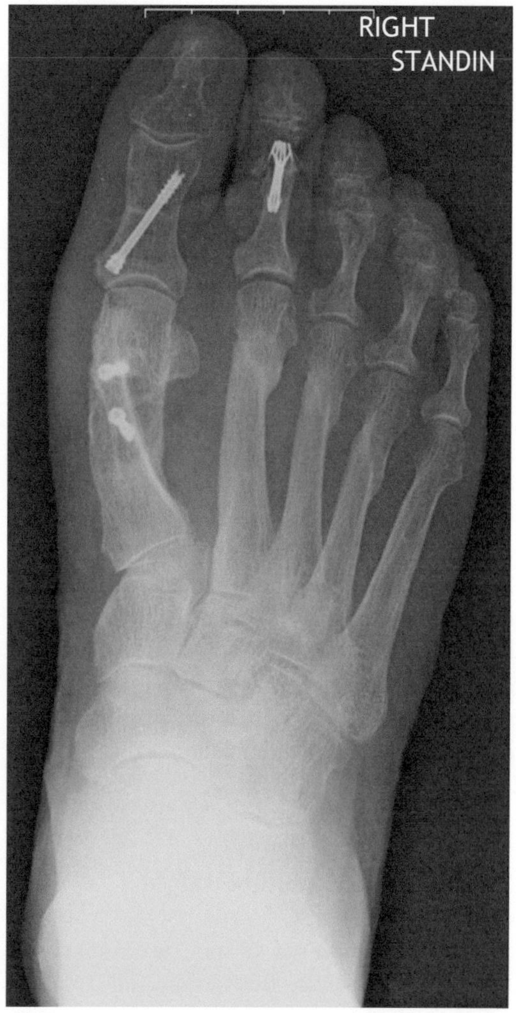

Fig. 25.14 Radiograph of DMMO in older adult. © Jean Yves Coillard 2015. All Rights Reserved

salgia. It appears clinically as a large, wide plantar callus (anterior round foot). Radiologically, the metatarsal parabola is often even. Obviously, the mechanical problems in the first ray must be solved completely and permanently as this contributes to lasting reduction. An osteotomy can be performed to correct the deformities, although an arthrodesis would be even more effective, either during the same session, or a second session.

In this indication, open surgical procedures are responsible for bone and skin complications that are by no means insignificant. In stark contrast, DMMO provides fast and reliable pain relief while avoiding the dreaded local complications. This scenario is the major indication for DMMO, and it applies to a very large number of patients (Figs. 25.13 and 25.14).

25.9.2 Recurring Metatarsalgia

DMMO has an out-sized role in this type of indication. After a Weil osteotomy, if the patient still has painful calluses and troublesome dorsal retraction due to inadequate shortening or lack of elevation, a standard surgical revision procedure is doomed to fail. Percutaneous surgery can be done with a minimal risk of elevating and shortening the metatarsal heads, without major risks and without working near the first surgical site. However, it is important to ensure the first ray is stable.

25.9.3 Propulsive Metatarsalgia

In this case, the indication is more controversial. These are younger patients with few plantar cutaneous signs or an isolated callus under M2, rarely more. Propulsive metatarsalgia is secondary to either an isolated bone anomaly (long M2) or ankle stiffness (joint or musculotendinous). If a conventional DMMO is proposed to these patients, the result may be less convincing, with persistent excess pressure under M2. In fact, while the DMMO displacement remains balanced, it retains the uneven M2 length and thus recurrence of the isolated propulsive metatarsalgia. In this scenario, one must find a way to shorten M2 more than the others when using a percutaneous technique. This can be accomplished by using a larger diameter burr only on M2. Another option is to change the orientation of the M2 osteotomy cut, for example, by making a very oblique DMMO which will allow more displacement (shortening). But some surgeons prefer ensuring the result by combining open M2 osteotomy with fixation and DMMO of the other metatarsals.

25.9.4 Isolated Metatarsalgia

Isolated metatarsalgia is not well suited to DMMO in principle. But despite this fact and given the lack of standardized treatment, some surgeons perform DMMO on several metatarsals or on a single metatarsal with the aim of shortening only that one. These cases are rare and all very different; thus, it is difficult to draw any conclusions.

25.9.5 Combinations

When faced with isolated M2 metatarsalgia or dislocation, some surgeons decide to shorten and elevate M2 very precisely based on millimeter-level calculations and then to fix it to ensure reduction while also performing DMMO on M3 and M4 or even M5 (Fig. 25.15). Others have proposed replacing the MTP2 joint with a silicone implant and performing DMMO on the other metatarsals to limit transfer metatarsalgia (Fig. 25.16). DMMO can provide spectacular correction of second toe supradductus (Fig. 25.17). All these combination techniques lead to good outcomes.

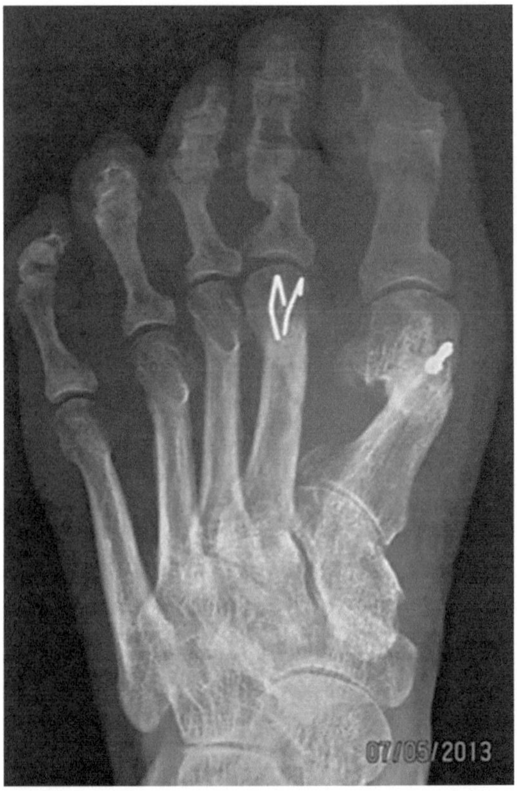

Fig. 25.15 Radiograph of combined M3, M4 DMMO, and M2-fixed osteotomy.

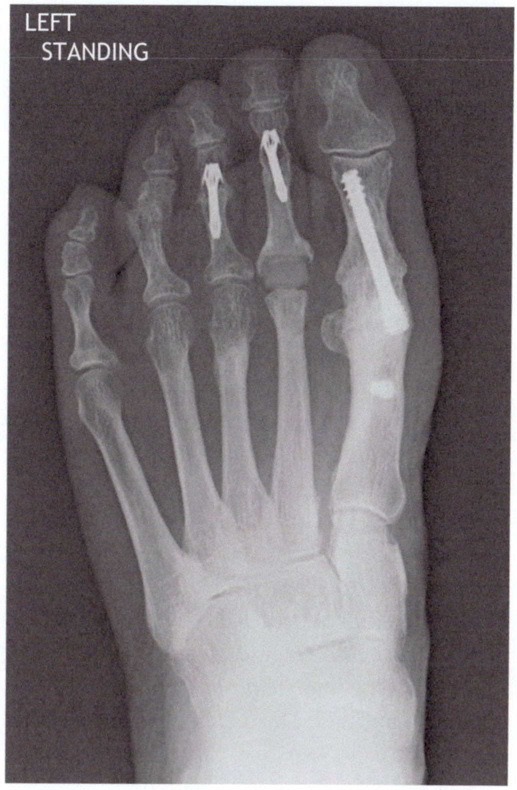

Fig. 25.16 Radiograph of combined M3, M4 DMMO, and silastic MTP2 implant. © Jean Yves Coillard 2015. All Rights Reserved

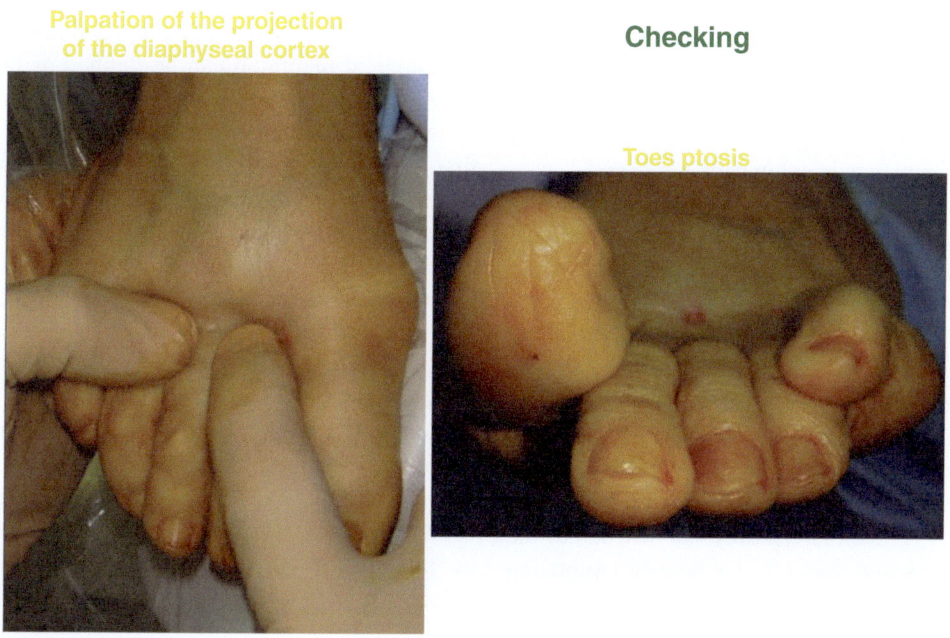

Fig. 25.17 Dramatic correction of second toe suppraductus can be achieved with DMMO. © Cyrille Cazeau 2015. All Rights Reserved

25.10 Specific Complications

We will only review the complications specific to DMMO.

The first specific complications are those inherent to the surgeon's learning curve. Skin burns, certainly the most frequent complication encountered by younger surgeons, must be immediately excised before closure; otherwise, there is a risk of having to deal with painstaking and ugly second-intention healing for several weeks.

One should also be aware of the possibility of *true* malunion due to the osteotomy being too proximal or the distal osteotomy not providing enough shortening.

The second type of specific complications is a consequence of minimally invasive surgery on the lateral metatarsals, for example, postoperative edema. This is partly the product of micromotion between fragments that persists for several weeks, until a fibrous callus locks the fragments together. This is not a serious complication, but it prevents the patient from wearing normal shoes for 2 or even 3 months.

Delayed union is also specific to non-fixed osteotomy procedures. Despite the absence of pain, a significant amount of time may elapse before a callus is visible on radiographs. Although we have observed this phenomenon regularly, we still do not have an explanation for it. We recommend doing nothing for 18 months, especially when the patient is not in pain.

Lastly, the third group of specific complications relates to true complications. By this, I mean nonunion, malunion, and synostosis.

True nonunion is rare. There is no sign of an initial bone callus; it remains painful and is accompanied by edema due to micromotion between fragments. On the contrary, most are tight nonunions, i.e., one that has a fibrous callus to stabilize the osteotomy site and limit edema and pain. Since these complaints are very rare, surgical revision is typically not scheduled; the surgeon should wait, not give in to the temptation of operating again (Fig. 25.18).

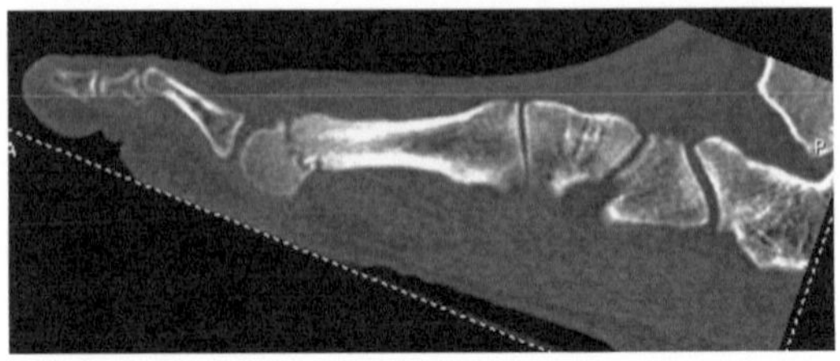

Fig. 25.18 M2 nonunion.

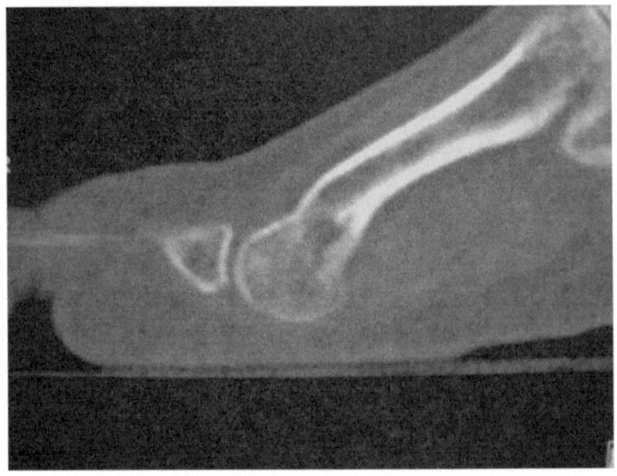

Fig. 25.19 Malunion in flexion.

It is difficult to describe a true malunion, since DMMO is a malunion by definition. A pathological malunion can be defined as bone union leading to direct (calluses) or indirect metatarsalgia (transfer metatarsalgia). In the first scenario, the cases we have encountered were due to insufficient displacement (under correction). The metatarsal head was jammed under the metatarsal neck, which had not been shortened enough. The logical consequence is recurrence of the plantar callus. The treatment consists of either a new minimally invasive osteotomy with intraoperative verification of sufficient shortening or performing an open technique. Indirect transfer metatarsalgia (overcorrection) could be due to excessive, overly proximal or isolated shortening. It must be treated with procedures on the impacted adjacent rays (Fig. 25.19).

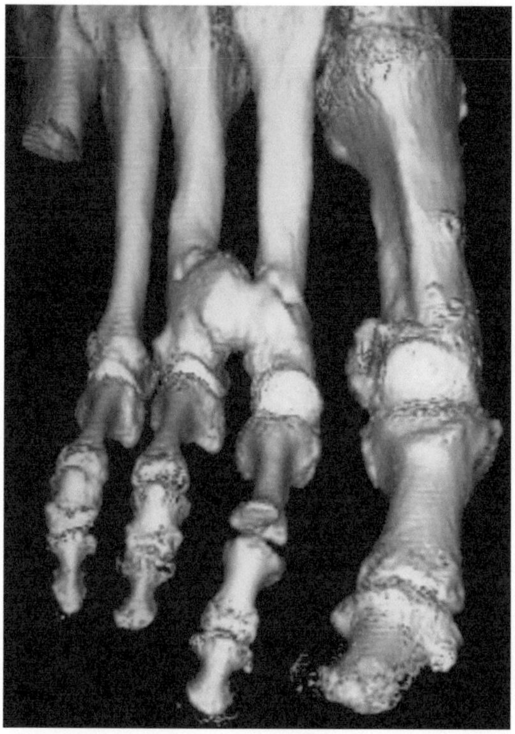

Fig. 25.20 Synostosis post-DMMO. © Jean Yves Coillard 2015. All Rights Reserved

Synostosis—a hypertrophic callus between two adjacent osteotomy sites—is very rare. If this bone bridge is painful, it can be easily excised like it would be for tarsal coalition (Fig. 25.20).

25.11 Postoperative Course

The postoperative course is straightforward and mainly depends on which procedures were done on the first ray. When done in isolation, the postoperative course for DMMO consists of the following:

- Regular medical follow-up for wound healing
- Immediate weight-bearing with partial unloading of the forefoot in the first days to limit pain and edema, which are consequences of micromotion at the osteotomy sites
- Standard analgesic and anticoagulant therapy based on the patient's risk factors
- Radiological monitoring until bone union is achieved

25.12 Conclusions

Percutaneous osteotomy of the lateral metatarsals is an invaluable option for the surgical treatment of mechanical metatarsalgia. The technique has been optimized, and its various modifications allow the DMMO to be adapted to every foot type. Complications are easy to manage. Published studies have confirmed the initial positive impression. Analyzing its problems has led to the development of useful technical modifications and confirmed the benefits of combining different procedures.

Sensing Without Seeing (C. Cazeau)

- Preloading in plantar flexion of the metatarsal head during the DMMO is accompanied by audible cracking when the last dorsal bone bridge gives way.
- DMMO is associated with metatarsal shortening and thus equal lengthening of the soft tissues. This is responsible for the initial, normal appearance of toe ptosis in the involved metatarsals (M2, M3, M4) (Fig. 25.21). This is a transient condition, which reverses itself within 21 days. The transient appearance of overlapping fifth toe is not a cause for concern; thus, tenotomy of the sole fifth ray extensor is ill-advised.
- After the procedure, direct palpation of the cortical dorsal diaphyseal projection of the metatarsal is proof the osteotomy was successful (Fig. 25.21).

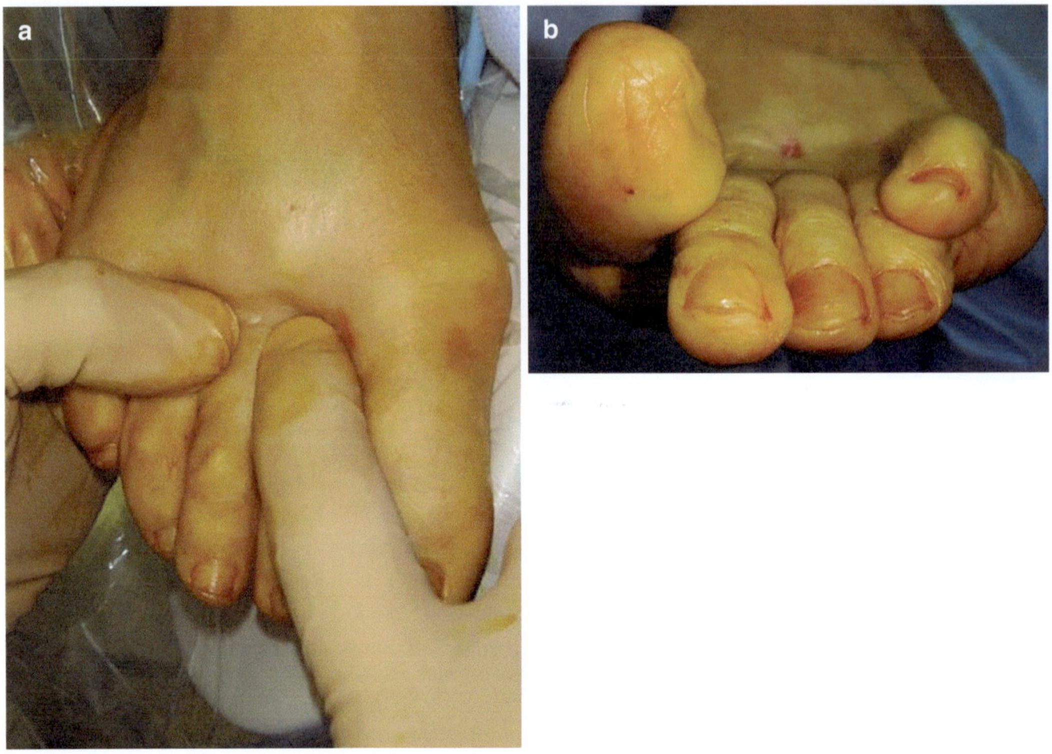

Fig. 25.21 (a) Palpation of the projection of the diaphyseal cortex; (b) toe ptosis. © Cyrille Cazeau 2015. All Rights Reserved

Editors' Point of View

DMMO is the queen of all percutaneous indications. It can be done early in one's learning curve, is easy to carry out, is fast, and generally does not cause MTP stiffness. It has many positive outcomes: suppression of metatarsalgia and correction of deviations or of second two supraductus. But it is critical that two types of mechanical loads be applied on the metatarsal heads immediately postoperative: a shortening force resulting from MPT flexion in the dressing and an elevation force due to the body's weight. The latter is more effective when gauze rolls are placed under the heads in the dressing to simulate the underhead element commonly found in insoles.

Suggested Reading

Cazeau C. Introduction. In: Cazeau C, editor. Chirurgie mini-invasive et percutanée du pied. Montpellier: Sauramps médical; 2009. p. 11–24.

Coillard J-Y. Traitement chirurgical des métatarsalgies statiques par ostéotomie mini-invasive (DMMO). In: Cazeau C, editor. Chirurgie mini-invasive et percutanée du pied. Montpellier: Sauramps médical; 2009. p. 127–34.

Darcel V, Villet L, Chauveaux D, Laffenêtre O. Prise en charge des métatarsalgies statiques par ostéotomies distales percutanées: suivi prospectif de 222 pieds. Monographie AFCP. Montpellier: Sauramps médical; 2009. p. 229–42.

Dhukaram V, Chapman AP, Upadhyay PK. Minimally invasive forefoot surgery: a cadaveric study. Foot Ankle Int. 2012;33:1139–44.

Henry J, Besse JL, Fessy MH, AFCP. Distal osteotomy of the lateral metatarsal: a series of 72 cases comparing the Weil osteotomy and the DMMO percutaneous osteotomy. Orthop Traumatol Surg Res. 2011;97(Suppl 6):57–65.

Roukis TS. Percutaneous and minimum incision metatarsal osteotomies: a systematic review. J Foot Ankle Surg. 2009;48:380–7.

Percutaneous Basal Elevation Osteotomy of the Metatarsals

26

Éric Toullec

26.1 Introduction

Basal elevation osteotomy of the metatarsals is best known as the BRT osteotomy because it was first described by L.S. Barouk, P. Rippstein, and E. Toullec in 2003 [1, 2].

Since the orientation of this osteotomy is opposite to the direction of the fixation screw, a sizeable approach is needed in an area of shoe contact, which can be detrimental. The principle of a dual percutaneous approach suitable for both procedures is attractive. However, since this is an experimental technique that has not been validated in a prospective clinical study, its indications are limited.

26.2 Principles of BRT Osteotomy

The BRT osteotomy is indicated for metatarsal elevation without shortening. The main indication is pes cavus with excessive plantar slope of the metatarsals.

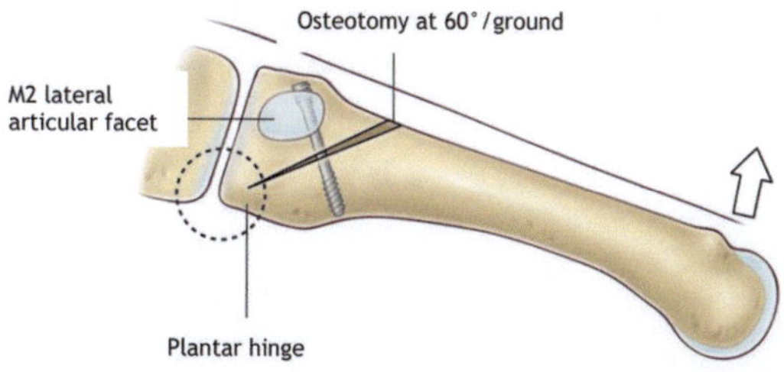

Fig. 26.1 BRT osteotomy in proximal metaphysis. © Éric Toullec 2015. All Rights Reserved

It is done in the proximal metaphysis area and requires that a plantar hinge be preserved to ensure stability (Figs. 26.1 and 26.5a). Correct burr positioning is essential to avoid damaging the intermetatarsal blood vessels and the intermetatarsal joints located on the dorsum of the metatarsal base.

A dorsal percutaneous approach could lead to the wrong metatarsal; for this reason, a fluoroscopy check is justified before performing the osteotomy.

We recommend performing the osteotomy on at least two or three metatarsals to prevent transfer metatarsalgia.

É. Toullec (✉)
Nouvelle Clinique Bordeaux Tondu, Floirac, France

C. Cazeau, Y. Stiglitz (eds.), *Percutaneous and Minimally Invasive Foot Surgery*,
https://doi.org/10.1007/978-3-030-98791-6_26

26.3 Percutaneous BRT Technique

The patient is positioned, so his foot rests on the fluoroscopy unit at the end of the table. We do not recommend using a tourniquet. Fluoroscopy is used to image the desired position of the metatarsal osteotomy by placing a Beaver blade or metal instrument in the field of view.

The incision is made with a Beaver blade in the middle of the metaphysis between the two extensors. Then, the lateral, medial, and dorsal sides of the metatarsal are roughened with a bone rasp. The burr (Shannon ∅2/L12 mm) is placed on the medial or lateral side of the metatarsal (Fig. 26.2) without going too deep. The burr is held at a 60° angle relative to the ground and 1.0–1.5 cm from the edge of the metatarsal base (Fig. 26.3). Unlike a DMMO, it is critical not to end up below the metatarsal because a plantar hinge must be preserved. Once the dorsal cut has been made, the possibility of metatarsal elevation is confirmed by pushing up under the metatarsal head. This displacement can also be verified on fluoroscopy.

If this displacement is not achieved, the burr is set a bit deeper in the middle of the osteotomy and the cut deepened by translating the burr medially to laterally. The procedure is repeated until enough metatarsal elevation is achieved (Fig. 26.4).

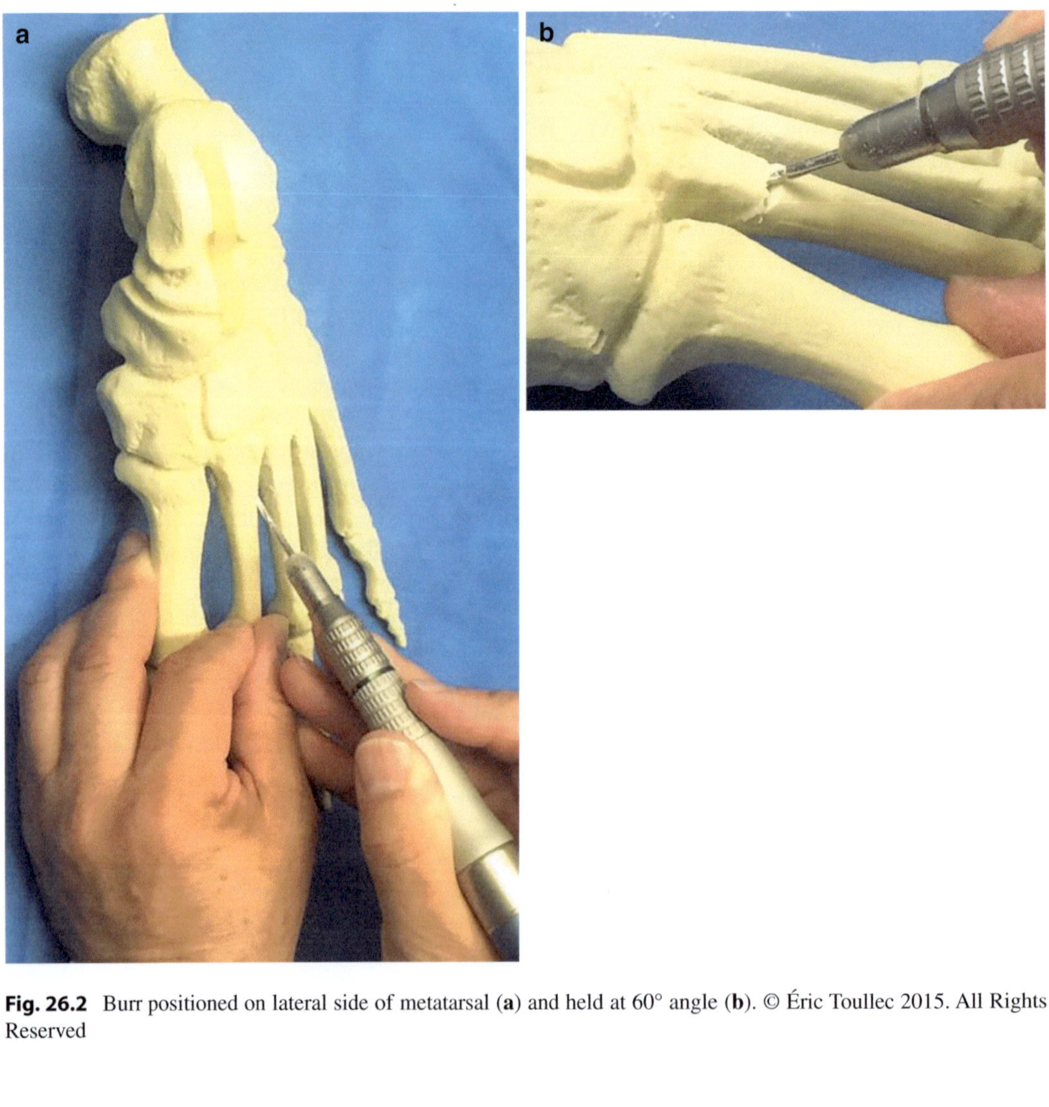

Fig. 26.2 Burr positioned on lateral side of metatarsal (**a**) and held at 60° angle (**b**).

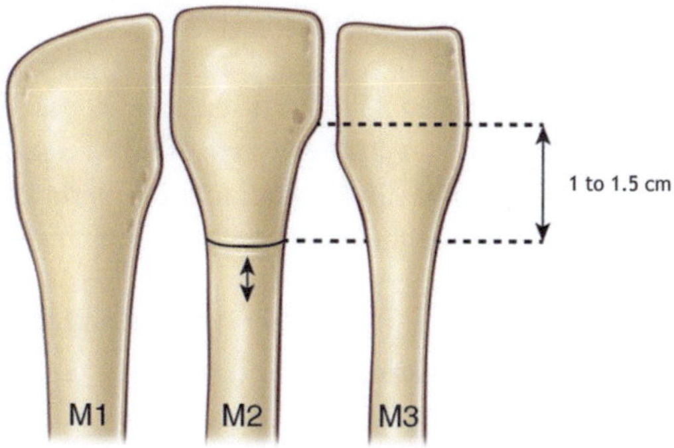

Fig. 26.3 Burr is positioned 1.0–1.5 cm from edge of metatarsal base. © Éric Toullec 2015. All Rights Reserved

Fixation is achieved with a dual-threaded 2.0- or 2.5-mm diameter screw (Fig. 26.5) inserted through a 1-cm miniature approach proximal to the dorsal portion of the osteotomy. The screw length is measured using a depth gauge over a K-wire as long as the surgeon's feels the opposite cortex, or by using fluoroscopy. The screw head must be fully embedded.

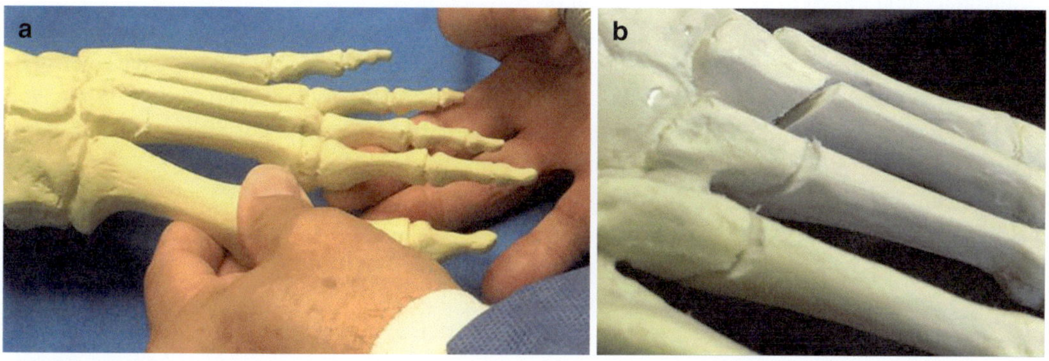

Fig. 26.4 Osteotomy cuts on the second, third, and fourth metatarsals (**a**); closing the osteotomy site will elevate the metatarsals (**b**). © Éric Toullec 2015. All Rights Reserved

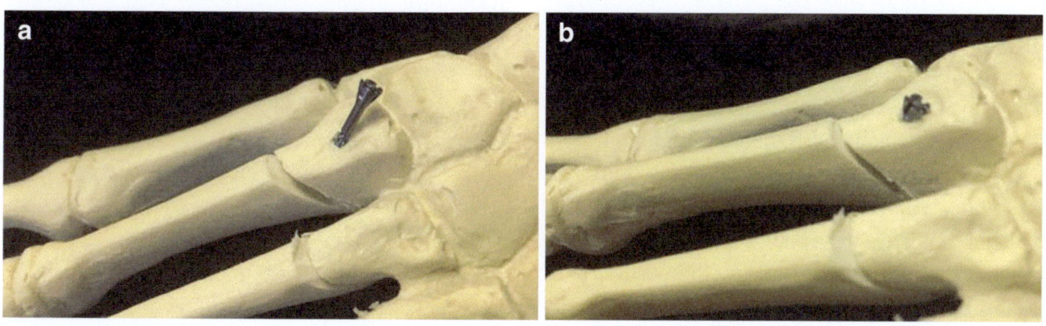

Fig. 26.5 Fixation with dual-threaded screw (**a**) with the head fully embedded (**b**). © Éric Toullec 2015. All Rights Reserved

26.4 Postoperative Course and Complications

Weight-bearing is allowed in a heel-contact shoe that unloads the forefoot for a minimum of 15 days. The initial dressing has a compressive action to limit hematoma development on the dorsum of the foot.

Among potential complications, a dorsal hematoma can interfere with wearing shoes and can also cause paresthesia in the territory of the superficial peroneal nerve or toe stiffness due to extensor tendon adhesions.

Incorrect setting of the osteotomy with transfer metatarsalgia linked to excessive elevation or recurrence of the excess plantar pressure due to insufficient elevation mostly occurs when the osteotomy was performed only on one ray.

Delayed union or nonunion occur in cases of plantar hinge fracture, overly distal osteotomy, overly distal screw placement, or poor pressure distribution. While the usual treatment is to redo the osteotomy and fixation with potential bone grafting, performing an osteotomy of one or more neighboring rays and temporary transverse pinning are also satisfactory solutions.

26.5 Discussion

26.5.1 Burr or Saw?

The development of minimally invasive techniques has gone hand-in-hand with the use of burrs. However, some surgeons prefer doing the osteotomy with a thin saw through a miniature incision. It is certainly easier to approach the metatarsal from the front with a saw than with a burr during BRT osteotomy. Also, since the distal elevation is multiplied threefold for the second metatarsal, it is more accurate with a 0.4-mm saw blade than a 2-mm burr.

26.5.2 Fixation or no Fixation?

Fixation requires an additional surgical approach with its associated risks: hematoma, screw migration or protrusion, and irritation of superficial peroneal nerve. On the other hand, the construct's stability and accuracy of the elevation appear to be more reliable with fixation. If no fixation is used, then stabilization with dressings or taping and a partial unloading shoe (with enough pressure to elevate the metatarsal heads) is needed.

26.5.3 BRT Indications

The BRT osteotomy is indicated in patients with excessive metatarsal slope in pes cavus, perforating ulcer of the foot, second ray syndrome, and certain cases of primary, post-traumatic, or iatrogenic metatarsalgia.

26.6 Conclusion

The BRT osteotomy is indicated for excess plantar slope of the first metatarsal and can be performed percutaneously with fewer wound healing risks. However, it requires ample training to avoid fracturing the plantar hinge that is crucial to stability.

Sensing Without Seeing (C. Cazeau)

It is fairly easy to make the metaphyseal plantar hinge; it is executed in the same way as in other percutaneous surgery sites. It is easy to alternate between the feelings of cortical osteotomy, then medullary, and then cortical while detecting the burr stopping against the intramedullary face of the hinge. However, in the percutaneous technique, it is impossible to directly view the dorsal bone resection area being closed during reduction maneuvers. As an indirect cue, it feels like the metatarsal head is missing on the plantar aspect. One must be vigilant when inserting the screw to make sure the head is completely buried, especially since the dorsal metatarsal base is subcutaneous.

Editors' Point of View

This basal elevation osteotomy for the metatarsals has proven itself over time. It is easiest to do percutaneously while preserving the plantar hinge. Fixation is not essential if immediate full weight-bearing is achieved.

References

1. Toullec E, Barouk LS, Rippstein P Ostéotomie de relèvement basal métatarsien BRT. Chirurgie de l'avant-pied. In: Valtin B, Leemrijse TH, editors. Cahier d'enseignement de la SOFCOT 2005. Paris: Elsevier; 2005. pp. 142–148.
2. Barouk LS. The BRT new proximal metatarsal osteotomy. In: Barouk LS, editor. Forefoot reconstruction. Paris: Springer; 2003. pp. 139–154.

Percutaneous Surgery for Bunionette

27

Eduard Rabat

27.1 Introduction

A bunionette is a very common deformity that involves the lateral side of the foot. It is particularly painful because it rubs inside footwear. This condition mainly affects women.

This deformity has several names, depending on the language, with most taking a cue from the similarities with hallux valgus. Also known as Tailor's bunion, it makes a historical reference to the cross-legged seated position on the ground of tailors, leading to direct impingement with the head of the fifth metatarsal.

In our opinion, the percutaneous surgical treatment described in this chapter is an indisputable indication given how simple it is to execute and how effective it is.

27.2 Description

The standard presentation is a bump at the head of the fifth metatarsal that is red and swollen from shoe rubbing (Fig. 27.1).

Four anatomical elements contribute to the pathology to varying extents (Fig. 27.2):

1. The intermetatarsal angle is increased between the fourth and fifth ray.

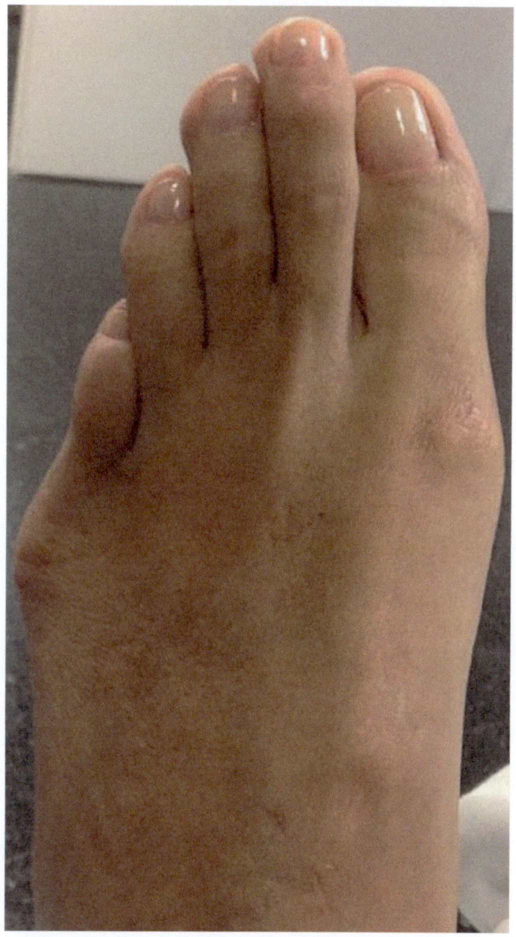

Fig. 27.1 Clinical presentation of bunionette. © Eduard Rabat 2015. All Rights Reserved

E. Rabat (✉)
Hospital Quirónsalud, Barcelona, Spain
e-mail: erabat@doctor-rabat.net

C. Cazeau, Y. Stiglitz (eds.), *Percutaneous and Minimally Invasive Foot Surgery*,
https://doi.org/10.1007/978-3-030-98791-6_27

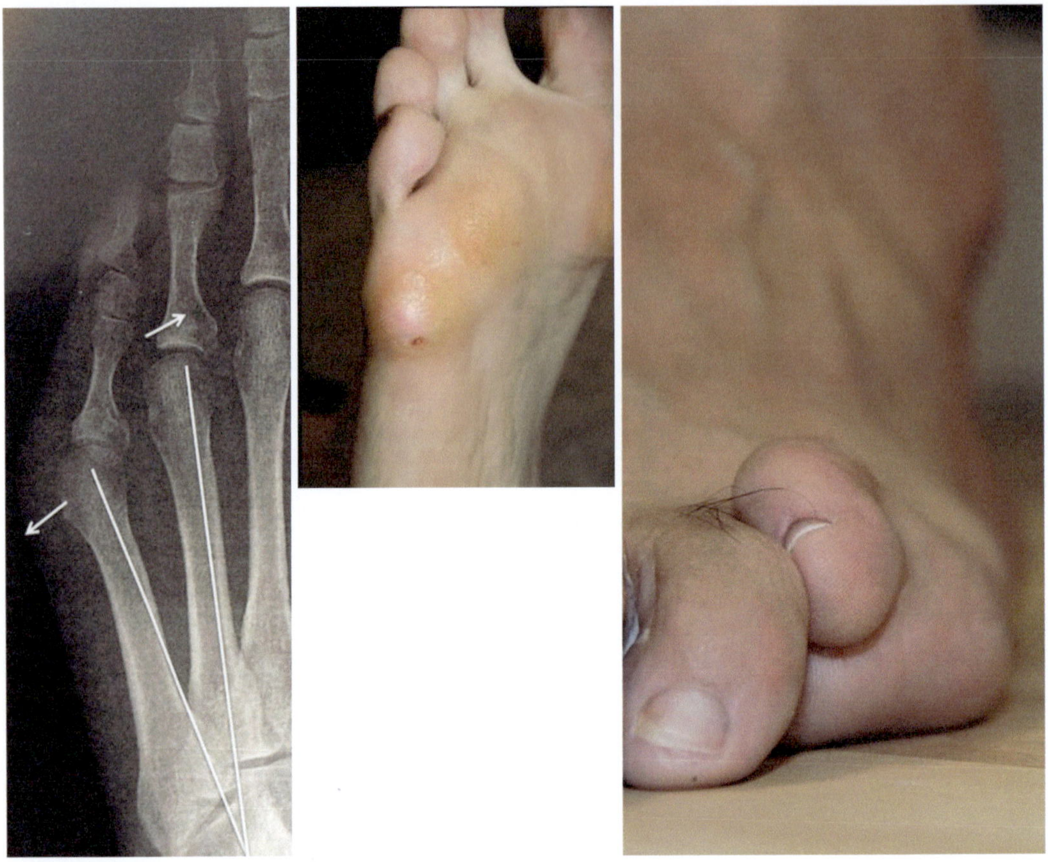

Fig. 27.2 Anatomical contributors to bunionette.

2. Development of an exostosis on the lateral side of the head of the fifth metatarsal
3. Varus position of the fifth toe
4. In some cases, painful hyperkeratosis is found under the head of the fifth metatarsal (M5).

A claw toe is also visible is some cases.

Coughlin described three types of bunionette (Fig. 27.3).

- Type 1: hypertrophy of the M5 head
- Type 2: lateral M5 deviation (bowing)
- Type 3: M4–M5 angle greater than 9°

The following are evaluated on radiographs:

- Size of the M5 head
- M4–M5 intermetatarsal angle
- Lateral deviation angle of M5 head

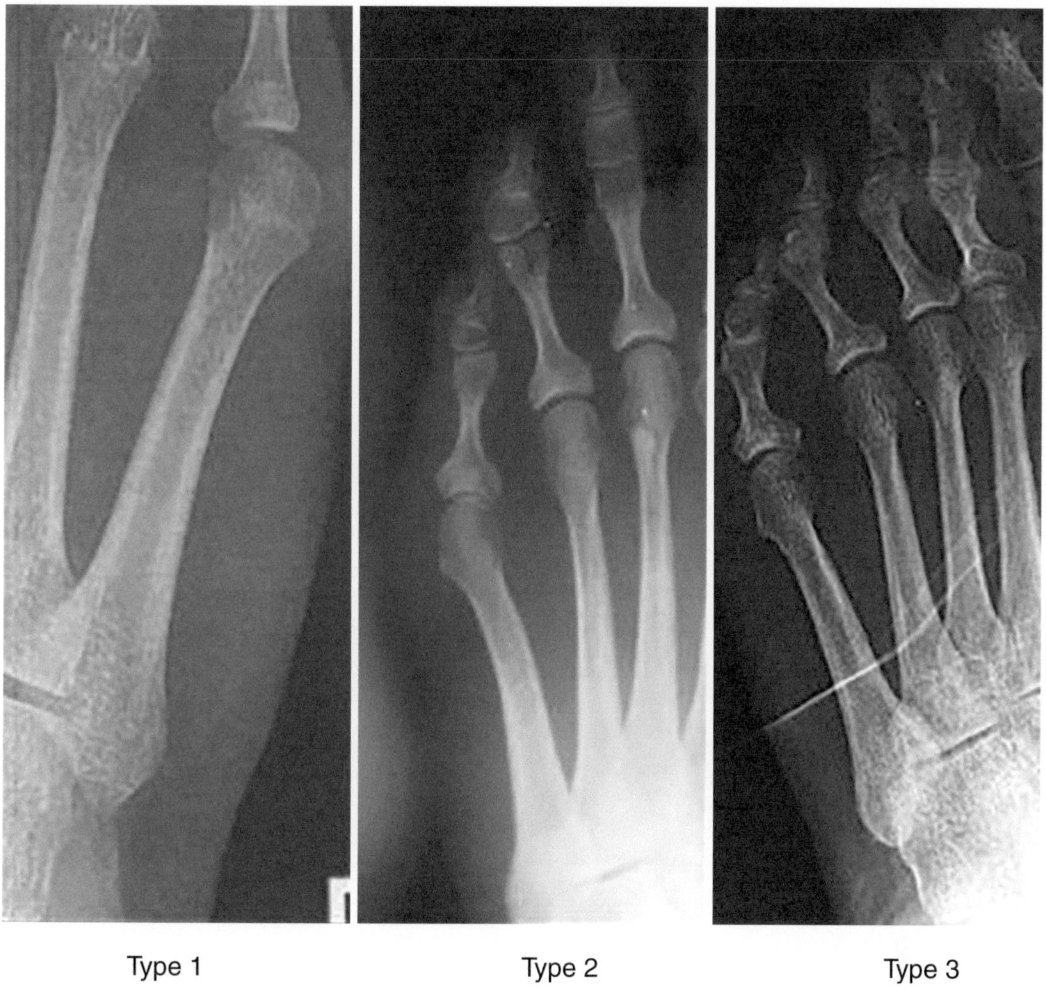

Fig. 27.3 Coughlin classification for bunionette. Type 1: large M5 head; Type 2: bowing metatarsal; Type 3: large M4–M5 intermetatarsal angle.

27.3 Main Surgical Procedures Used

27.3.1 Standard Technique: Procedures on Fifth Metatarsal

The core procedure consists of M5 osteotomy, which can be either proximal, distal, or diaphyseal.

We recommend doing an osteotomy of the distal third of M5, which allows every type of deformity to be corrected without bone fixation, unlike a proximal osteotomy which has a risk of secondary displacement thus requires fixation (Fig. 27.4).

We only perform diaphyseal osteotomy when treating plantar diabetic ulcers allowing considerable elevation of M5. While it may be excessive, given the seriousness of the condition, it allows for healing without any bone union problems (Fig. 27.5).

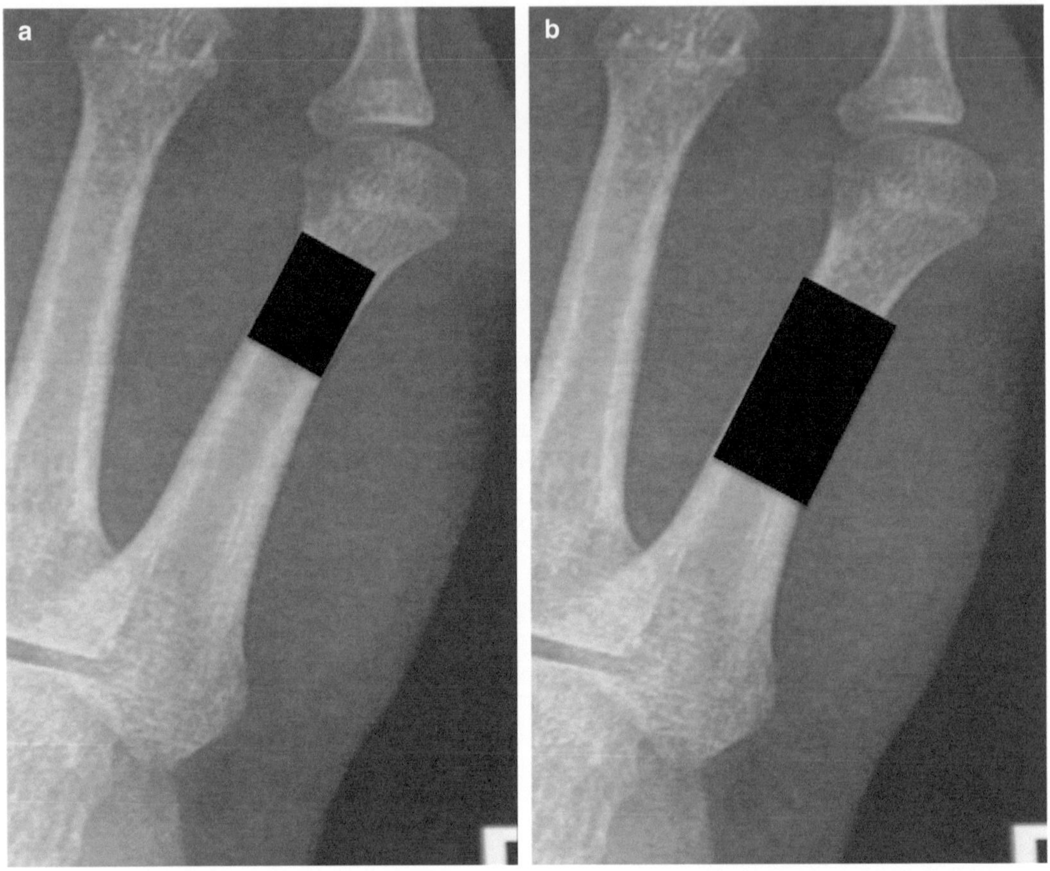

Fig. 27.4 Location of osteotomy at the distal third of M5 (**a**) and in its more proximal portion (**b**). © Eduard Rabat 2015. All Rights Reserved

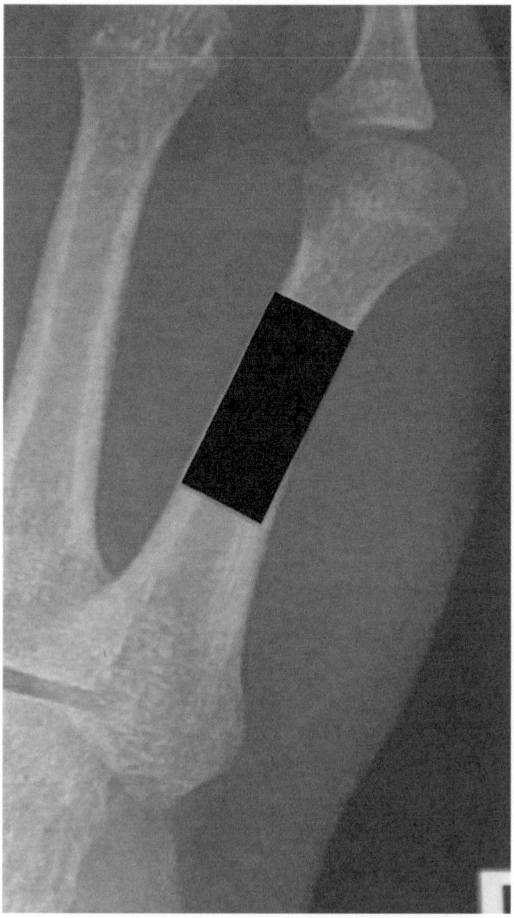

Fig. 27.5 Diaphyseal osteotomy for treating plantar diabetic ulcers. © Eduard Rabat 2015. All Rights Reserved

27.3.2 Potential Additional Surgical Procedures

Exostectomy and osteotomy of the base of the proximal phalanx of the fifth toe and medial soft tissue release can be performed as needed.

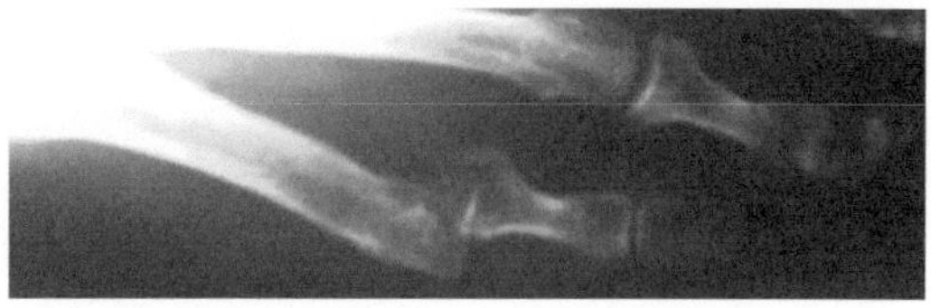

Fig. 27.6 Dislocation of fifth metatarsophalangeal joint. © Eduard Rabat 2015. All Rights Reserved

27.3.2.1 Exostectomy

This surgical procedure is useless in most cases, given that the M5 osteotomy is performed distally. This corresponds to Coughlin stage 1, which combines an enlarged metatarsal head with a small M4–M5 angle. Lateral rubbing in shoes is eliminated. One must be careful not to overdo it, as this can result in dislocation of the fifth metatarsophalangeal joint (Fig. 27.6). The latter is even more difficult to treat when medial soft tissue release has been done.

Dis

27.3.2.2 Closing Wedge Osteotomy of the Proximal Phalanx Base

This is often called an "Akinette" given its resemblance with the Akin osteotomy for hallux valgus. This procedure is very useful in most cases, not only because it improves the foot's appearance but because it also separates the fourth and fifth toes, preventing the development of corn between these toes (Fig. 27.7).

27.3.2.3 Medial Soft Tissue Release

We believe this procedure is also useless. The M5 osteotomy completely corrects the deformity;

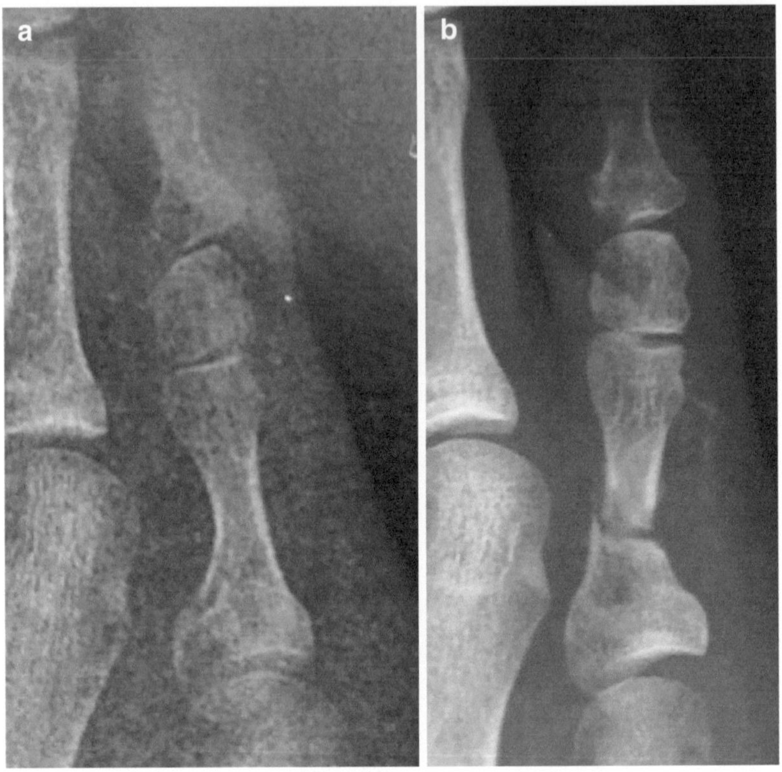

Fig. 27.7 Preoperative (**a**) and postoperative view of percutaneous unfixed Akinette osteotomy (**b**). © Eduard Rabat 2015. All Rights Reserved

thus any soft tissue release increases the risk of dislocation, especially if exostectomy was also performed.

27.4 Surgical Technique

All these techniques have been described by Mariano de Prado. The principles that he set out must be followed closely.

27.4.1 Osteotomy at Distal Third of M5

While the osteotomy site is in the distal third of the bone, the exact location of the procedure will depend on the nature of the deformity.

In cases of a large intermetatarsal angle (Couglin type 3) or fifth toe bowing (type 2), the osteotomy is made in the most proximal part of the distal third. For a lesser deformity, it can be done more distally.

The broad "distal third" concept allows this procedure to the adapted to all the pathological situations encountered.

In particular, it is possible to induce varus in M5 and to elevate it by removing the painful plantar callus. This also means that M5 does not need to be shortened, thereby preventing load transfer to M4 and resolving intertoe callus problems.

We perform this using a long Shannon burr (12 × 2 mm) with fluoroscopy guidance.

The approach starts by making a small 0.5-cm incision in the fourth intermetatarsal space, medial to the M5 head, immediately behind the interdigital space, and then driving the blade down until it contacts the medial side of M5. Like is typically done in percutaneous surgery, a working space is created with an elevator (Fig. 27.8).

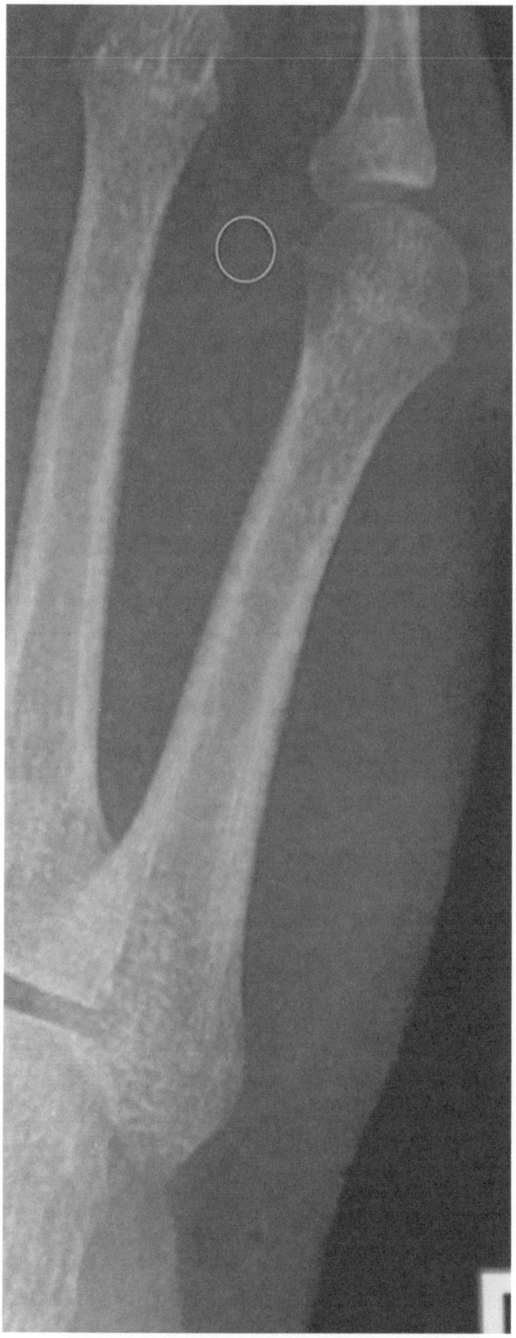

Fig. 27.8 Approach for distal third osteotomy. © Eduard Rabat 2015. All Rights Reserved

The osteotomy consists of a mediolateral plantar oblique cut, always starting under the M5 head.

This procedure results in a medial closing wedge, which corrects the metatarsus valgus. A lateral bone hinge can be preserved, or a full osteotomy done to achieve greater correction (Fig. 27.9).

It is important to remove the bone debris produced by the osteotomy.

27.4.2 Closing Wedge Osteotomy at the Base of Proximal Phalanx

Here, a short Shannon burr is used (8 × 2 mm). The approach is located dorsolateral or plantar midline. If the patient has a fifth claw toe, we also perform tenotomy of the flexors, thus carry out a transverse osteotomy. In all other cases, a dorsolateral approach is used. The osteotomy cut is made lateral to medial to produce a closing wedge and correct the deformity. The bone wall on the opposite cortex may or may not be retained (Fig. 27.10).

27.4.3 Exostectomy

An incision is made between the dorsal and planter skin behind the M5 head by inserting a Beaver blade through the bursa until it contacts the bone, and then the working space is created with an elevator. A gradual back-and-forth maneuver is used with a Shannon burr. The dorsal side of the head must not be forgotten, as it also rubs in footwear.

With the techniques described above, excellent correction can be achieved in all cases.

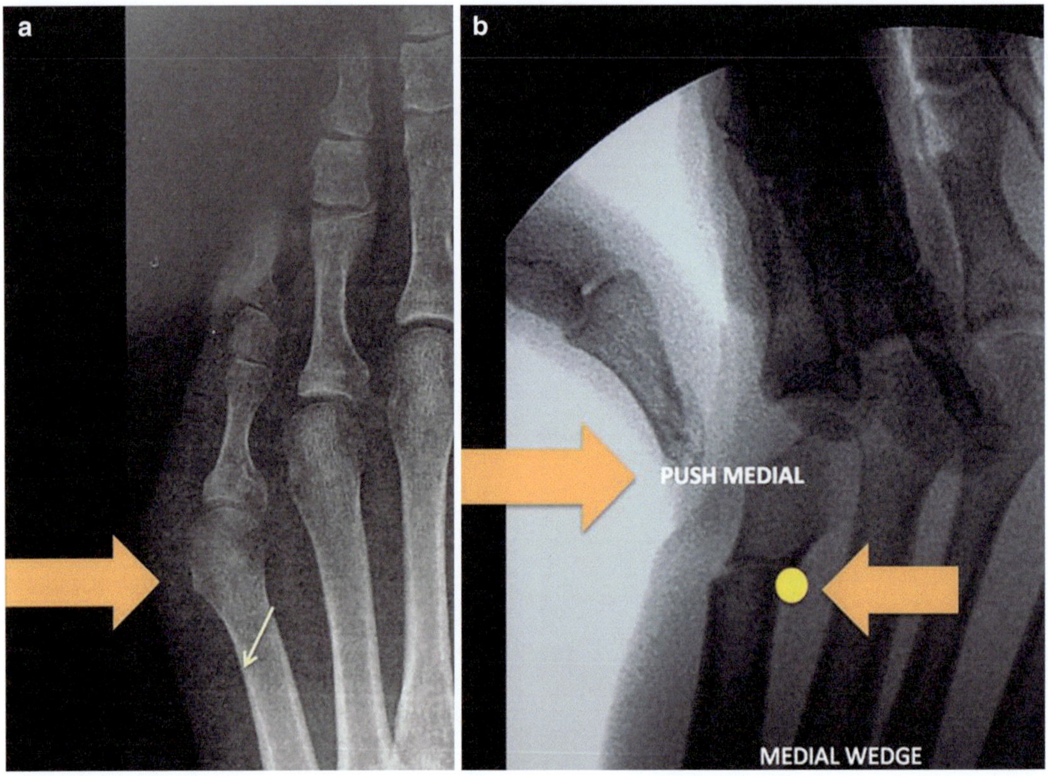

Fig. 27.9 Location of planned osteotomy (**a**) and fluoroscopy view of medial closing wedge osteotomy being performed (**b**).

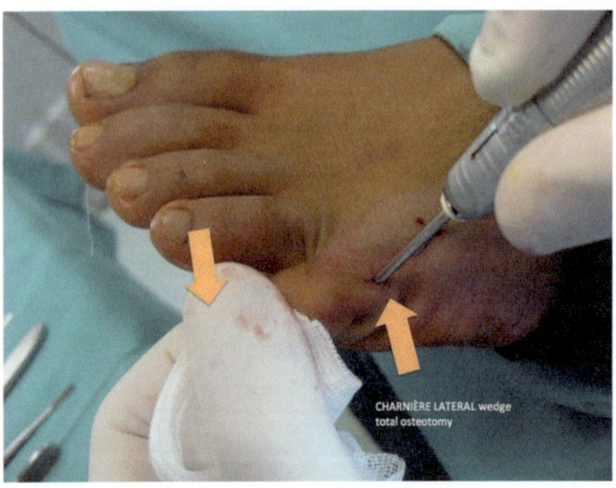

Fig. 27.10 Medial closing wedge osteotomy and lateral mobilization of the fifth toe.

27.5 Postoperative Care

The initial postoperative dressing holds M5 and the fifth toe; it is worn for 1 week. Immediate full weight-bearing is allowed using a flat rigid-soled postoperative shoe.

The sutures are then removed. A new dressing is applied to immobilize M5 transversely and to immobilize the fifth toe in an appropriate position using compresses placed in an angled overlap configuration (Fig. 27.11).

This bandage will be worn until week 4, at which point the patient will be allowed to wear comfortable street shoes.

Bone union occurs during the second month on average; until this occurs, the patient may feel slight but non-disabling pain at the bone callus. Nonunion is very rare.After 3 months, the patient can resume all sports activities.

Editors' Point of View

This is another surgical indication that is better suited to percutaneous than open surgery. Fixation is not essential if M5 is shortened and full weight-bearing is encouraged.

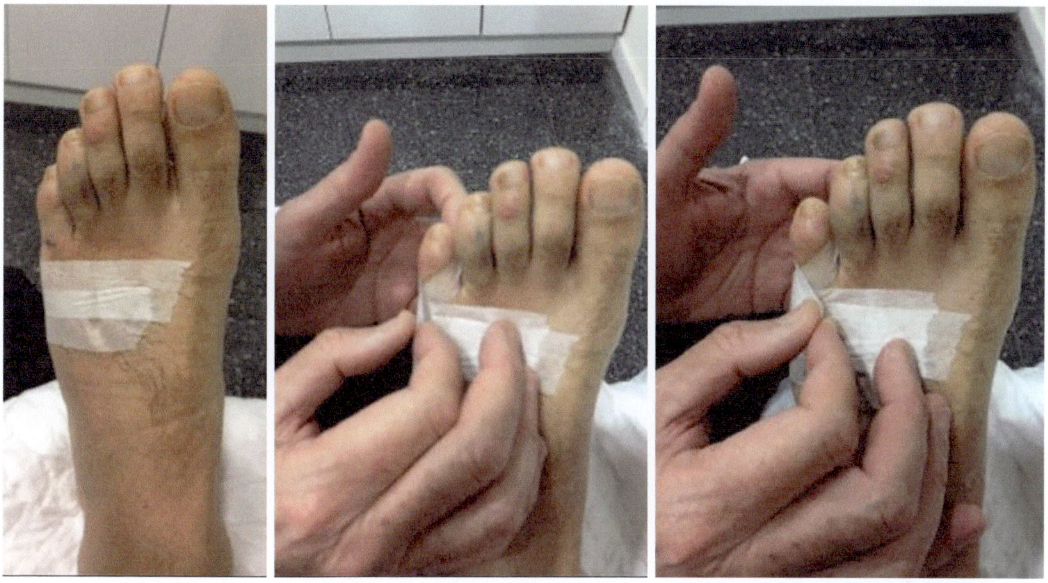

Fig. 27.11 Dressing applied to immobilize M5 and the fifth toe. © Eduard Rabat 2015. All Rights Reserved

Percutaneous Treatment of Fifth Ray Deformities (Other Than Bunionette)

28

Eduard Rabat and Olivier Laffenêtre

We will describe the percutaneous treatment of the following deformities: fifth toe supraductus and infraductus varus, fifth hammer and claw toe, and soft corns between toes. Percutaneous bunionette surgery is featured a dedicated chapter of this book.

28.1 Anatomical Considerations

The fifth ray consists of three phalanxes: proximal, middle, and distal. The latter two are often fused.

While the anatomy of the fifth toe resembles that of the other toes, there are a few important differences. First, it has no extensor digitorum brevis tendon. Second, it has a muscle that the other three lateral toes do not—the abductor digit quinti—which inserts distally on the lateral part of the base of the proximal phalanx (it is analogous to the abductor hallucis). Lastly, there are no dorsal interossei muscles; however, there is a plantar interossei muscle—the third one—that inserts on the plantar and medial side of the base of the proximal phalanx. All these attachments on the base of the phalanx means that contracture of the extensor digitorum longus in dorsiflexion also contributes to contracture of the flexor digitorum longus and brevis and thereby to claw toe development (Fig. 28.1).

E. Rabat (✉)
Hospital Quirónsalud, Barcelona, Spain
e-mail: erabat@doctor-rabat.net

O. Laffenêtre
Institut de la Cheville et du Pied, Paris, France

C. Cazeau, Y. Stiglitz (eds.), *Percutaneous and Minimally Invasive Foot Surgery*,
https://doi.org/10.1007/978-3-030-98791-6_28

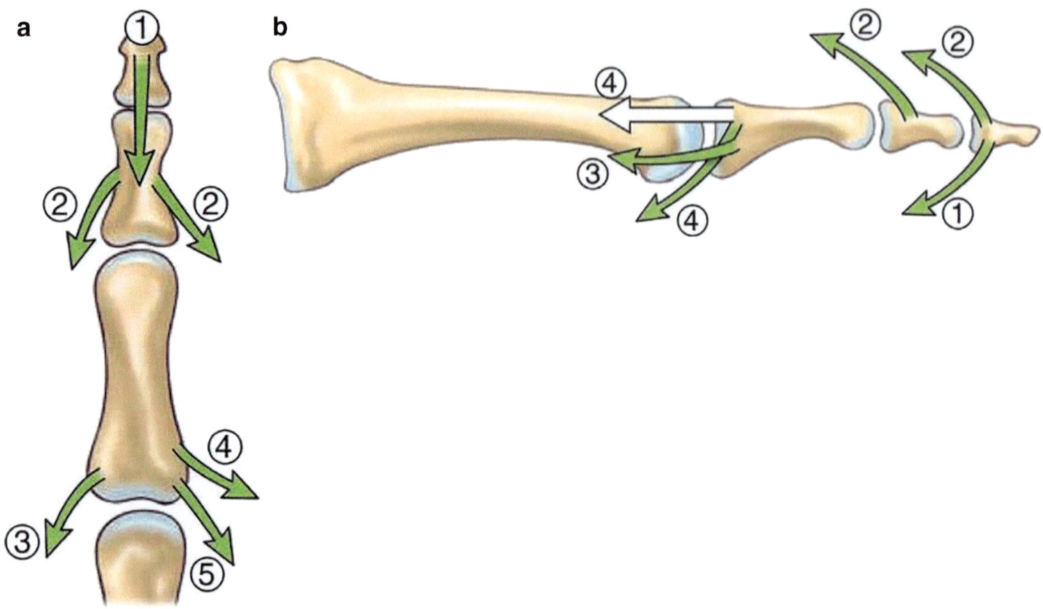

Fig. 28.1 Tendon insertions on the fifth toe. Plantar view (**a**); lateral view (**b**). © Eduard Rabat 2015. All Rights Reserved

28.2 General Parameters

The fifth ray deformities described in this chapter are the least disputed indications for percutaneous surgery, making it an appealing option, especially for surgeons who do not use these techniques to treat other forefoot deformities.

However, it does not mean this surgery ignores the general rules of foot surgery, and even less, those of percutaneous surgery. We are required to evaluate each case independently and not to apply the same treatment to every patient, especially that the deforming forces are not always the same.

During the all-important clinical examination of the foot, one cannot ignore the remainder of the forefoot nor the hindfoot. We already know that many cases of fifth ray pain are due to a problem at the first ray such as hallux rigidus or other conditions that cause patients to walk with more foot supination to relieve their pain. As for the hindfoot, it is typically varus that overloads the fifth ray, although this can be treated surgically at the forefoot.

Most of these cases can be easily resolved; however, the most severe cases tend to recur and become quite challenging for orthopedic surgeons to treat.

Let's take a historical detour. During the first half of the twentieth century, the most common treatment for severe fifth toe deformities, or even that of the middle toes, was amputation. In some cases, this procedure was performed at birth to treat overriding fifth toe, which was well tolerated from a mechanical point of view.

Thanks to research by Dr. J.C. Gonzalez-Casanovas, we now have access to a historical document—the keynote speech given by Dr. Alvaro Esquerdo at the Royal College of Surgery of Barcelona in 1897 titled *Conservative Foot Surgery* in which he brilliantly summarizes the ideas of that era related to surgery of the foot and lesser toes. He said:

> Diseases, trauma or neoplasia of the fingers of the foot can require a sacrifice. While in some instances I did a resection or grinded down the irritated phalanges to preserve the shape of the foot, I am now convinced that procedures requiring a high degree of surgical skill are not necessarily in the

best interest of the patient... due to slow healing... because ankylosis may develop... it is difficult to avoid deviations... this may make it uncomfortable to wear shoes or walk. Not having one toe, even if it is not the big toe... or even two toes... does not hinder walking...

28.2.1 Basic Surgical Techniques

We will describe the most used percutaneous techniques.

28.2.1.1 Soft Tissues

This consists of tenotomy of the extensor digitorum longus (Fig. 28.2) and flexor digitorum longus and brevis of the fifth toe (Fig. 28.3) and metatarsophalangeal capsulotomy.

28.2.1.2 Exostectomy

Dorsal cheilectomy (Fig. 28.4) is performed at the proximal interphalangeal joint for fifth toe varus, dorsal exostosis of the fifth toe, and interdigital callus.

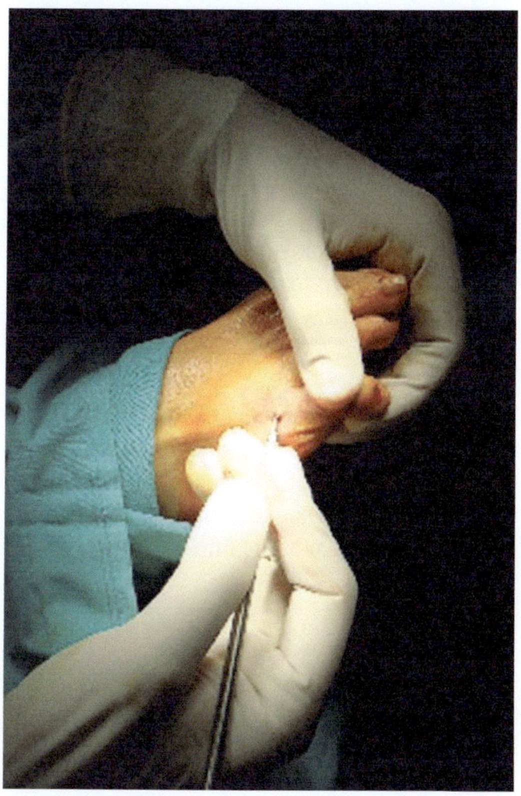

Fig. 28.2 Tenotomy/capsulotomy of the extensor digitorum longus.

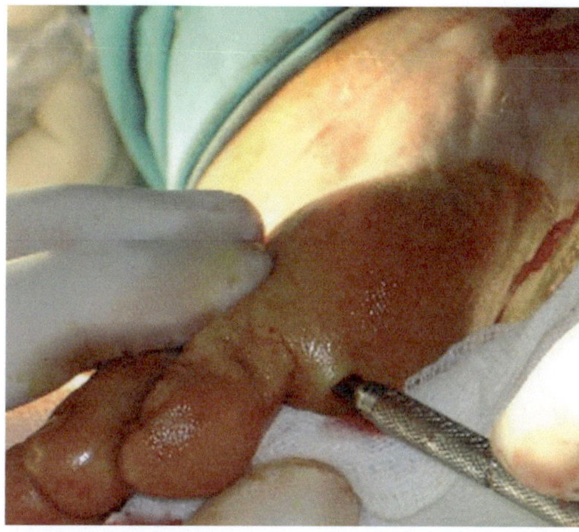

Fig. 28.3 Tenotomy of the flexor digitorum longus and brevis.

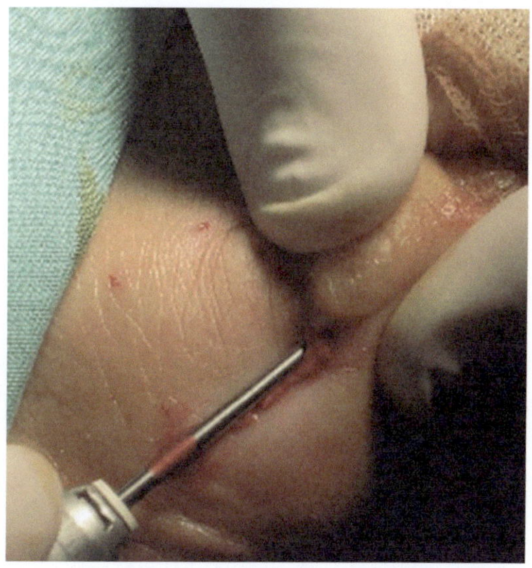

Fig. 28.4 Dorsal cheilectomy of the fifth toe.

28.2.1.3 Osteotomy

Osteotomy of the proximal phalanx of the fifth toe (Fig. 28.5) may consist of a plantar closing wedge to produce toe flexion, or dorsal wedge to elevate it. Any of these can be combined with a lateralization procedure when the toe is in valgus.

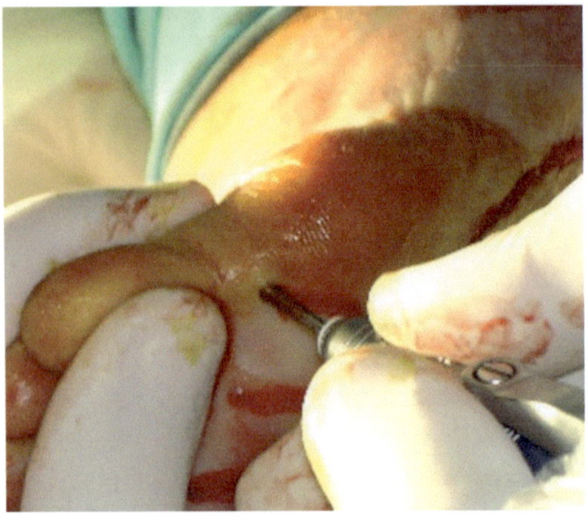

Fig. 28.5 Osteotomy of the base of the proximal phalanx.

Distal shortening osteotomy of the fifth metatarsal, in cases where excessive length requires complete correction of a hammer toe, is the only type of osteotomy that we perform at this level.

28.2.2 Powered Tools: Burrs and Instruments

The specific tools and instruments described in a previous chapter of this book are required. We use a short Shannon burr for proximal phalanx osteotomy and corn removal procedures on the dorsal side of the toe. A straight Shannon burr is used for distal osteotomy of the fifth metatarsal.

28.3 Fifth Toe Supraductus Varus

Fifth toe supraductus varus is typically a congenital deformity (overriding fifth toe) although it can also have a postural origin. It is important to highlight that, in the first 3 months of life, excellent correction can be achieved by simply applying Steri-Strip™ adhesive skin closures.

The architect of the deformity is the extensor digitorum longus (Fig. 28.6), which applies traction dorsally and medially; its contracture is propagated to the dorsal metatarsophalangeal joint capsule and to the skin itself.

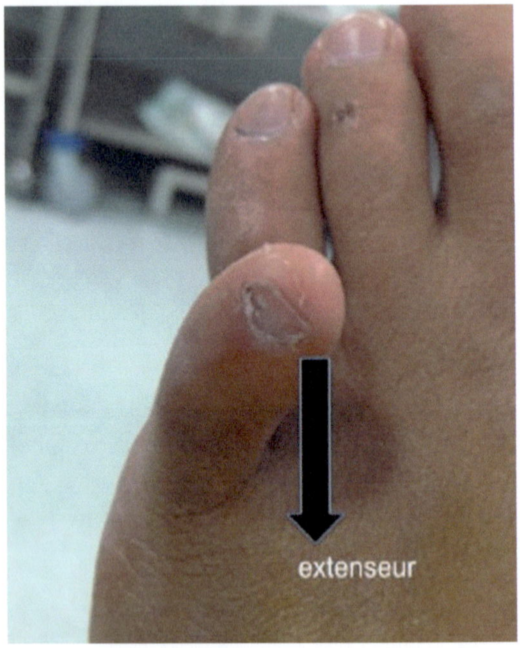

Fig. 28.6 Fifth toe supraductus varus.

28.3.1 Percutaneous Treatment

We use the following strategy to return (lower) the toe to its natural position:

- Tenotomy of extensor digitorum longus
- Dorsal capsulotomy
- Osteotomy of proximal phalanx, with lateral plantar base (lowering and valgus-producing effects)

In some cases, tenotomy of the flexor digitorum longus and brevis can be used to correct the deformity. In cases of recurrence or that are difficult to correct, a plantar skin graft can be used to lengthen the base of the fifth toe.

28.3.2 Dressings

The postoperative dressings are crucial as with any percutaneous surgery. They must hold the toe in its new position and isolate it from the neighboring toes if other procedures were done on the

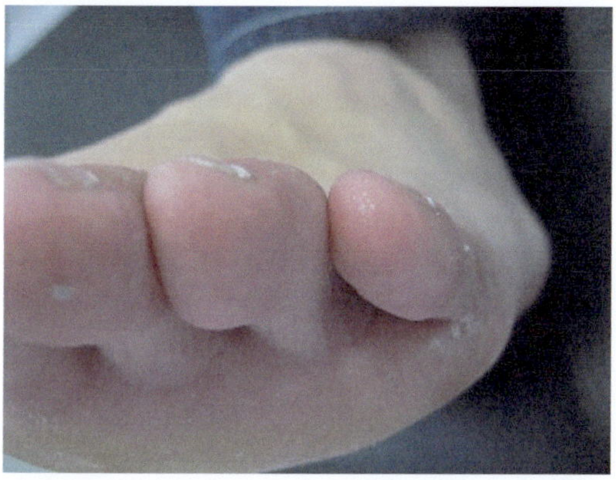

Fig. 28.7 Results of percutaneous treatment of fifth toe supraductus varus.

forefoot. Surgical dressings will be used for at least 1 month to allow the osteotomy to heal (Fig. 28.7).

28.4 Fifth Toe Infraductus Varus

The infraductus version of the varus deformity is less common (Fig. 28.8). It is often congenital, but we also see it occur concurrently with other (severe) deformities of the same forefoot.

The main initiators are the flexor digitorum longus and brevis tendons of the fifth toe that have been contracted for many years in an infraductus position passing under the fourth toe (Figs. 28.9 and 28.10).

28.4.1 Percutaneous Treatment

Percutaneous treatment (Fig. 28.11) consists of the following:

- Tenotomy of the flexor digitorum longus and brevis tendons of the fifth toe
- Osteotomy of the proximal phalanx of the fifth toe with a dorsal and lateral base (elevation and valgus-producing effects)

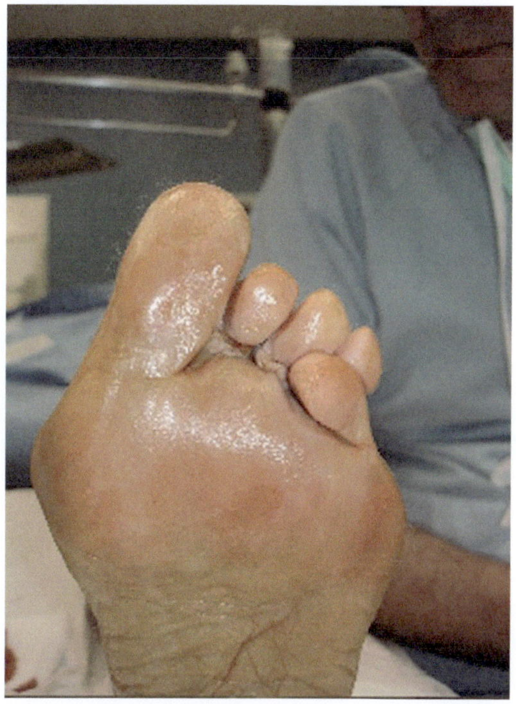

Fig. 28.8 Fifth toe infraductus varus.

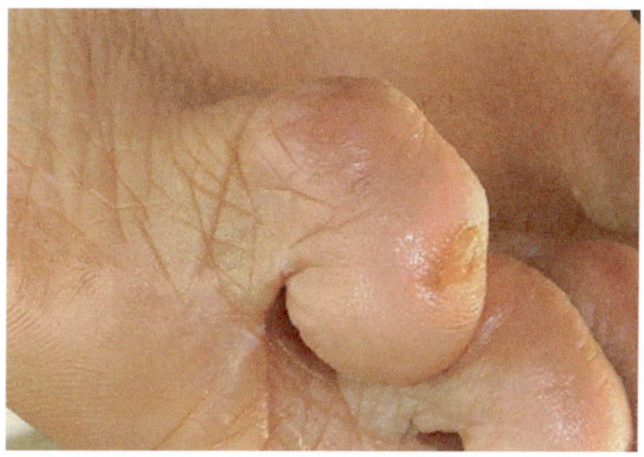

Fig. 28.9 Elements contributing to the deformity.

28.4.2 Dressings

It is the same principles as described above.

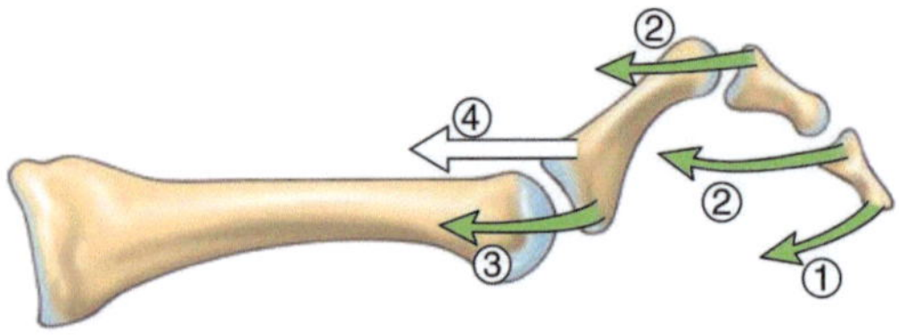

Fig. 28.10 Elements contributing to the deformity.

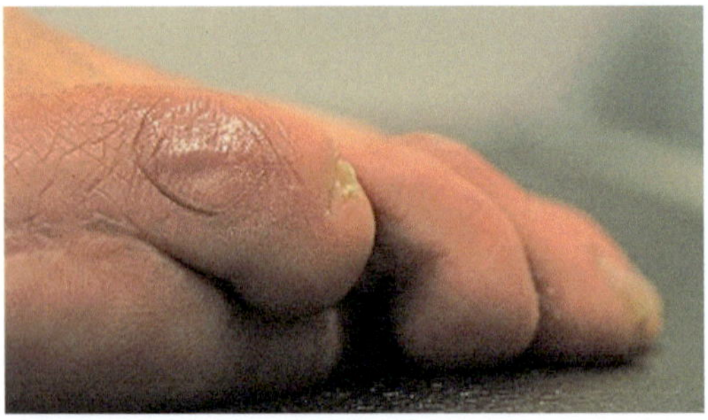

Fig. 28.11 Results of percutaneous treatment.

28.5 Fifth Hammer and Claw Toe

This is one of the most common toe deformities and also one of the most painful because the toe rubs on the lateral part of shoes. This deformity may not respond to treatment, especially if all the forces that contributed to the deformity are not eliminated. It is vital to look at the fifth toe's length; when it is very long, it acts as a triggering factor because it generates tendon contracture and because reduces space, made worse by narrow shoes.

The main initiator is contracture of the extensor digitorum longus, which impacts the distal and middle phalanges. As this action gets worse, the third plantar interossei muscle contributes to dorsiflexion of the toe. This brings on gradual contracture of the flexor digitorum longus and brevis, which is a consistent finding in the most severe cases.

Clinical examination of the patient and determining the degree of toe flexibility while looking for flexor contracture are very important.

28.5.1 Percutaneous Treatment

Without Flexor Contracture

1. Tenotomy of the extensor digitorum longus combined with wide capsulotomy including the interossei muscle
2. Proximal osteotomy of the proximal phalanx with plantar base to lower the toe and reposition it correctly
3. Dorsal exostectomy

   In this presentation, the flexor digitorum longus and brevis contribute to the lowering; thus it is not logical to perform tenotomy on them.

With Flexor Contracture

1. Tenotomy of the extensor digitorum longus and capsulotomy
2. Tenotomy of the flexor digitorum longus and brevis
3. Dorsal exostectomy
4. Proximal phalanx osteotomy with plantar base (short Shannon burr)

Persistent Dorsal Subluxation

In the rare instance when the dorsal subluxation persists, it means the fifth metatarsal and the fifth toe are too long. A percutaneous distal oblique osteotomy, from dorsal-distal to plantar-proximal, may need to be done to shorten the fifth metatarsal.

1. Tenotomy of the extensor digitorum longus followed by capsulotomy
2. Tenotomy of the flexor digitorum longus and brevis
3. Dorsal exostectomy
4. Proximal phalanx osteotomy with plantar base (short Shannon burr)
5. Distal percutaneous shortening osteotomy of the fifth metatarsal (large Shannon burr)

28.5.2 Dressings

The surgical dressing is initially not very restrictive; it corrects the deformity and is replaced after 7 days (suture removal). At this point, it is important to apply a new dressing that will hold the toe in the desired position for at least 1 month—the time needed for the osteotomy to heal.

In the most severe cases, and beyond 1 month, the patient is taught how to bandage his/her toe and instructed to continue using the dressings to prevent recurrences.

28.6 Soft Corn between Toes

These are soft, humid, and very painful calluses that form between the fourth and fifth toes, due the latter contacting the fourth. They are easy to distinguish from the typically hard calluses formed on the dorsal side of the foot. This condition is related to secondary hyperkeratosis due to bone impingement, which remains soft because it occurs in the moist space between toes.

There are two presentations:

- Type 1: corn due to varus deformity of the fifth toe that causes bone-to-bone contact at the lateral condyles of the phalanges (Fig. 28.12)
- Type 2: corn due to exostosis on the medial side of the phalanges of the fifth toe

28.6.1 Percutaneous Treatment

Type 1 Soft Corn

It is essential to correct the fifth toe's malposition by performing proximal phalanx osteotomy with lateral base while preserving a medial hinge to separate the two toes.

Type 2 Soft Corn

In this scenario, we approach the exostosis with a short Shannon burr over the most prominent part of the toe, more toward the end, then grind away the bump. It is important not to take too much away, as the joint could be damaged. Removing the exostosis is generally enough to resolve this problem. The resulting bone paste is extracted using a dedicated rasp.

28.6.2 Dressings

For *type 1*, the toe must be strapped with adhesive plaster until the osteotomy has healed, thereby ensuring the osteotomy remains in the correct position. Later, a silicone spacer can be used by the patient for a certain period of time.

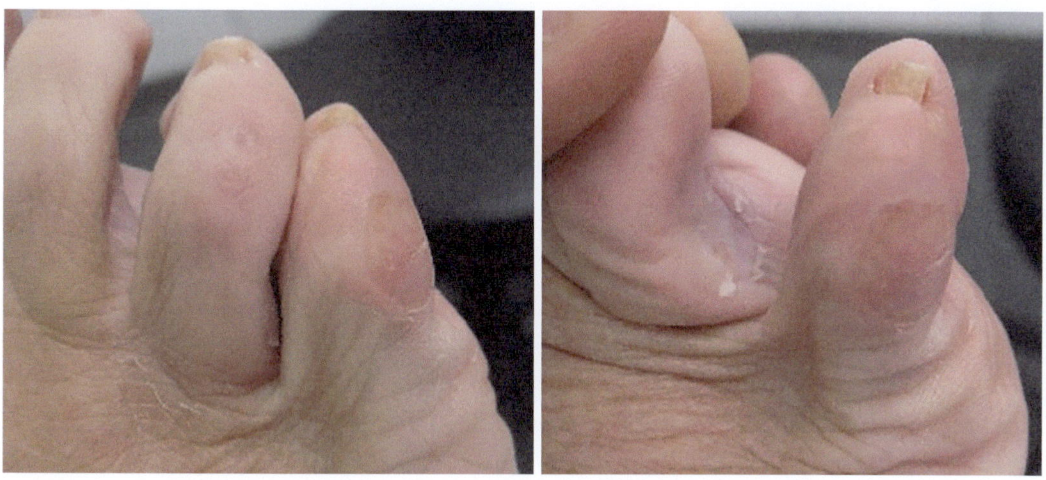

Fig. 28.12 Type 1 soft corn. © Eduard Rabat 2015. All Rights Reserved

For *type 2*, only a simple, soft dressing is needed while the postsurgical swelling resolves; this leads to spectacular results.

Editors' Point of View

Percutaneous surgery of fifth ray deformities is much less aggressive than open surgery, because Z-shaped skin flaps are no longer necessary. Like for hammer toe, the procedures can be done on either the bone, joint, or tendons. It is preferable to keep the flexor digitorum longus, along with the lumbricals and interossei to preserve toe curling. Treatment of soft corns and callus between toes will remove rubbing; the risks are minimized by making the incision away from the area of concern.

29 Percutaneous Surgery of Lateral Toe Deformities

Barbara Piclet Legré

Abbreviations

DIP	Distal interphalangeal
e	Extension
f	Flexion
l	Lateral
m	Medial
MTP	Metatarsophalangeal
PIP	Proximal interphalangeal

29.1 Introduction

Percutaneous surgical techniques are particularly well-suited to correcting lesser toe deformities since they reduce the risk of vascular and skin complications (contracture, necrosis), and the procedures can be tailored to the deformities present. This involves performing targeted bone and tendon procedures that are selected based on the type of deformity and its reducibility. The potential time savings should not factor in the decision; while a flexible deformity can be treated very quickly, it may take as long or longer to correct a fixed deformity and/or dislocation percutaneously than with an open technique.

29.2 Pathophysiology

The extensor only has a strong effect on the first phalanx (P1), and the flexors only have strong effects on the second and third phalanges (P2, P3). The balance is restored by the interossei and lumbricals (atrophied due to footwear choices and being sedentary) (Fig. 29.1).

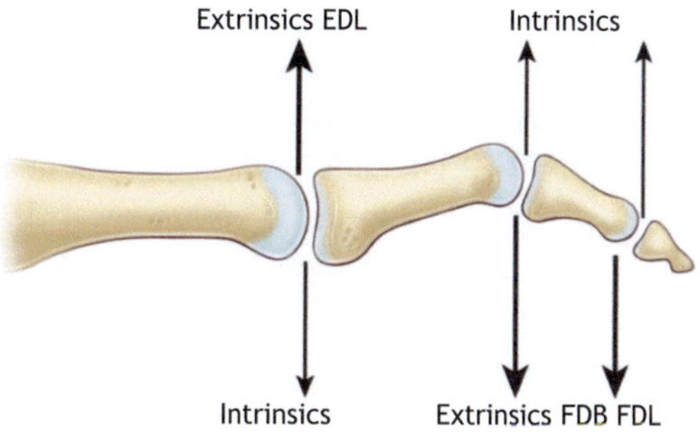

Fig. 29.1 Pathophysiology: extrinsic muscles are much stronger than intrinsic ones. © Barbara Piclet Legré 2015. All Rights Reserved

B. P. Legré (✉)
Centre du Pied, Marseille, France

C. Cazeau, Y. Stiglitz (eds.), *Percutaneous and Minimally Invasive Foot Surgery*,
https://doi.org/10.1007/978-3-030-98791-6_29

29.2.1 Extrinsic Muscles

The extensor digitorum longus (EDL) does not insert on P1. The extensor digitorum brevis (EDB) joins the fibular side of the corresponding EDL at the metatarsophalangeal (MTP) joint of the second, third, and fourth toes. The extensor tendon mechanism is attached at the MTP joint and P1 by a fibrous aponeurosis having proximal and distal segments. The proximal sling has transverse fibers. This sling arises from the lateral and medial edges of the extensor expansion, spreads around the MTP capsule, and integrates itself downward into the plantar plate, the transverse intermetatarsal ligament, and the flexor tendon sheath. This solid expansion stretches out distally to the base of P1. The distal wing segment has oblique fibers. This grouping of extensor tendons splits three-ways on the back of P1: one central slip that inserts on the back of P2 and the PIP capsule; two lateral slips which, after having received contributions from the medial-sided lumbrical and lateral-sided EDB, converge progressively on the dorsum of P2 and form one common terminal tendon that inserts on the dorsal capsule of the distal interphalangeal (DIP) joint and the P3 base. The triangular area between the lateral tendons is filled by a fascial structure, the triangular lamellae. The main function of the extensor complex is P1 dorsiflexion through a sling effect: the EDL pulls on the sling. Minimal loads are transferred to the interphalangeal (IP) joints. The extensor complex becomes an extensor of the proximal IP joint (PIP) only when the MTP joint is in neutral or plantar flexion. The PIP joint is neutralized when the MTP is in dorsiflexion; when a deformity with P1 in dorsiflexion occurs, the EDL cannot extend the IP joints.

The extrinsic flexor digitorum longus (FDL) (Fig. 29.3) and intrinsic flexor digitorum brevis (FDB) (Fig. 29.2) do not insert on P1. The FDB inserts on P2 and flexes the PIP joint, while the FDL inserts on P3 and flexes the DIP joint. At P1, the FDB divides into two slips which allows the FDL to pass through it and become more superficial as it inserts on P3. The two FDB slips insert together on the plantar side of the P2 base, near the edges. The flexors have a minimal effect on plantar flexion of P1. The flexors are stretched when the MTP joint is in dorsal flexion. This exerts passive traction on the IP joints. Thus, when P1 is in dorsal flexion, the toe contracts because there is no major antagonist against the flexors. The deformity appears after a certain amount of time due to stiffening in this position. Passive traction of the flexors creates a significant plantar flexion force on the IP joints, although the primary function of the flexors occurs during the stance phase of gait: large plantar flexion force exists on the IP joints, but

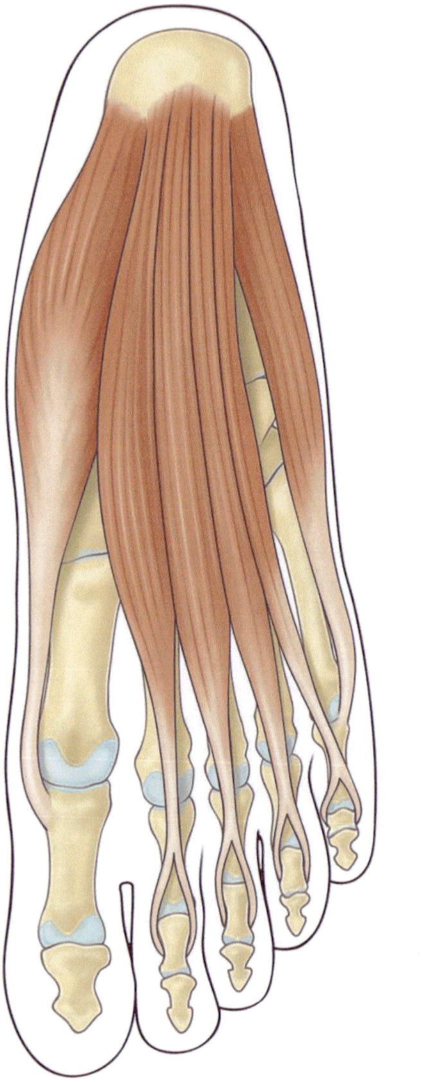

Fig. 29.2 Superficial muscles on plantar surface of foot: FDB 2345 and abductor 5. © Barbara Piclet Legré 2015. All Rights Reserved

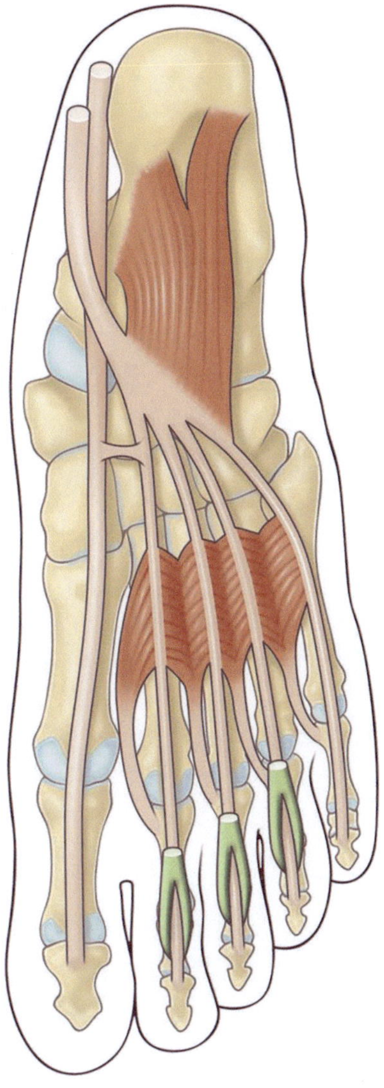

Fig. 29.3 Deep muscles on plantar surface of foot: FDL lumbricals.

since the toes cannot cross the ground, the retrograde ground reaction force can cause significant dorsal flexion in the MTP joints.

29.2.2 Intrinsic Muscles

Along with the FDB, the other intrinsic muscles consist of four dorsal interossei, three plantar interossei, and four lumbricals. The interossei pass dorsally at the transverse intermetatarsal ligament. Since the functional axis of the foot passes through the second toe, abduction and adduction are relative to this axis: the dorsal interossei are abductors and the plantar interossei are adductors. The second toe has two dorsal interossei muscles. There is no dorsal interossei muscle on the fifth ray. The interossei insert distally on the deep transverse intermetatarsal ligament, the medial or lateral MTP capsule, the plantar plate, and the P1 base. The interossei muscles (Figs. 29.4 and 29.5) produce plantar flexion of P1 and provide transverse stabilization. The lumbricals pass plantar to the transverse intermetatarsal ligament and reside on the tibial side of the toe. They insert distally on the wing and on the medial and central slips of the trifurcation of the extensor mechanism. The lumbricals (Fig. 29.3) produce plantar flexion of P1 and dorsal flexion of the PIP and DIP joints.

They have a small adduction component. Their additional force comes from the mobile proximal insertion (FDL): when a muscle contracts, loads are applied in both directions. When the lumbricals contract, loads are applied to the FDL on one hand, and on the P1 base and extensor mechanism on the other. Thus, the musculotendinous complex is stretched proximally and relaxed distally. This creates play in the distal FDL.

29.2.3 Plantar Plate

During walking, the MTP goes into flexion. The static resistance of the plantar plate combined with the dynamic loads of the intrinsic muscles keeps P1 in a neutral position. If the hyperextension forces become chronic, these structures stretch out and become less effective (intrinsic muscles that pull at a 90° angle are less effective at flexing P1). Consequently, when the P1 is dorsiflexed chronically, the EDL loses its tenodesis effect on the IP joints, allowing P2 and P3 to flex. When P1 stretches, the flexors (FDL, FDB) are under a lot of tension, which contributes to PIP joint flexion. The only forces that oppose this flexion are from the lumbricals and interossei, which are easily exceeded by the flexors. The muscular activity is balanced when the plantar flexion—coordinated at the MTP by the action of the interossei, lumbricals, and plantar fascia—prevents hyperextension of the MTP, which then allows the EDL and EDB to extend the PIP and DIP, and the FDL and FDB act like toe flexors joined with the MTP to grip the ground. It is important to remember that these deformities are most often generated by muscle imbalances (Fig. 29.1) because in practice, the extrinsic muscles dominate the intrinsic muscles.

The second toe has two dorsal interossei muscles but no plantar ones (Figs. 29.4 and 29.5). The dorsal interossei balance each other out in their medial and lateral adduction and abduction forces. They cause plantar flexion of P1. The extension merges with the sling and creates an extension load on the IP joints.

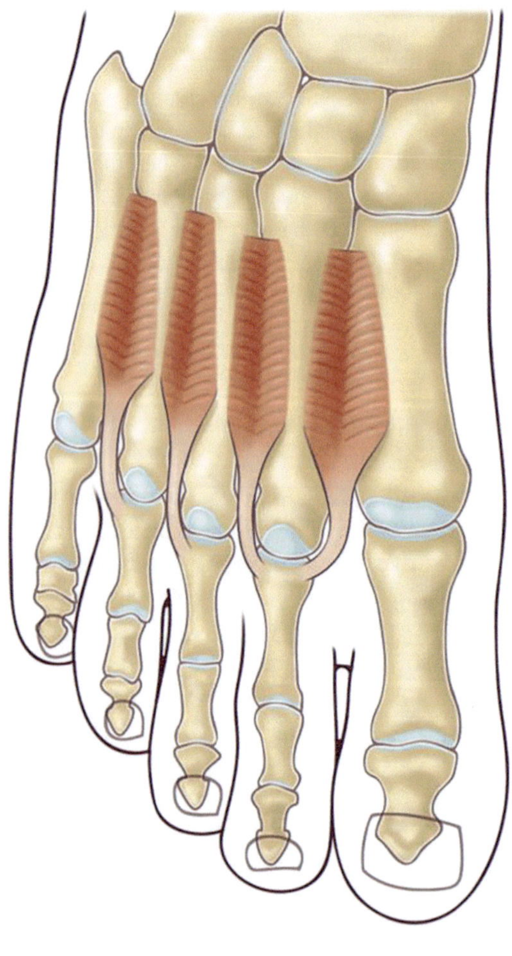

Fig. 29.4 Dorsal interossei. © Barbara Piclet Legré 2015. All Rights Reserved

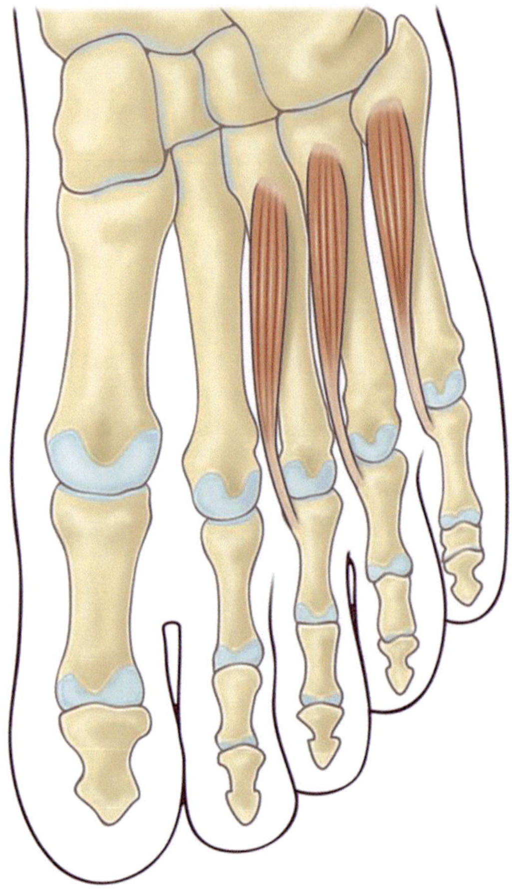

Fig. 29.5 Plantar interossei muscles. © Barbara Piclet Legré 2015. All Rights Reserved

The lumbrical adducts the second toe, without a force opposed by its insertion on the medial portion of the sling. Its main function is to flex P1 and to extend the IP joints. Typically, with an intact lateral capsule and thanks to the second interossei, lumbrical adduction does not cause medial deviation of the second toe because this muscle is so small. However, if the collateral ligament is torn or the lateral capsule and second interosseous muscle are defective, the relatively small lumbrical can exert enough adduction to deviate the second toe.

One must remember that the P1 position on the metatarsal head is the location of antagonism between the powerful extensor system (its slip mechanism in opposition to the weak intrinsic muscles and capsule) and the plantar fascia. The positions of P2 and P3 are subjected to the flexor loads directly opposed to the weak intrinsic muscles (Fig. 29.1). There is an ongoing competition at each joint, and the extrinsic muscles usually win out. Excessive dorsal flexion of P1 is the definite trigger for most of these deformities.

29.3 Classifications of Toe Deformities

The term "claw" is used in a general manner. Nevertheless, the true definition of a claw in zoology corresponds to the most common form of nail, which bends toward the subungual space and is pointed, curved, and sometimes retractable. While a vast majority of mammals have claws, only primates have true flat nails. Birds and reptiles also have them. This term is used in certain arthropods (scorpions, crabs, crawfish) because of popular imagery.

The etymology of claw brings the notion of being able to grab. In fact, this word is not used in an anatomical or functional sense but in a creationist one.

In the literature, the description of lesser toe deformities is sparse and inconsistent. There are various misleading name-based classification systems (hammer toe, claw toe, swan-neck, camptodactyly, clinodactyly), etiology-based classifications (although these deformities are most often idiopathic), and anatomical classifications (proximal, distal, total, reversed).

We believe morphological criteria are the determining factor when deciding which percutaneous surgical procedure is most appropriate.

An anatomical classification based on the position of the deformity in the joints was proposed by P. Plante [1]. He defined three types of claw toes:

1. Extension flexion-flexion
2. Extension flexion-extension
3. Flexion flexion-flexion

However, the deformities are more varied than this…

Our team has proposed a new classification system to describe all these deformities in various planes while using the international abbreviations. The description is clinical and reinforced by radiographic findings. It starts at the proximal seat of the deformity:

- The MTP (metatarsophalangeal) joint can be in extension, MTP (default case); in flexion, MTPf; in lateral deviation, MTPl; or in medial deviation, MTPm
- The PIP (proximal interphalangeal) joint can be in flexion, PIP (default case); in extension, PIPe (rare); in lateral deviation, PIPl; or in medial deviation, PIPm
- The DIP (distal interphalangeal) joint can be in flexion, DIP (default case); in extension, DIPe (rare); in lateral deviation, DIPl; or in medial deviation, DIPm

The location of the deformity is followed by the number of the toe in question:

- MTP = MTP extension; for example, MTP2
- PIP = PIP flexion (Fig. 29.6); for example, PIP2, PIP3, and PIP4 (Fig. 29.7)
- DIP = DIP flexion (Fig. 29.8)

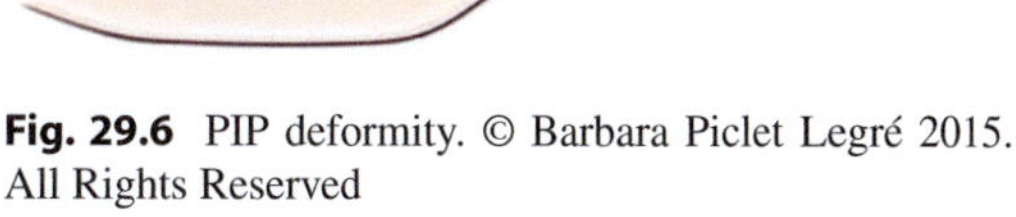

Fig. 29.6 PIP deformity. © Barbara Piclet Legré 2015. All Rights Reserved

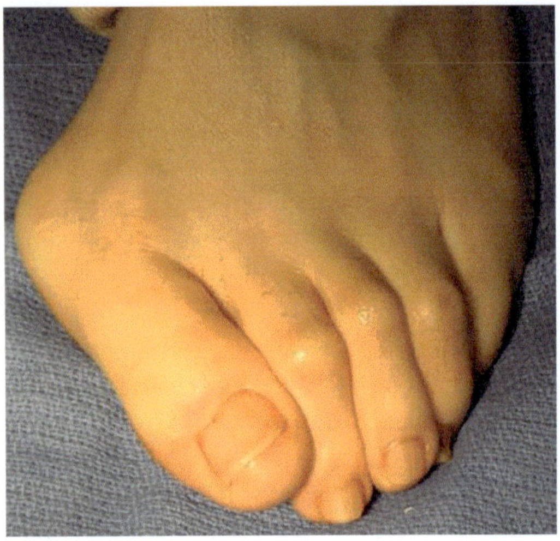

Fig. 29.7 PIP2, PIP3, and PIP4. © Barbara Piclet Legré 2015. All Rights Reserved

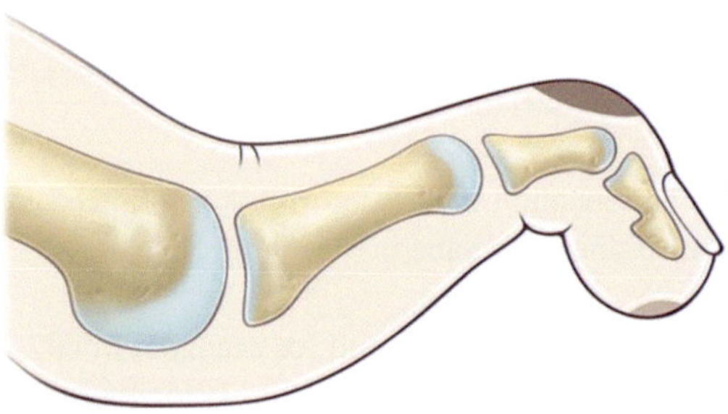

Fig. 29.8 DIP deformity. © Barbara Piclet Legré 2015. All Rights Reserved

- DIP sagittal: DIP, DIPe; for example, DIP2 (Fig. 29.9)
- DIP horizontal: DIPl, DIPm; for example, DIPl2 (Fig. 29.10), DIPm4 (Fig. 29.11)

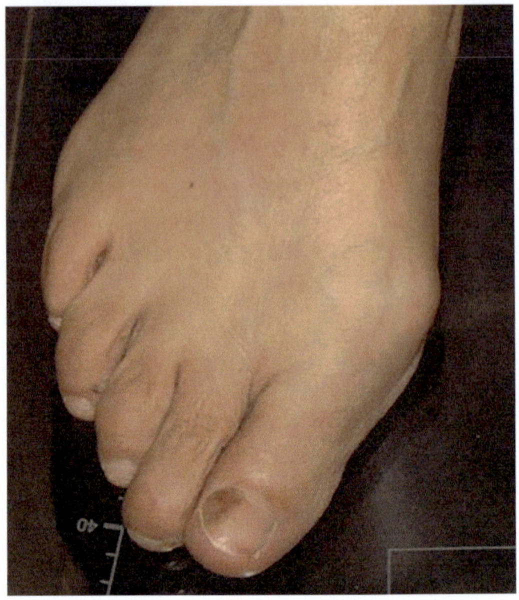

Fig. 29.9 DIP2. © Barbara Piclet Legré 2015. All Rights Reserved

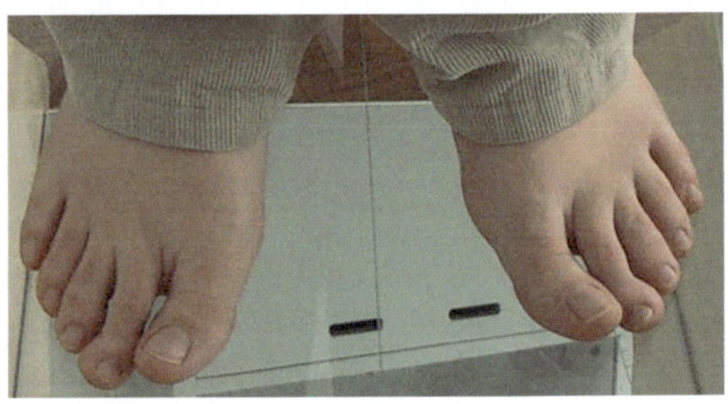

Fig. 29.10 DIPl2. © Barbara Piclet Legré 2015. All Rights Reserved

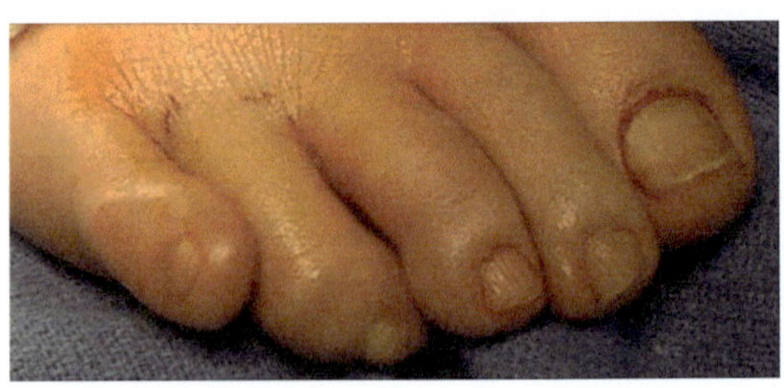

Fig. 29.11 DIPm4. © Barbara Piclet Legré 2015. All Rights Reserved

29.4 Combinations

Combinations of MTP, PIP, and DIP deformities are defined by the orientation of the deformity at each level. PIP deformity often occurs in combination with MTP deformity:

- MTP PIP (MTP extension) (Fig. 29.12); for example, MTP PIP2 (Fig. 29.13).

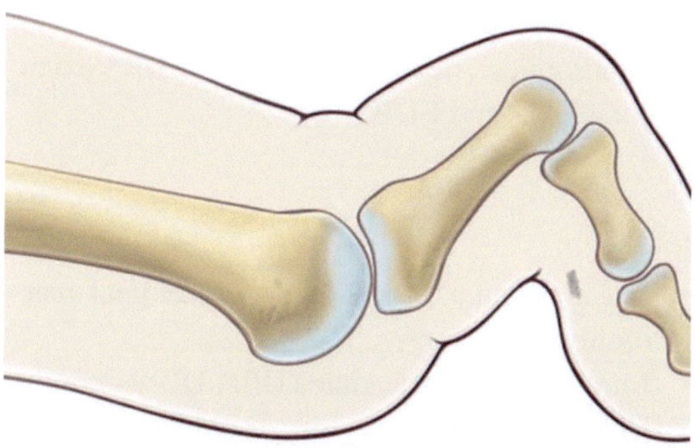

Fig. 29.12 MTP deformity in dorsal flexion and PIP in flexion. © Barbara Piclet Legré 2015. All Rights Reserved

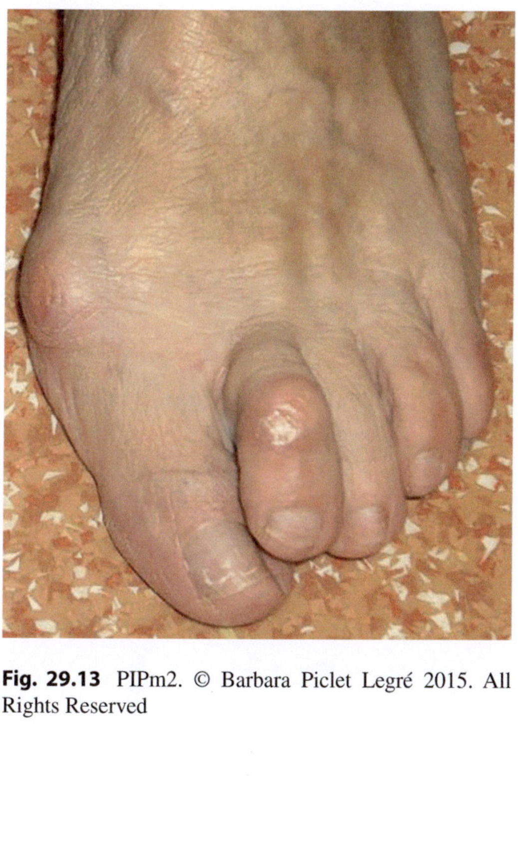

Fig. 29.13 PIPm2. © Barbara Piclet Legré 2015. All Rights Reserved

- MTP + PIP (MTP subluxation or dislocation, for example, MTP + PIP2
- MTPl PIP (MTP lateral subluxation); for example, MTPl, PIP3
- MTPm, PIP (MTP medial subluxation); for example, MTPm, PIP4

Other examples are as follows: PIPDIP2 (Fig. 29.14), PIPDIPe3 (Fig. 29.15), PIPDIPl3, PIPDIPm4, PIPDIPl2, MTPlPIPDIP3, MTPlPIPDIP2, MTPmPIPDIP4, etc.

A reducibility criterion can be added after the morphology criteria (f = flexible, sr = semi-rigid, r = rigid), for example, PIPsr2.

However, it is better to place the etiology criterion before the morphology one (rh = rheumatism, pt. = post-traumatic, nr = neurological, ic = iatrogenic); for example, rhPIP2.

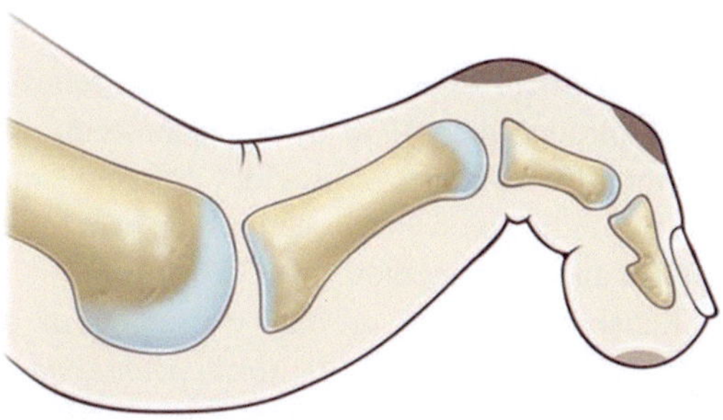

Fig. 29.14 PIP DIOP. © Barbara Piclet Legré 2015. All Rights Reserved

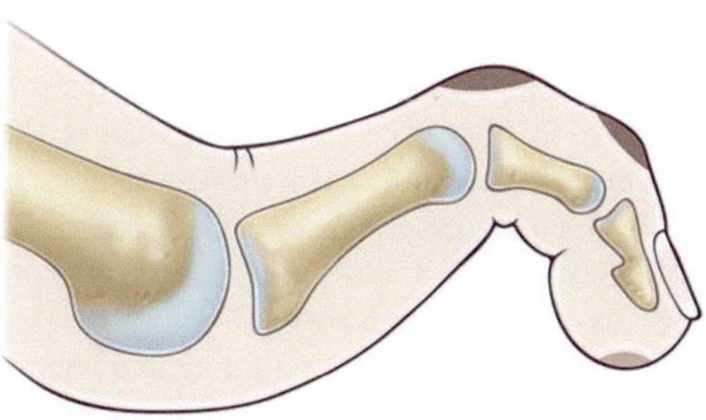

Fig. 29.15 PIP DIPe. © Barbara Piclet Legré 2015. All Rights Reserved

29.5 Clinical Consequences of Lateral Toe Deformities

The most common complaint is dorsal rubbing in shoes, although there may also be excessive pulp pressure or metatarsalgia due to vertical pressure on the metatarsal head. These three symptoms can appear in combination to various degrees.

29.6 Conservative Treatment of Lateral Toe Deformities

Conservative treatment consists of the patient wearing toe wedges and foot orthotics. A more rigid, nighttime brace helps to prevent stiffening of a semi-rigid deformity, although it is mainly used during the late postoperative period when a toe does not respond to strapping.

The Kinesio® taping method is a bandaging technique that uses colored adhesive elastic bands to orient or reduce mobility and relieve pain. Introduced in 1970 by a Japanese chiropractor—Kenso Kase—it provides different support depending on which directions the bands are applied and/or their color.

Rehabilitation can prevent worsening of a flexible deformity. This is the *strain counterstain* principle developed by Lawrence Jones [2] of the American Academy of Osteopathy, which was taken up by Dr. Michel Maestro. It consists of passively positioning the deformed toe in the position of most comfort, relieving pain by reduction and stopping the inappropriate activity of the proprioceptors that allow the somatic dysfunction to persist. By passively reproducing the initial position of tension, the patient moves the joint into a comfortable position, which shortens the overactive muscles as much as possible. Holding it for 90 s allows the bundle to slow down its afferent overactivity.

Slowly and deliberately returning to a neutral position prevents the previously spasmed muscle from being excited again, which is the Kusunose technique [3]. For a proximal deformity, the patient applies light traction in the toe axis and then holds the first phalanx in slight plantar flexion for 90 s.

29.7 Percutaneous Surgical Treatment of Lateral Toe Deformities

Intraoperative fluoroscopy is needed during the learning phase or when a specific procedure is indicated. Surgical procedures are performed on the soft tissues and bones.

Soft Tissues

- Joint procedures: MTP or plantar PIP release
- Tenotomies: flexors: FDL and FDB; extensors: EDL and EDB

Bones

- Extra-articular procedures—phalangeal osteotomy (P1, P2)
- Intra-articular procedures (PIP, DIP)—condylectomy, arthroplasty

29.7.1 Flexor Tenotomy

- *Tenotomy of the FDB only* on a toe carefully positioned in plantar flexion (Fig. 29.16) during the entire procedure to avoid damaging the plantar collateral nerve. The incision is made proximal to the PIP (Fig. 29.17), laterally or medially, depending on the operated foot and the surgeon's dominant hand, located over the posterior portion of the

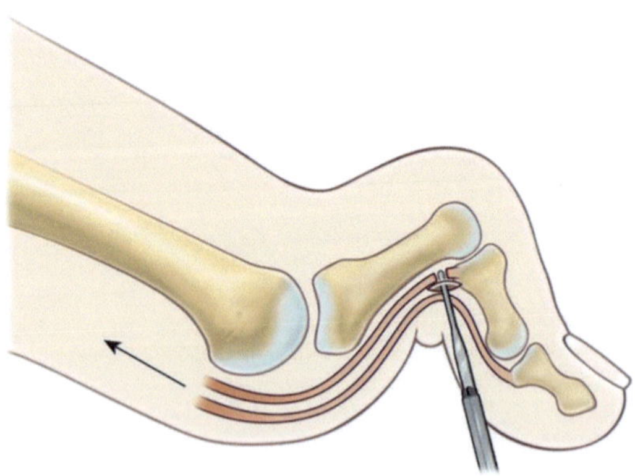

Fig. 29.16 FDB tenotomy. © Barbara Piclet Legré 2015. All Rights Reserved

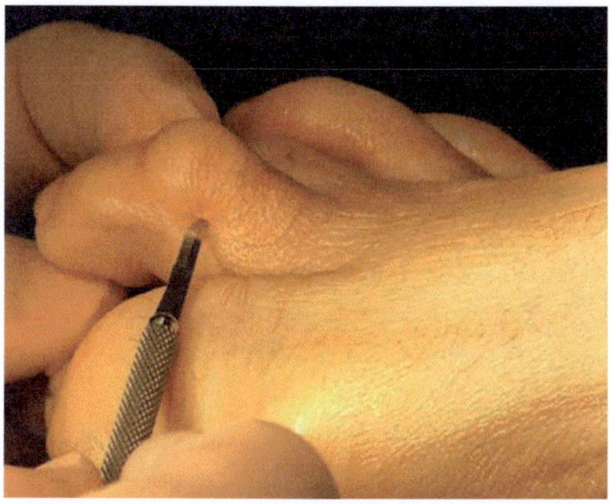

Fig. 29.17 FDB tenotomy.

tuberosity of the distal P1 epiphysis that the surgeon palpates with the thumb of the hand not holding the Beaver blade. The blade is introduced directly again to the bone on the plantar side of the P1 neck and must remain in contact with the bone toward the plantar side of the P1 epiphysis in order to arrive at the plantar side of the P2 base. At this point, a rotational movement is used to cut the plantar PIP capsule to the P2 base, and then in a second step (and more distally), the two FDB digitations (Fig. 29.18). A bone rasp is then inserted to verify that both FDB digitations were cut completely by carefully palpating the entire plantar side of the P2 shaft, including its lateral and medial edges. The diaphysis can only be reached with the bone rasp after the interphalangeal capsule is detached. In practice, this procedure is necessary given the distal insertion of the two digitations relative to the capsule. The toe is released and then placed in dorsal flexion using a passive maneuver to verify that the PIP flexion deformity has been corrected.

One can also carry out the isolated FDB tenotomy through a plantar approach at the P1 base, where the FDB is superficial, although there is a higher risk of not being selective. In addition, plantar PIP release is very helpful for correcting the deformity.

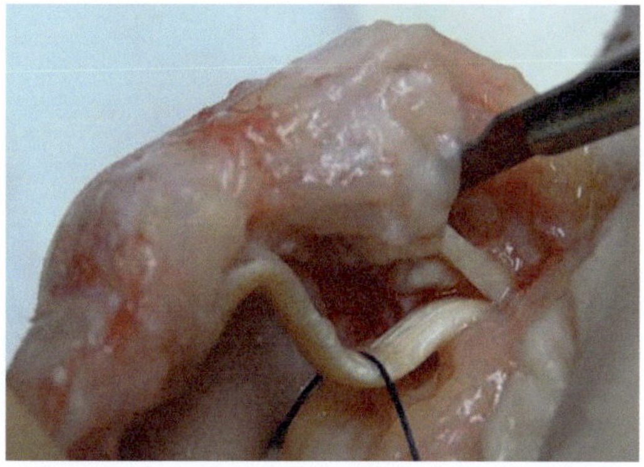

Fig. 29.18 FDB slips.

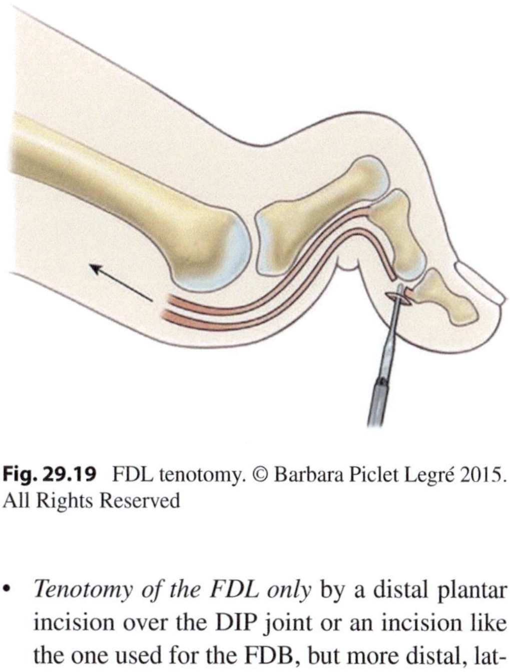

Fig. 29.19 FDL tenotomy.

- *Tenotomy of the FDL only* by a distal plantar incision over the DIP joint or an incision like the one used for the FDB, but more distal, lateral, or medial, depending which foot is being operated and which hand is the surgeon's dominant one, in order to reach the plantar side of the P3 base (Fig. 29.19).
- *Complete tenotomy* as taught to us by Mariano de Prado by a plantar incision at the base of the toe, over P1, identical to the approach of the first phalanx (Fig. 29.20), which makes it possible to transect the FDL and FDB tendons. The effectiveness is gauged by a simultaneous dorsiflexion maneuver of the toe.

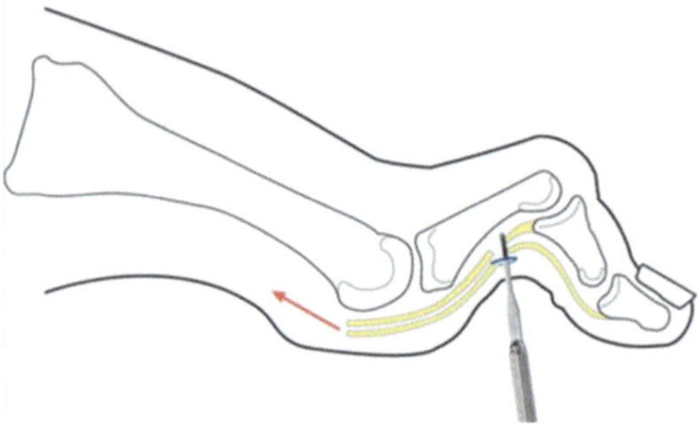

Fig. 29.20 Complete FDL + FDB tenotomy.

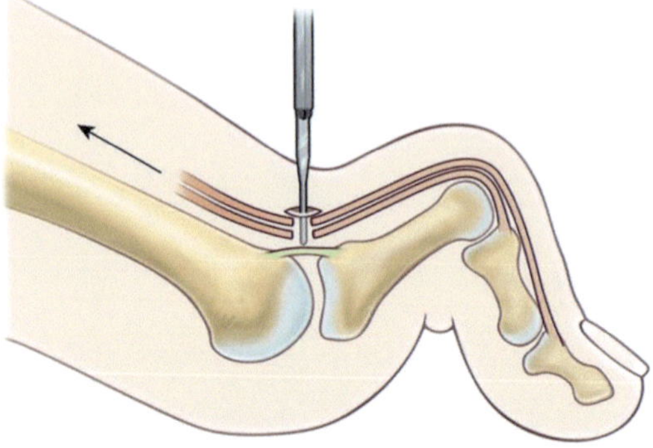

Fig. 29.21 EDL and EDB tenotomy.

29.7.2 Extensor Tenotomy

Extensor tenotomy is not performed in every case. It is performed in the zone where the two tendons (extensor and foot) are individualized (Fig. 29.21), i.e., at the level of the fibrous sling over the MTP joint, which helps to preserve the hood or sling effect (anchoring of the EDL to the plantar side of the metatarsal head and the base of the plantar plate) and to prevent proximal contracture of the tendons with toe drop. To confirm the procedure was successful, plantar flexion is applied simultaneously to the toe in question.

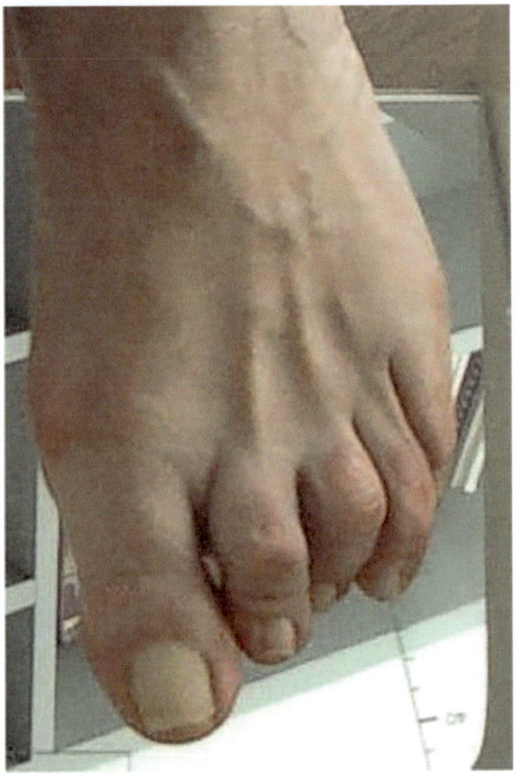

Fig. 29.22 Visible extensors.

The success criteria are both tactile—with the disappearance of tendon tension—and visual (although inconsistent depending on the patient's morphology) (Fig. 29.22).

- This additional procedure is only done when the MTP joint is extended.
- Dorsal MTP release is the logical extension of extensor tenotomy into the deep layers, although these tendons may be offset laterally. Applying traction on the toe helps to separate the joint and makes it easier to insert the Beaver blade in certain cases of dislocated toes.

29.7.3 Osteotomy of First Phalanx (P1)

P1 osteotomy is done through a plantar approach at the base of the toe, over the proximal P1 metaphysis (Fig. 29.23), while keeping the flexor tendons intact. The incision is made while maintaining the operated toe in dorsiflexion before inserting the Beaver blade longitudinally until it contacts the bone between the toe's plantar fold and the projection of the metatarsal head. Fluoroscopy checks are only needed in the early cases. This incision passes on the medial or lateral face depending on which foot is being operated and the surgeon's dominant hand. A bone rasp in then introduced to prepare the working space in which a suitable burr starts the osteotomy on the edge of the phalanx and continues while staying in contact with the bone.

The best placement for this osteotomy is the proximal metaphyseal portion of P1 as this optimizes the time to union. It can be either:

- *Unicortical*, which is sufficient to achieve plantar flexion in moderate deformities and to correct medial or lateral MTP deformity (Fig. 29.24)
- *Bicortical*, which used most often because it is simpler and provides the shortening needed for lasting correction in the most severe deformity cases, or when the toe is too long (Fig. 29.25)

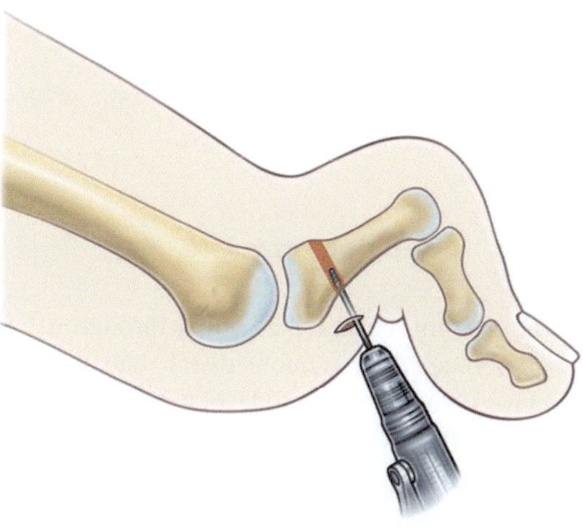

Fig. 29.23 P1 osteotomy.

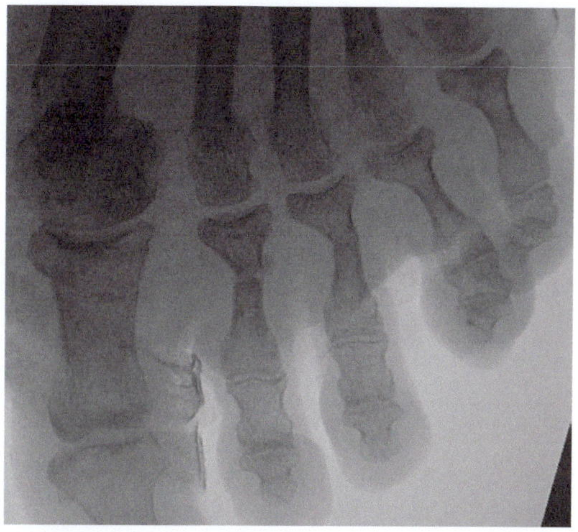

Fig. 29.24 P1 unicortical.

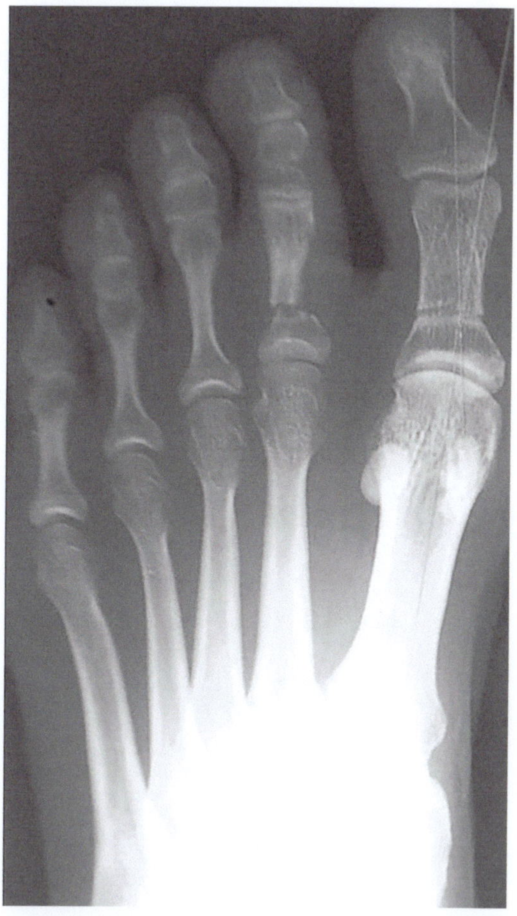

Fig. 29.25 P1 bicortical.

29.7.4 Osteotomy of Second Phalanx (P2)

P2 osteotomy is performed through a medial or lateral approach depending on which foot is being operated and which procedure will be performed. It is done mid-shaft to avoid joint penetration (Fig. 29.26) and can be either:

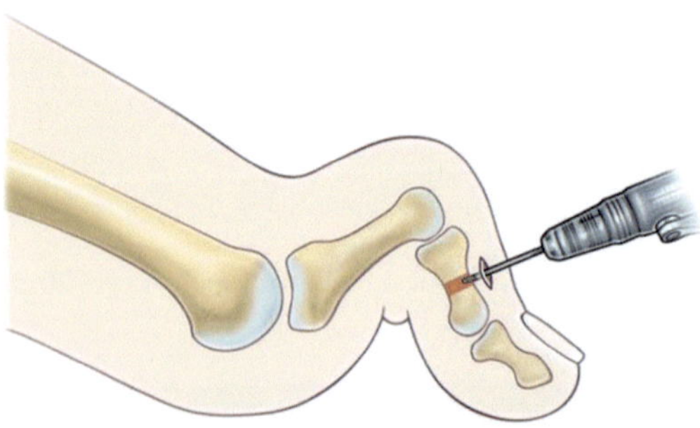

Fig. 29.26 P2 osteotomy. © Barbara Piclet Legré 2015. All Rights Reserved

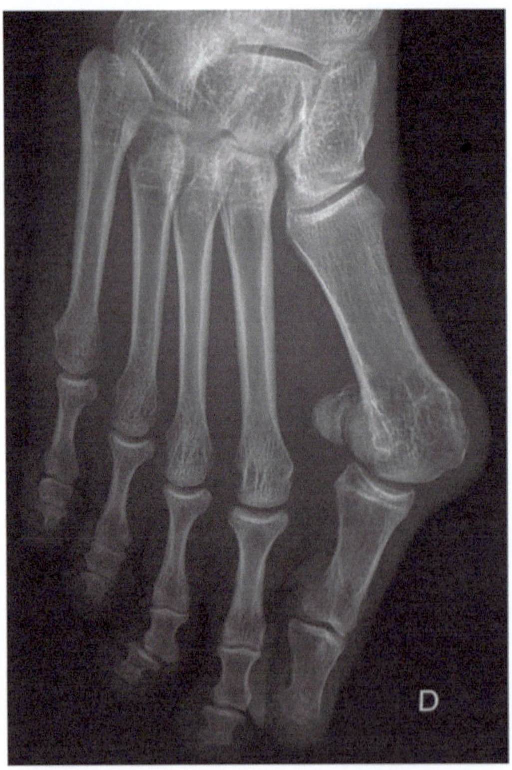

Fig. 29.27 DIPI3. © Barbara Piclet Legré 2015. All Rights Reserved

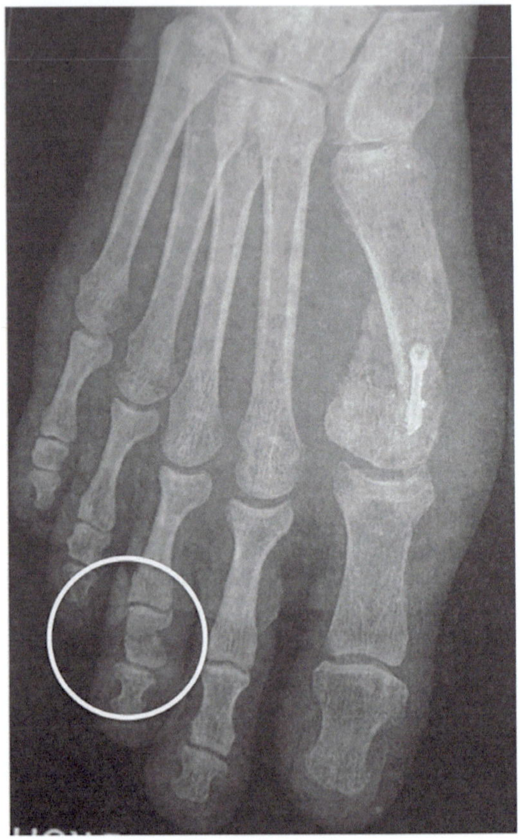

Fig. 29.28 P2O3 without DIP release. © Barbara Piclet Legré 2015. All Rights Reserved

- *Unicortical* to allow dorsal flexion or correction of a lateral or medial DIP deformity. This osteotomy allows reduction of DIP lateral or medial subluxation without having to perform DIP release (Figs. 29.27 and 29.28).
- *Bicortical* to shorten an overly long second phalanx.

29.7.5 Condylectomy

Condylectomy can be performed through a lateral approach that is more distal than the one used for P2 osteotomy and level with the P2 neck (Fig. 29.29). It is used to ream the dorsal protruding portion of the P1 head, along with a portion of the P2 base (Fig. 29.30). Bone debris is removed by applying pressure around the incision; this is most effective when no tourniquet is

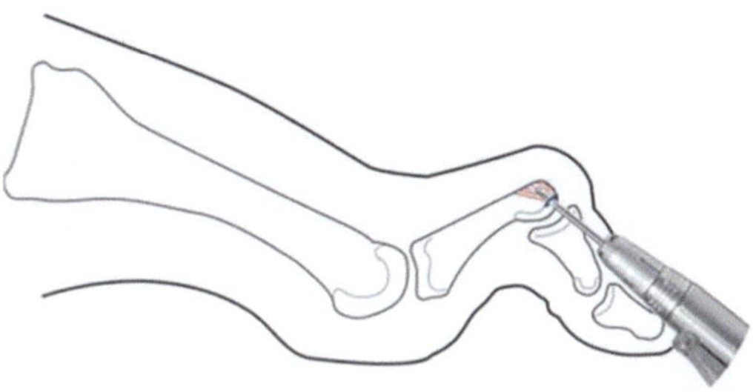

Fig. 29.29 Condyloplasty level with P2 neck.

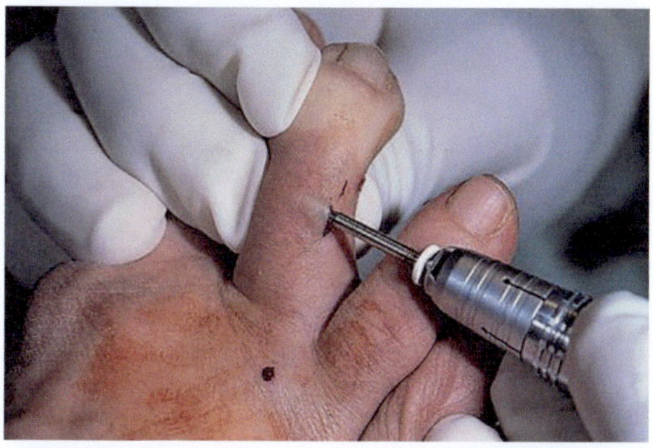

Fig. 29.30 Condyloplasty as described by M. de Prado.

used. The risk of leaving some bone debris is not zero despite fluoroscopy checks and can cause discomfort later on when the patient wears shoes. This condyloplasty is sometimes easier through a distal dorsal approach at the level of the P2 base, with the toe flexed.

29.7.6 Full Procedure

The full procedure described by M. de Prado (Fig. 29.31) can be broken up into a sequence of procedures on soft tissues and bone procedures selected based on the location, magnitude, and reducibility of the deformity.

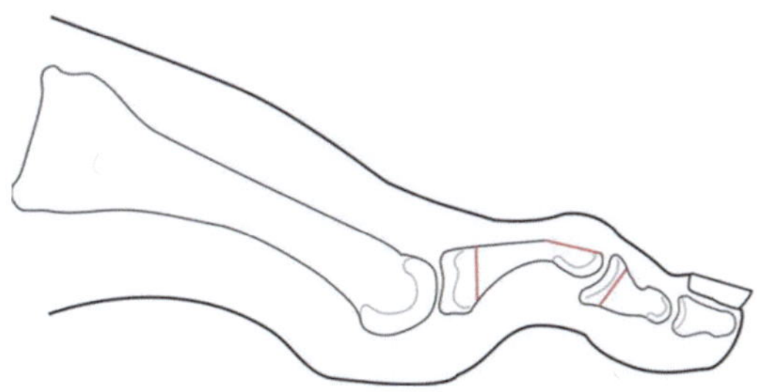

Fig. 29.31 Full procedure as described by M. de Prado.

29.8 Surgical Indications

The new classification that we have proposed allows us to customize which percutaneous surgical procedure will be done. Tenotomies and osteotomies are performed based on several criteria.

29.8.1 Morphological Criteria

PIP deformity is the most common. Appropriate percutaneous procedures are selective tenotomy of the FDB combined with plantar PIP arthrolysis to achieve full release of PIP flexion. P1 osteotomy ensures long-lasting correction. Additional P2 osteotomy can be useful when the toe deformity is not sufficiently corrected. Condyloplasty is the final procedure when the PIP has residual flexion deformity. We have few indications for it. It sometimes becomes an arthroplasty when faced with a very rigid toe or one that has been previously operated on.

For the MTP and PIP, extensor tenotomy is needed along with the procedures described for the PIP. MTP + PIP is treated the same way with the option to combine it with MTP release and osteotomy of the metatarsal neck (DMMO).

Dorsal MTP release can be dangerous if it is not justified. In fact, a subluxed toe can become a

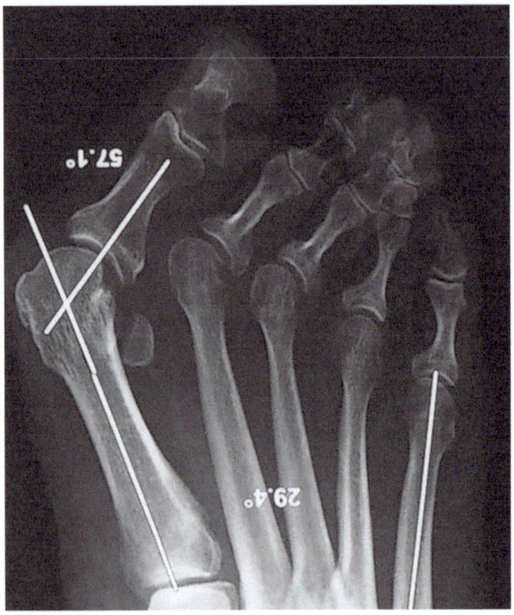

Fig. 29.32 MPI23. © Barbara Piclet Legré 2015. All Rights Reserved

dislocated toe after MTP release. We recommend being very careful with the indications for this procedure; we only use it with dislocations.

Certain lateral or medial MTP deformities can justify a targeted MTP release with meticulous postoperative dressing application to hold the toe in plantar flexion or in neutral position. However, this release is not often necessary (Figs. 29.32 and 29.33).

The DIP joints are corrected using P2 osteotomy and/or selective FDL tenotomy (Figs. 29.34 and 29.35).

Complex deformities (PIPDIP, MTP + PIPDIP) are operated with targeted surgical procedures. For example, MPf PIPDIP will be treated by complete flexor tenotomy (FDB, FDL).

29.8.2 Reducibility Criteria

A flexible deformity will likely not need a tendon procedure since the deformity corrects itself with a simple phalanx osteotomy. However, a rigid deformity may require a combination of tendon and bone procedures to correct it.

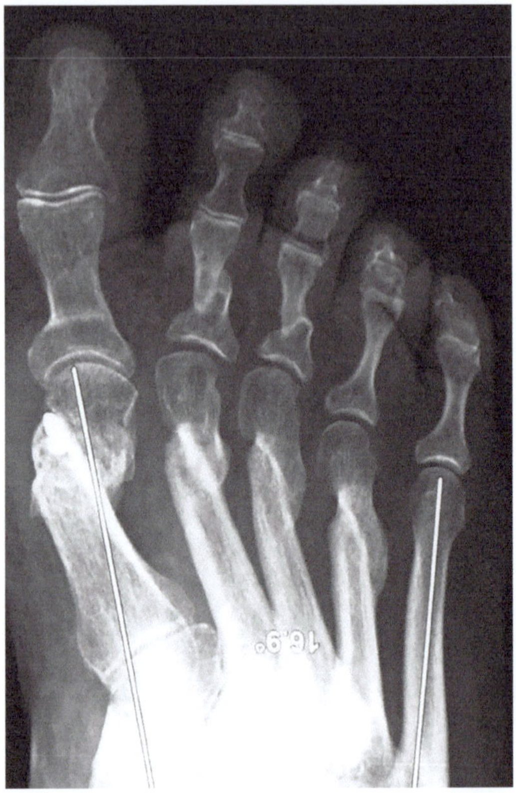

Fig. 29.33 DMMO 234 P1023. © Barbara Piclet Legré 2015. All Rights Reserved

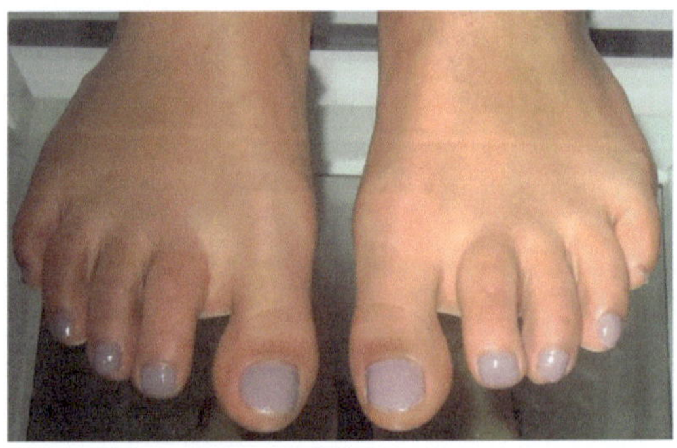

Fig. 29.34 Clinical case No. 2 at 6 months. © Barbara Piclet Legré 2015. All Rights Reserved

29.8.3 Etiology Criteria

Even though lateral toe deformities generally have a mechanical origin, the etiology can guide the choice of treatments. It is easier to do a tenotomy for a neurological deformity. Radiographs will be examined

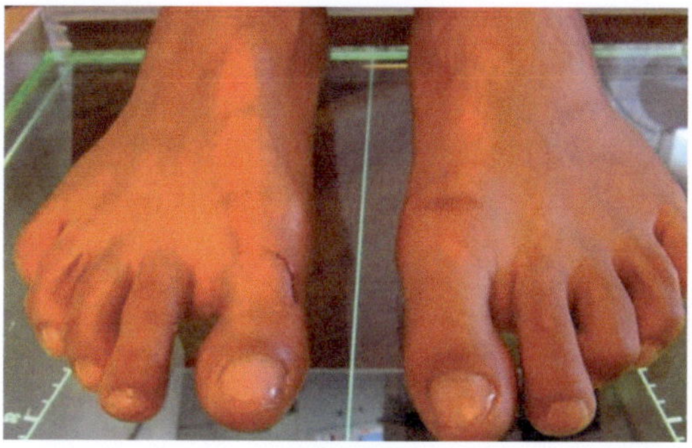

Fig. 29.35 Clinical case No. 2 at 3 years postoperative.

in minute detail in patients with arthritis-related deformities to remove any potential osteophytes.

29.9 Specific Cases

29.9.1 Without Osteotomy

- Flexible distal deformities can benefit from an isolated FDL tenotomy
- Neurological deformity is often satisfactorily resolved by complete flexor tenotomy (FDL, FDB)
- Isolated extensor tenotomy is sometimes indicated when the toe has its MTP in dorsal flexion with PIP deformity
- Once tenotomy has been performed; the surgeon determines whether an additional P1 osteotomy is necessary

29.9.2 Without Tenotomy

- Lateral MTP toe deformity without plantar flexion of the PIP benefits readily from P1 osteotomy, often in combination with percutaneous DMMO (Figs. 29.32 and 29.33)
- Isolated P1 osteotomy for a flexible deformity (Figs. 29.37 and 29.38) (for the third and fourth toes)
- Isolated P2 osteotomy for distal horizontal deformity (Figs. 29.27, 29.28, and 29.36)
- Iatrogenic or post-traumatic feet with toe overlap in which osteotomy of multiple phalanges can help to realign the forefoot to make it easier to wear shoes

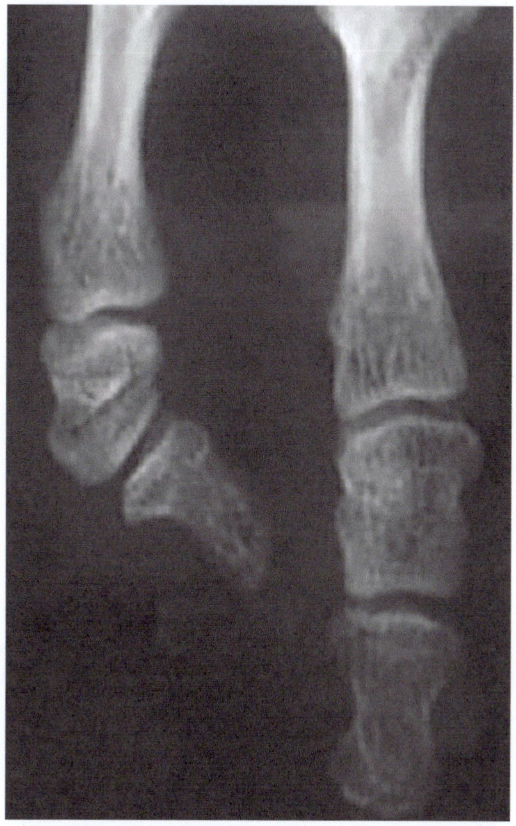

Fig. 29.36 P2 unicortical osteotomy.

29.10 Clinical Cases to Illustrate the Indications

Case No. 1 Woman, 65 years of age, hallux valgus pain, corn on the PIP of the second, third, and fourth toes with metatarsalgia. Lateral MTP3 subluxation visible on radiographs. Her second toe was MTP PIPsr; toes 3 and 4 were PIPs. We performed minimally invasive M1P1; DMMO 234 for the lateral subluxation of the third ray and metatarsalgia; tenotomy of EDL, EDB, and FDB of the second toe; and P1 osteotomy at second to fourth toe (Figs. 29.37 and 29.38).

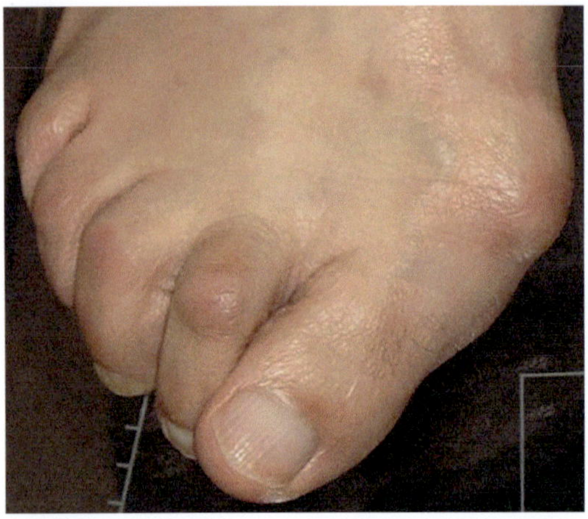

Fig. 29.37 MTP PIP2, PIP34.

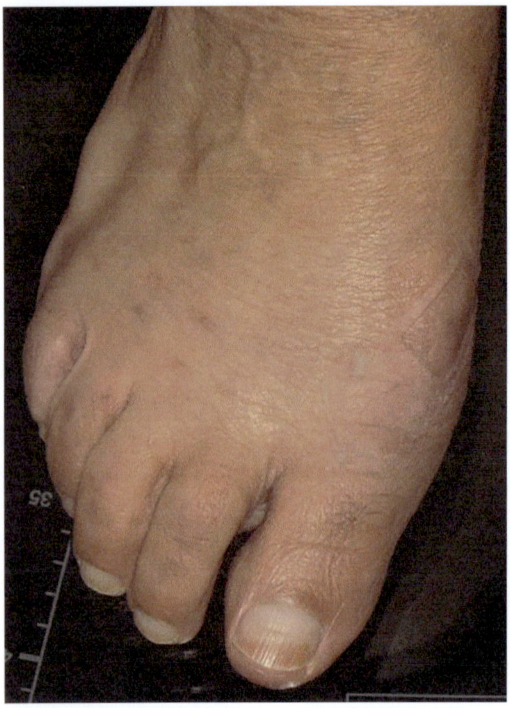

Fig. 29.38 PIPs34 without tenotomy.

Case No. 2 Woman, 32 years of age, lateral 2345 toe impingement when wearing shoes. We found PIPs2 and DIPms345 deformities. We performed tenotomy of FDB2, FDL345, P1 osteotomy in the second to fifth toes and P2 osteotomy in the third and fourth toes (Figs. 29.34 and 29.35).

References

1. Plante P. Le Médecin du Québec. 2009;44(4):69–72.
2. Jones LH. Strain and counterstrain. New York: American Academy of Osteopathy; 1981.
3. Kusunose RS. Technique du strain counterstrain (tension contre tension). www.jiscs.com/PDFs/Chapter13FRENCH08.pdf.

Haglund's Syndrome: Percutaneous Calcaneal Resection

30

Yves Stiglitz and Christophe Piat

30.1 Introduction

In the standard description of Haglund's syndrome, the hypertrophic posterosuperior corner of the calcaneus rubs against the shoe's heel counter. This brings on hyperkeratosis, or even true fluid bursitis, which causes pain on the posterior aspect of the heel.

This somewhat theoretical description is based on radiographic analysis and does not take into account two important aspects that drive the surgical treatment:

- Most often, the bone hypertrophy is located not only on the posterior calcaneus but also extends laterally and/or medially. The bone resection step must take this into account (Fig. 30.1).
- Achilles tendinopathy is often also present; the surgeon must partition the symptoms to clearly establish which pathological unit is responsible for the current symptoms and then treat each separately.

It is appropriate to propose a percutaneous surgical solution to the patient, resulting from miniaturization of the surgical approaches.

Y. Stiglitz (✉) · C. Piat
Clinique Victor Hugo, Paris, France

C. Cazeau, Y. Stiglitz (eds.), *Percutaneous and Minimally Invasive Foot Surgery*,
https://doi.org/10.1007/978-3-030-98791-6_30

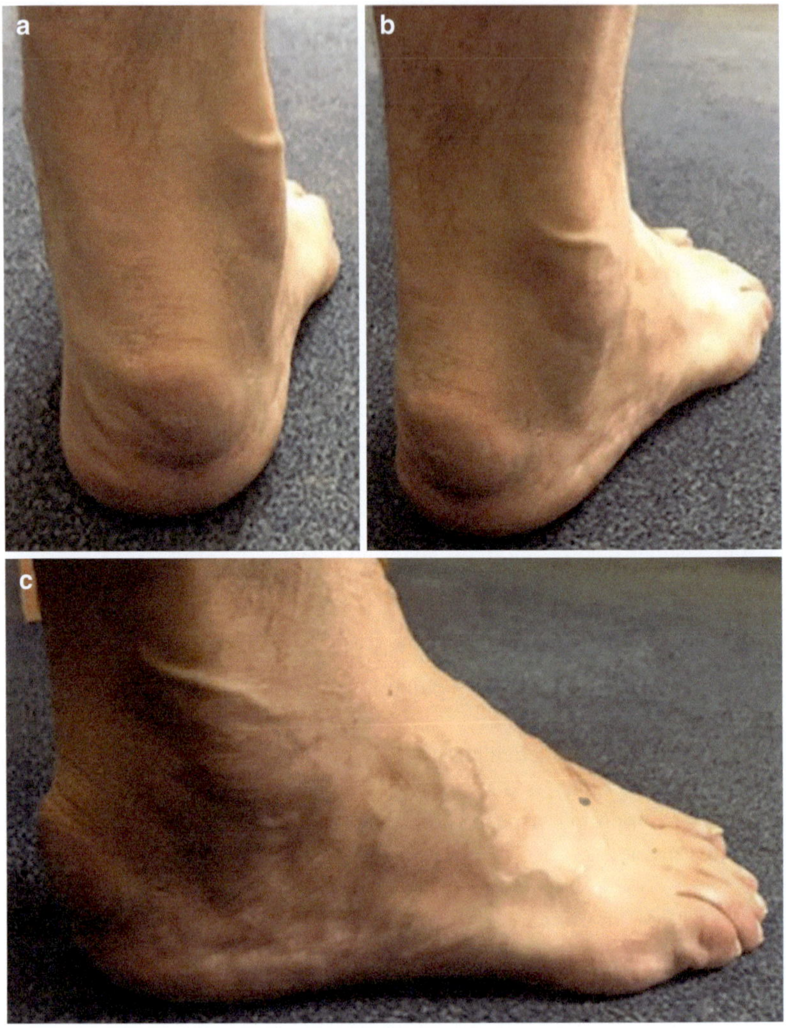

Fig. 30.1 Posterior (**a**), posterolateral (**b**), and lateral view (**c**) of a right foot affected by a large inflamed bursa on the posterolateral aspect of the heel. The area of rubbing is not limited to the posterior aspect of the heel and extends laterally. © Yves Stiglitz 2015. All Rights Reserved

30.2 Surgical Technique

30.2.1 Instrumentation

The standard instruments used in percutaneous foot surgery must be available: Beaver blade, periosteal elevator, bone rasp, and angled rasp.

The rotation speed of any powered surgical tools is set to 8000 rpm in order to prevent bone and skin burns. It is also equipped with a 4:1 speed limiter, which reduces the speed by a factor of 4 and increases the torque coupling, to prevent jamming of the burr within the bone being resected. Bone resection is performed with a burr of a size suitable for the bone volume. Long thin burrs tend to break; thus it is preferable to use thicker wedge-type burrs that are 3 mm in diameter.

Lastly, fluoroscopy is essential for guiding this procedure and to evaluate in real time how much bone has been removed and how much still needs to be removed. In the ideal case, the fluoroscopy system is one designed for surgery on the extremities, as it will be easier to manipulate, especially when taking lateral views. The images can also be obtained using a standard fluoroscopy system by placing it on the side opposite to the operated limb (Fig. 30.2).

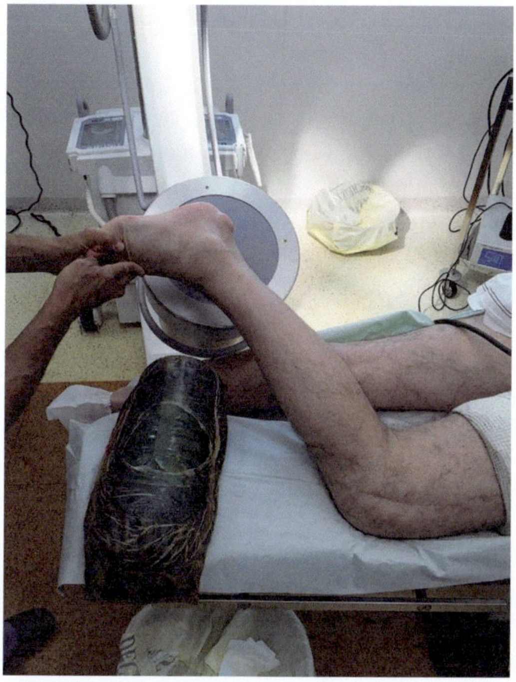

Fig. 30.2 Fluoroscopy unit is positioned at the end of the table on the side opposite to the operated limb. A lateral view is obtained with the knee flexed and hip rotated laterally.

30.2.2 Patient Set Up

The procedure is done with the patient prone. The foot hangs over the edge of the table and is nearly vertical with the ground; the ankle should make an almost 90° angle. The lower limb often externally rotates by itself. This must be countered by supports placed in areas that will not interfere with bone resection. They are placed under the contralateral wing of the ilium to counter excess external rotation and under the ipsilateral ilium to counter excess internal rotation. Lastly, to allow enough clearance for the motorized handpiece, we suggest raising the operated leg using a cushion and if possible, lowering the contralateral leg (Fig. 30.3).

30.2.3 Surgical Approaches

Bone resection is required not only on the posterosuperior corner of the calcaneus but also on its lateral (and/or medial) side, over the Achilles tendon insertion. The incisions are positioned to address the areas of interest identified during the preoperative assessment.

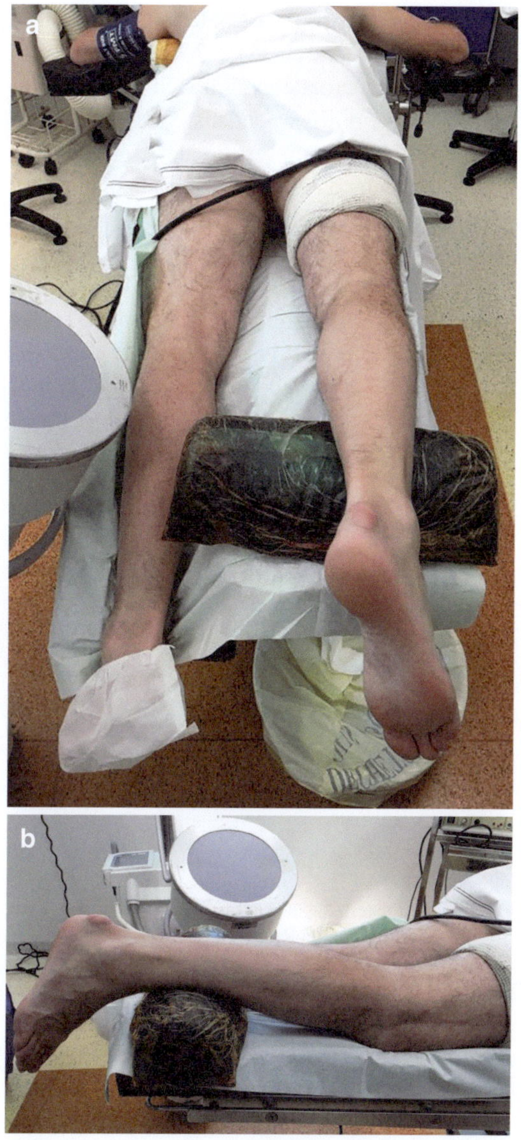

Fig. 30.3 Patient is prone, foot hanging off edge of table with the ankle at nearly 90 degrees. The contralateral leg is offset downward, and the operated leg is shifted upward. (**a**) Superior view (**b**) lateral view.

30.2.3.1 Postero-Superolateral Approach

The postero-superolateral approach is located on the lateral side of the calcaneus, 5–10 mm above the Achilles tendon's insertion and 10–15 mm in front of its lateral edge (Fig. 30.4). It must be posterior enough to ensure the sural nerve is not damaged during the procedure.

Through this approach, the burr will be able to reach the posterosuperior and lateral bone resection areas. However, it is vital to verify the position of the Beaver blade on fluoroscopy before making the incision (Fig. 30.5). The planned maneuver is then carried out.

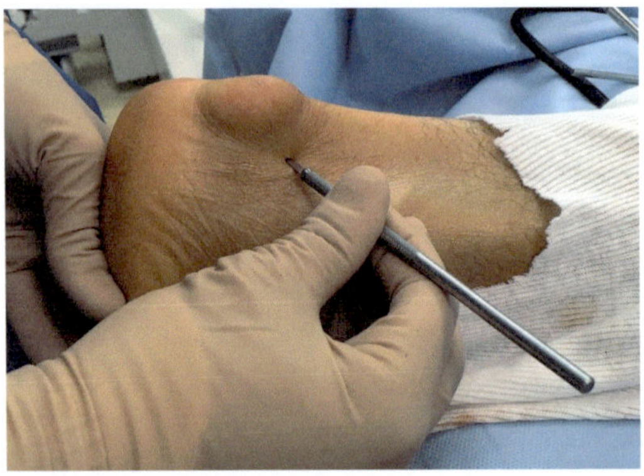

Fig. 30.4 Postero-superolateral approach. © Yves Stiglitz 2015. All Rights Reserved

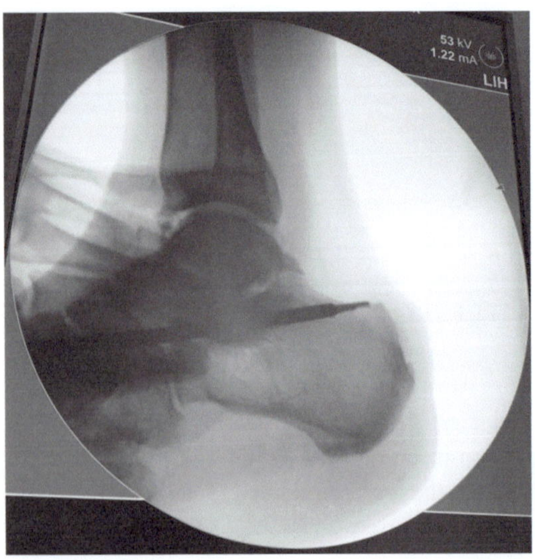

Fig. 30.5 Fluoroscopy used to check the postero-superolateral approach, which must be aimed correctly to reach the bone resection area. © Yves Stiglitz 2015. All Rights Reserved

30.2.3.2 Postero-Supero-Medial Approach

The postero-supero-medial incision is made on the medial side of the calcaneus, in a location that mirrors the lateral one. While there is no danger of damaging critical structures, the blade's position should still be verified by fluoroscopy to ensure it will provide definite access to the bone resection area.

30.2.4 Procedure

The first (and typically only) approach is made laterally, as described above. If needed, a medial incision is added by reaming on the medial side of the calcaneus, like the lateral one.

A percutaneous bone rasp (Fig. 30.6) is introduced to create the working space needed to reduce the risk of damaging soft tissues during burr maneuvers. Periosteum is removed from the calcaneus on its superior, posterior, and lateral sides (Fig. 30.7) until the planned resection limits are reached.

A 3- or 4-mm-diameter wedge burr (Fig. 30.8) is placed on the motorized handpiece and then applied against the bone (Fig. 30.9). The surgeon must not apply direct pressure with the burr on the bone, as this could create a bone rail that will be problematic for the rest of the procedure.

On the lateral side of the calcaneus, it is preferable to ream the bone layer by layer, from

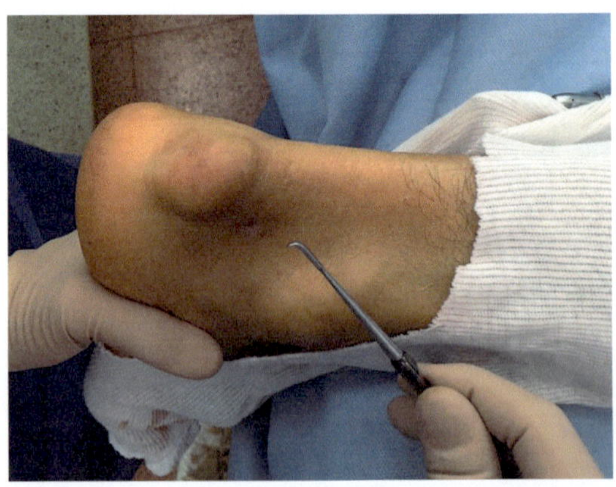

Fig. 30.6 Percutaneous bone rasp used to create working space under fluoroscopy guidance. © Yves Stiglitz 2015. All Rights Reserved

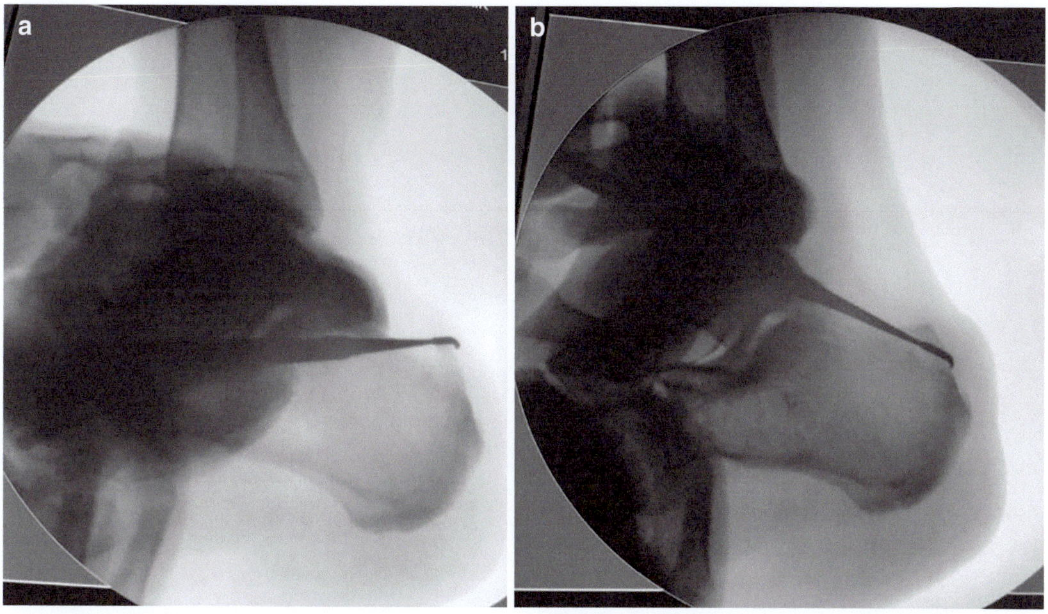

Fig. 30.7 Fluoroscopy used to check the bone rasp's position during periosteum removal. The instrument is introduced through the lateral incision to access the superior (**a**) and posterior (**b**) bone hypertrophy areas.

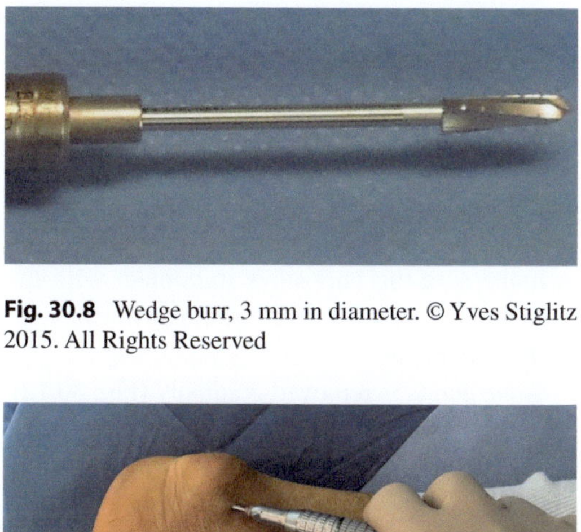

Fig. 30.8 Wedge burr, 3 mm in diameter.

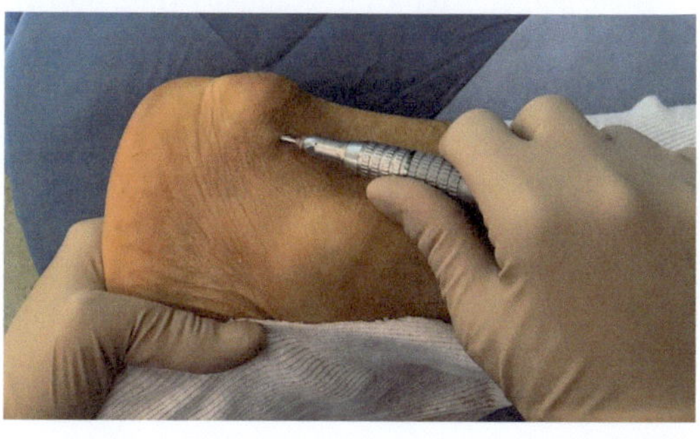

Fig. 30.9 Introducing the burr after it has been assembled with the motorized handpiece.

superficial to deép, using a windshield wiper movement of the wrist with the incision as the rotation point. Externally, the surgeon's wrist will follow a plane symmetric to the one the burr will make against the bone (Fig. 30.10a).

The most delicate portion of the procedure occurs when burring in front of the Achilles tendon. The ankle is dorsiflexed to tension the tendon. The burr is inserted perpendicular to the skin—still using the same lateral approach—until it is located anterior to the tendon. It will contact the anterior part of the tendon and superior edge of the hypertrophied calcaneus. This position corresponds to the posterior point of Kager's triangle, which will be the posterior limit of burring since the risk of tendon damage is high. At this point, we recommend confirming the positioning with fluoroscopy (Fig. 30.10b). The burr is translated anteriorly by about 10 mm before powering it up. The bone is carefully resected by doing back-and-forth motions from front to back, while always keeping the burr in contact with the bone (Fig. 30.11).

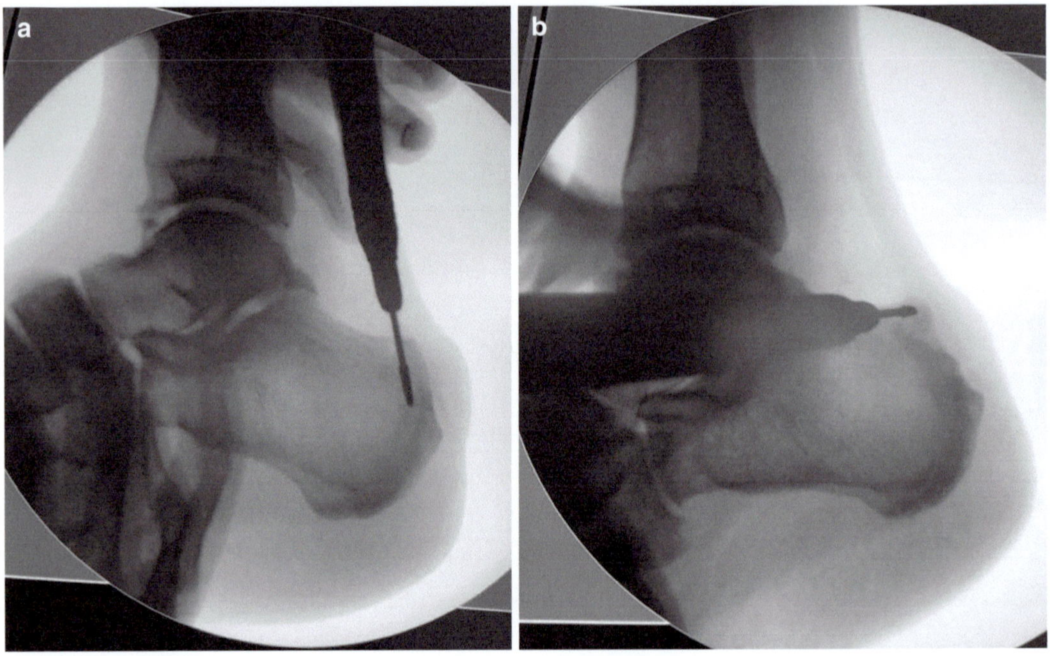

Fig. 30.10 Fluoroscopy used to verify the burr's position at each step. Resection on lateral side of calcaneus (**a**). Resection of posterosuperior corner, forward of anterior edge of the Achilles tendon (**b**. © Yves Stiglitz 2015. All Rights Reserved)

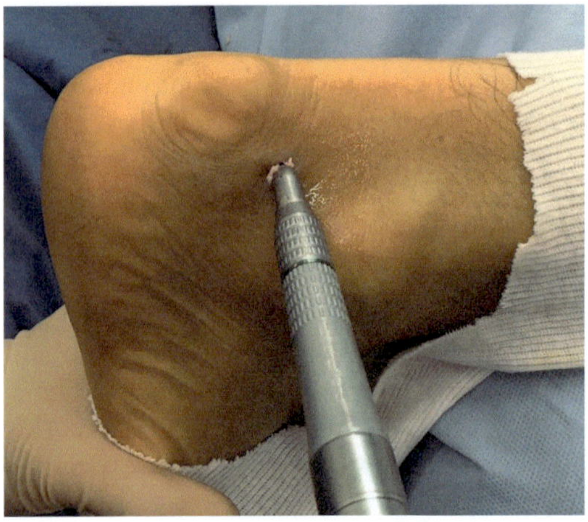

Fig. 30.11 Resection of the posterosuperior corner of the calcaneus. The handpiece is introduced perpendicular to the axis of the Achilles tendon and the burr activated anteriorly to this structure. © Yves Stiglitz 2015. All Rights Reserved

Some surgeons recommend releasing the tension on the Achilles tendon to protect it during burring. In our experience, keeping moderate tension on the tendon allows the surgeon to perceive a posterior abutment. If there are any doubts whatsoever, fluoroscopy should be used to make sure the burr stays in contact with the bone and is located in front of the posterior edge of the calcaneus.

Bone debris is removed gradually (Fig. 30.12), either by finger pressure or by using a rasp to bring to the surface any deep bone that was burred. Injecting 10 or 20 cc of saline can sometimes help to extract any bone that is solidly compacted.

At the end of the procedure, fluoroscopy is used to confirm that enough calcaneal bone has been resected and that all bone debris has been removed (Fig. 30.13).

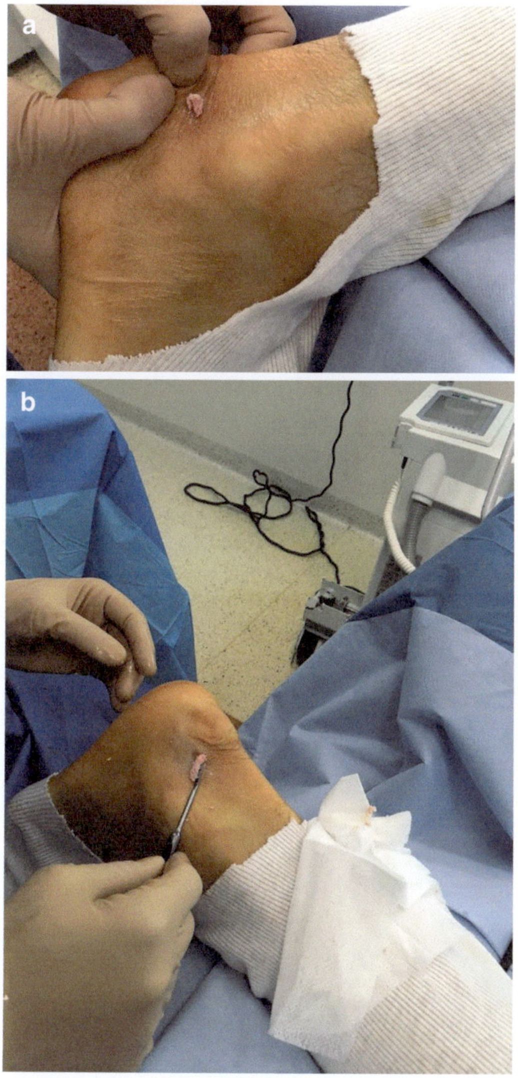

Fig. 30.12 Removal of bone debris, either by finger pressure (**a**) or using a rasp (**b**) to bring up any deep bone that was burred. © Yves Stiglitz 2015. All Rights Reserved

The incision is closed without a drain using one throw of nonabsorbable suture, which is less inflammatory than absorbable suture. A dry, lightly compressive dressing is placed over the site.

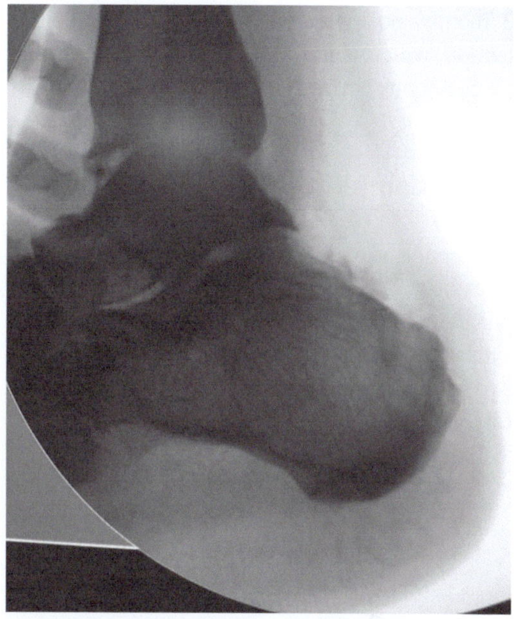

Fig. 30.13 Final fluoroscopy check to evaluate the amount of bone resected and to make sure all the bone debris has been removed. © Yves Stiglitz 2015. All Rights Reserved

30.3 Postoperative Care

Full weight-bearing is allowed immediately, although crutches are used to protect the foot for the first few days postoperative. The patient is free to decide when the crutches are no longer needed.

Step 1 and 2 analgesics are prescribed and used in combination with NSAIDs. We recommend that patients take all these medications for the first 2 days and then use them only as needed to control pain. Nursing care is prescribed for about 2 weeks, which consists of short-term wound care and daily injection of anticoagulants to prevent deep vein thrombosis.

Rehabilitation can be prescribed if the patient has trouble recovering ankle dorsiflexion. No sports participation is allowed for the first

3 months postoperative to protect the Achilles tendon, which could have been damaged during percutaneous burring.

30.4 Complications

We cannot provide information on complication rates because there are no published studies on percutaneous calcaneal resection in Haglund's syndrome, as far as we know. Theoretically, the two most worrisome complications would be as follows:

- Lesion of sural nerve, which is why the lateral approach must be made sufficiently posterior
- Lesion of the Achilles tendon from burr contact; this can be prevented by taking several fluoroscopy images during the procedure to verify the burr's position, especially as a surgeon is learning this technique.

Conversely, the percutaneous procedure has a lower risk of wound healing disturbance than an open procedure, as long as the burr is used at low speeds and it does not come into contact with skin.

30.5 Conclusion

Percutaneous posterior calcaneus resection for Haglund's syndrome is simple to implement but is technically demanding. It has serious theoretical risks that are harder to control than in an open procedure. Nevertheless, its many advantages mean that experienced surgeons can use it to simplify the postoperative course.

Editors' Point of View

The percutaneous technique is very elegant and much less aggressive than the open one. The main pitfall is weakening the Achilles tendon, which can be protected by placing a small Pauwels blade against it.

Plantar Fasciitis

31

Mariano De Prado and Manuel Cuervas-Mons

31.1 Introduction

Plantar fasciitis is a widespread foot condition and one of the most common reasons for medical visits at foot and ankle clinics [1]. It presents as pain in the heel with an insidious onset, which increases during walking and when standing for long periods of time. It is estimated that 10% of the population suffers from this disorder [1], with a peak in the incidence at 40–60 years of age, but no gender predominance.

This disorder was first described by Wood in 1812; the radiological finding of *calcaneal spur* was attributed to him in 1900. A biomechanical mechanism for this condition was finally proposed in 1940 [2]. Since 1950, several treatments have been proposed—both conservative and surgical—with plantar fasciotomy being the most widely used surgical treatment [3].

31.2 Etiology

The plantar fascia is a thick aponeurosis whose function is to maintain the longitudinal arches of the foot [4]. The repeated microtrauma that occurs during walking and standing can contribute to degeneration of its collagen fibers, mainly in the middle portion of the central band, at the calcaneal insertion [2]. If these events exceed the body's regenerative capacities, the plantar fasciitis will become symptomatic [5], with the appearance of insidious and exquisite pain that increases during walking or standing.

Although 85% of cases have no identifiable trigger [1]; the etiological factors can be divided into two groups: mechanical and systemic. Mechanical alterations can contribute to the plantar fasciitis due to direct or indirect overloading of the calcaneal insertion. Risk factors are obesity, lack of flexibility with foot stiffness, or the opposite—having flat feet [1].

As for systematic causes, talalgia can be a local manifestation of inflammatory arthropathy (ankylosing spondylitis, reactive arthritis, etc.) or a metabolic (gout, diabetes), neurological, and vascular disease. We will only focus on mechanical causes in this chapter.

The foot's longitudinal arch is maintained statically by the plantar aponeurosis and dynamically by the flexor digitorum brevis, abductor hallucis, and abductor digiti quinti muscles. Static overloading (flat foot, cavus foot, Achilles tendon shortening, limited subtalar joint motion, etc.) and dynamic overloading (sports or occupational activities) can increase the tension on the fascia and the muscle attachments, eventually leading to symptoms of plantar fasciitis.

When these situations become chronic, signs of enthesitis can appear, along with periostitis of

M. De Prado (✉)
Hospital Quirón, Murcia, Spain
e-mail: marianodeprado@yahoo.es

M. Cuervas-Mons
e-mail: manuel.cuervasmons@gmail.com

C. Cazeau, Y. Stiglitz (eds.), *Percutaneous and Minimally Invasive Foot Surgery*,
https://doi.org/10.1007/978-3-030-98791-6_31

the medial process of the calcaneal tuberosity. Repeated microtears and small contusions contribute to the development of calcifications that make up the calcaneal spur.

31.3 Clinical Findings

The main clinical feature is pain—usually on the medial side of the heel—that radiates along the plantar fascia. It typically occurs after a period of rest, often overnight. While it is very intense initially, it decreases with walking but then reappears at the end of the day [6]. However, this symptom-free period may not be present, with the pain being continuous instead, especially in the initial stages. It can be intense and feel like one has walked on a nail. The patient will point to the calcaneal spur as the source.

The pathophysiology of this pain is well known. During the day, while walking or standing for long periods of time, the fascia is continuously loaded. When sitting or lying down, the patient holds their foot with the ankle slightly plantar flexed to relieve pain, which shortens and contracts the plantar fascia. When the foot is reloaded, the first few steps place tension on the fascia and triggers pain. The pain disappears as the aponeurosis gets stretched but then reappears as the stretching continues.

31.4 Diagnosis

The diagnosis is based on the patient's history and on palpation reproducing the symptoms.

31.4.1 History

It is important to ask the patient for details about the pain, location, intensity, radiation, and associated symptoms. One must determine if the pain is isolated or associated with signs of inflammatory or systematic disease. The patient's occupation and sports activities must be documented.

31.4.2 Clinical Examination

The patient is examined when standing and sitting, and then during walking, including looking for asymmetric wear in their shoes. The patient's weight and any leg misalignment are documented.

Objective signs of plantar fasciitis are reproduction of the pain upon palpation of the medial process of the calcaneal tuberosity. The location of the pain at the medial and inferior process of the calcaneus where the abductor hallucis inserts has led some authors to state that this disorder is an insertional enthesopathy, like epicondylitis.

The exact location of the pain (Fig. 31.1) is identified, along with any areas of excess pressure and paresthesia or dysesthesia, indicative of potential entrapment neuropathy.

31.4.3 Supplemental Examinations

Since the diagnosis is above all clinical, any other examinations mainly contribute to identifying the cause. Plain radiographs are useful for identifying calcaneal fractures. They can also be used to look for a potential calcaneal spur (Fig. 31.2), which reinforces the diagnosis of plantar fasciitis. The best views are dorsoplantar, lateral, and three-quarters with loading, along with retrocalcaneal.

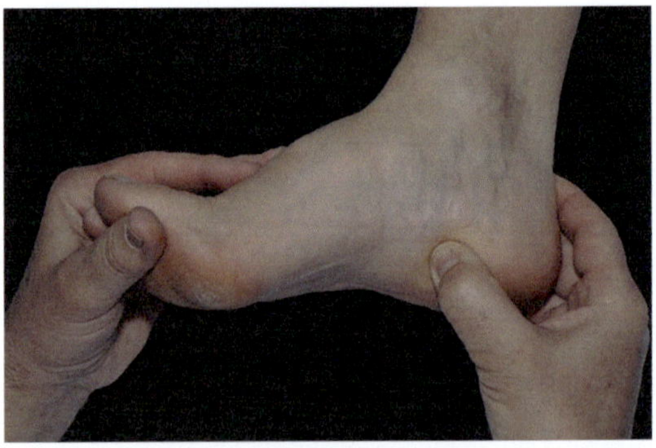

Fig. 31.1 Location of pain is determined by palpation.

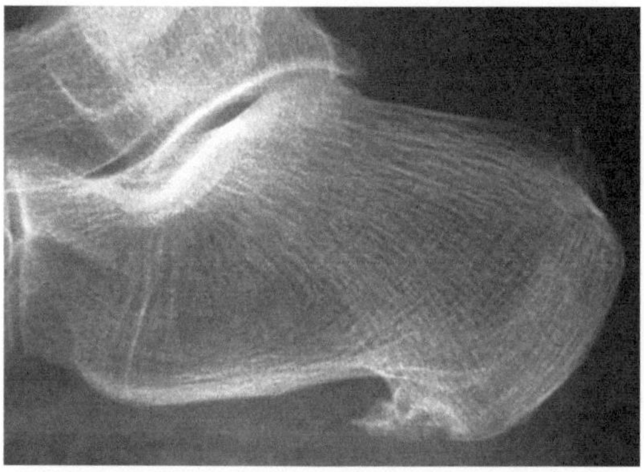

Fig. 31.2 Lateral view of a calcaneal spur. © Mariano De Prado 2015. All Rights Reserved

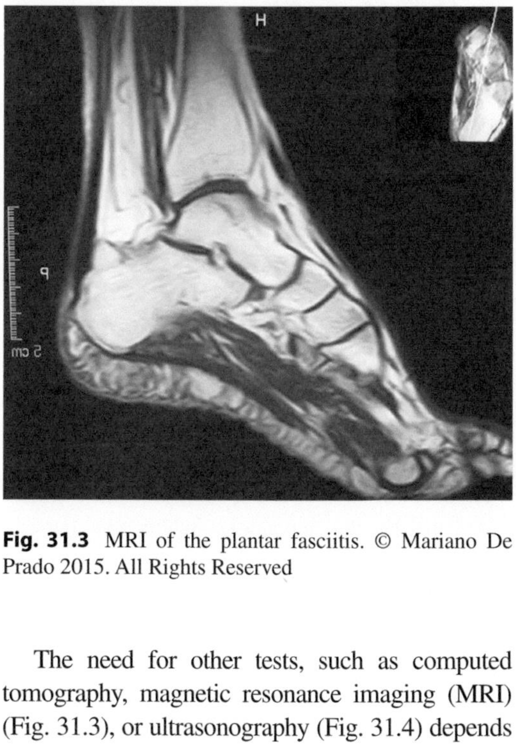

Fig. 31.3 MRI of the plantar fasciitis. © Mariano De Prado 2015. All Rights Reserved

The need for other tests, such as computed tomography, magnetic resonance imaging (MRI) (Fig. 31.3), or ultrasonography (Fig. 31.4) depends on whether the diagnosis is still uncertain at this point [7].

In some situations, we will look for signs of an inflammatory arthropathy (HLA-B27, etc.). Electromyography is useful for detecting entrapment neuropathy, and a bone scan can be ordered to look for a calcaneal bone lesion that is not visible on standard radiographs.

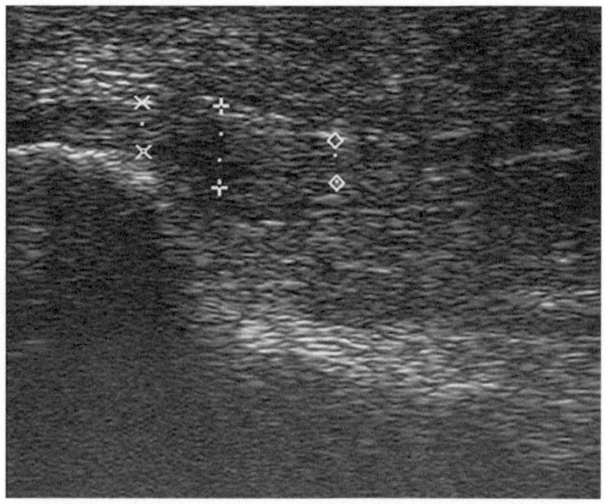

Fig. 31.4 Ultrasound imaging of the plantar fasciitis. © Mariano De Prado 2015. All Rights Reserved

31.5 Treatment

The patient is initially treated conservatively, with surgical treatment reserved for those whose condition worsens. Most patients improve greatly with conservative treatment [7], with up to 95% of them better at 6 months [8].

31.5.1 Conservative Treatment

Conservative treatment is mandatory for at least 6 months. It consists of stretching the plantar fascia, insoles, night-time splinting, bandaging, physical therapy and shockwave therapy, anti-inflammatory drugs, and corticosteroid injections. However, corticosteroid injections are controversial, especially in athletes because of the risk of aponeurosis rupture.

31.5.2 Surgical Treatment

Surgery is the final step [1] and is needed in about 10% of patients [4]. The indication is the presence of disabling symptoms, during sports or work-related activities, after 6 months of comprehensive conservative treatment and ultrasonography findings of the fascia being ≥6 mm thick. Surgery is contraindicated in cases of instability and ligament laxity.

Several surgical techniques are used currently. The standard procedure is an open complete or partial fasciotomy with or without excision of the calcaneal spur. The aggressiveness of this technique and its consequences is the main argument for pursuing the conservative treatment to the limit. It also led to the development of new, less aggressive techniques, such as endoscopic or percutaneous fasciotomy and minimally invasive surgery.

31.5.3 Authors' Preferred Method

We prefer using minimally invasive surgery. Percutaneous fasciotomy was described in 1983 by Pilzer [9], and it has been used by many surgeons over the past 30 years with a wide range of outcomes [10, 11]. We believe it allows us to perform the procedure with less damage to soft tissues and contributes to faster functional recovery. Once the surgical approach is determined, the next questions are:

31.5.3.1 Complete or Partial Fasciotomy?

Some authors recommend doing partial plantar fasciotomy, solely on the medial bundle. However, we have adopted the standard reasoning for treating enthesopathies, namely complete fasciotomy in order to prevent recurrences.

31.5.3.2 Resection of Calcaneal Spur?

Some surgeons believe that resecting the calcaneal spur is not indicated, as it is not responsible for the patient's symptoms. Unlike them, we recommend that it be resected because it has a major psychological effect on the patient, who continues to worry when the spur is still visible, especially since this surgical procedure is not very aggressive.

31.5.4 Surgical Technique [12, 13]

31.5.4.1 Instrumentation

The typical instrumentation used for minimally invasive surgery is used here:

- No. 64 Beaver-type scalpel blade
- Long Shannon burr No. 44
- Small and large rasps
- Fluoroscopy system

31.5.4.2 Patient Setup

The patient is positioned supine, with his foot on the image intensifier and resting on its lateral side (Fig. 31.5a, b).

31.5.4.3 Anesthesia

Regional anesthesia of the posterior tibial nerve is performed; however, some of the sensory branches to the heel may not be affected; thus, a subcutaneous injection of the posterior tibial nerve on its medial side and the saphenous nerve on its lateral side is also required.

31.5.4.4 Locating the Entry Point

The entry point (Figs. 31.6, 31.7, 31.8, and 31.9) for this technique is crucial because the motorized instruments must remain tangential to the plantar cortex of the calcaneus. If the approach was perpendicular to the cortex, it could weaken and fracture the calcaneus when the patient resumes weightbearing.

Fluoroscopy is used to pinpoint the location. A line is traced on the skin on the medial side of the heel, over the plantar side of the calcaneus, and extended to reach the edge of the foot. The entry point is marked on the sole of the foot with a skin marker 10 mm lateral to the line reaching the edge of the foot.

31.5.4.5 Fasciotomy

With the foot on its lateral side, the plantar fascia is placed under tension by pressing under the metatarsal heads (Fig. 31.10).

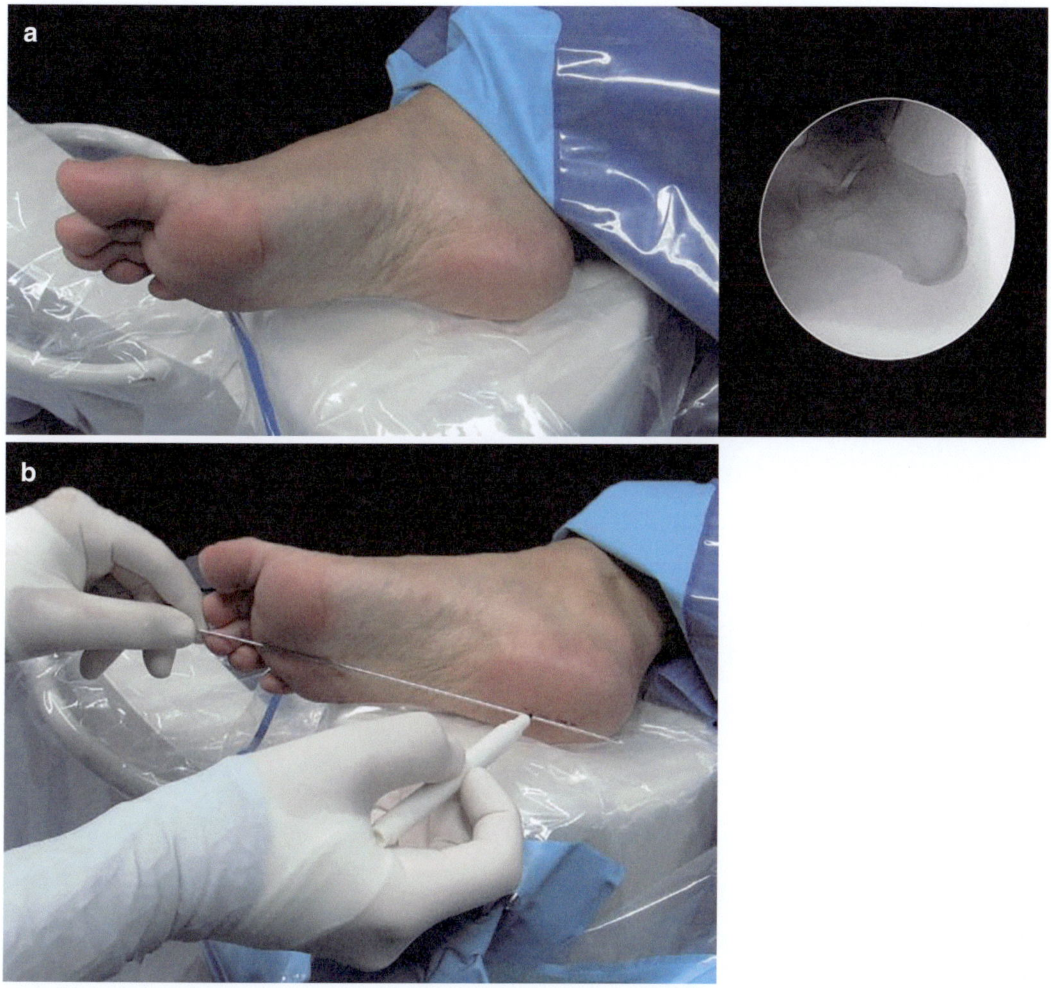

Fig. 31.5 Patient's foot resting on image intensifier (**a**); a line is traced on the sole of the foot (**b**).

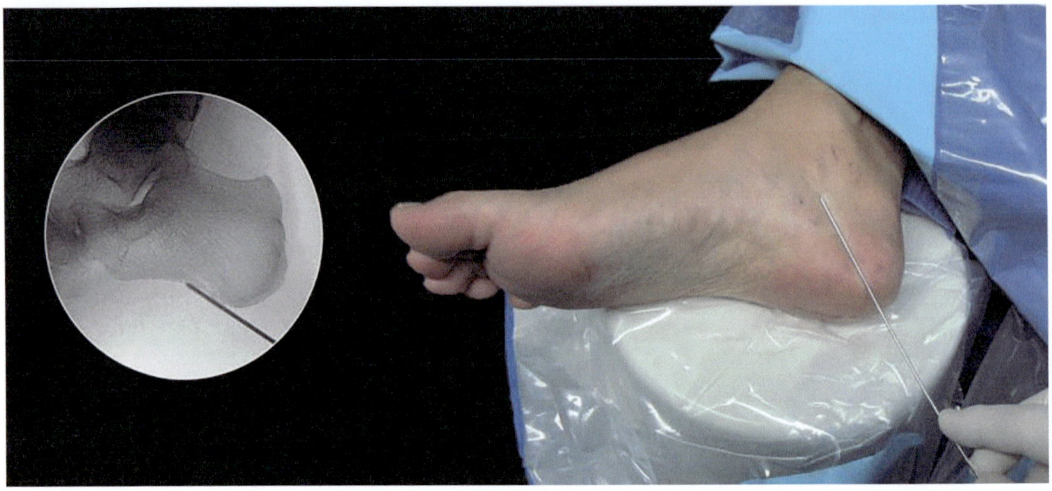

Fig. 31.6 K-wire used to locate plantar cortex of calcaneus. © Mariano De Prado 2015. All Rights Reserved

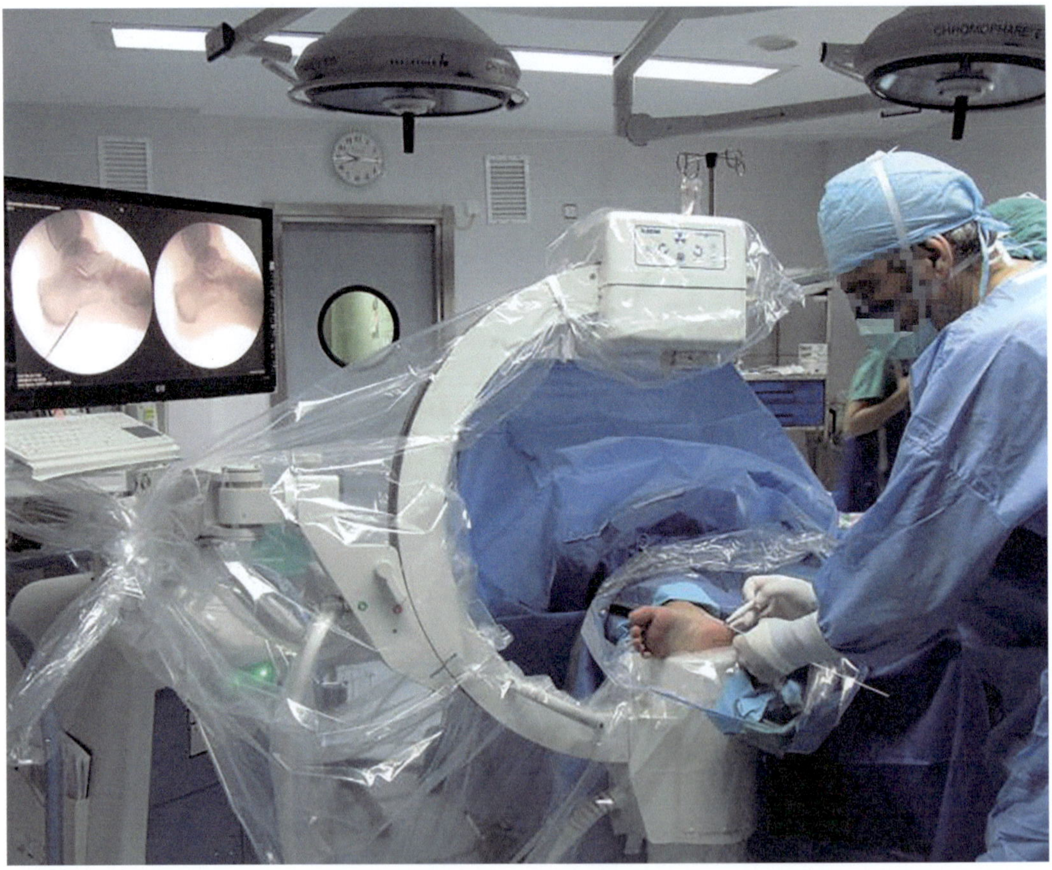

Fig. 31.7 Surgeon using fluoroscopy to locate entry point. © Mariano De Prado 2015. All Rights Reserved

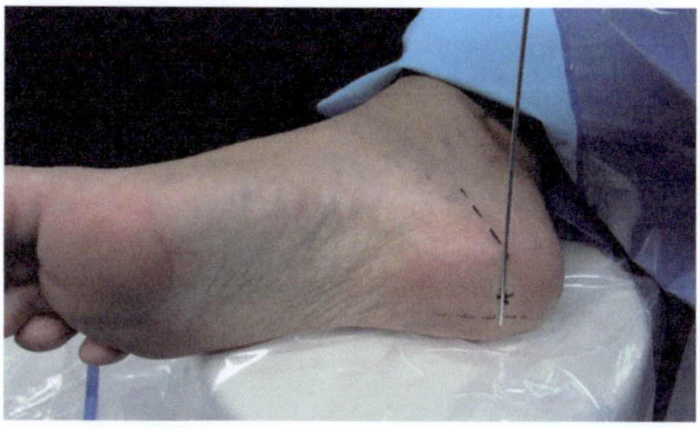

Fig. 31.8 Line traced on the medial side of the heel.

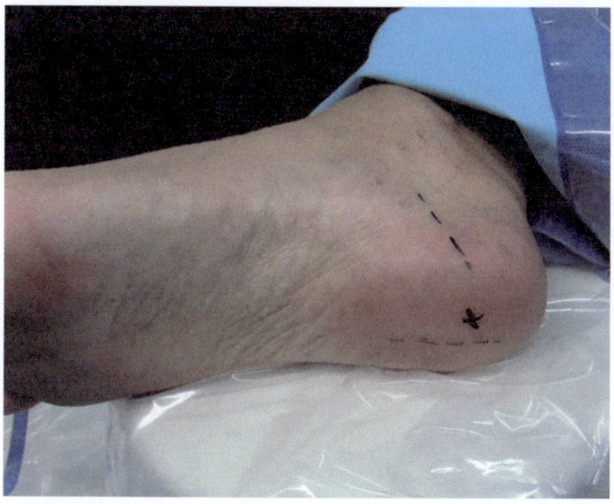

Fig. 31.9 Entry point (x) is located 10 mm from the edge of the foot.

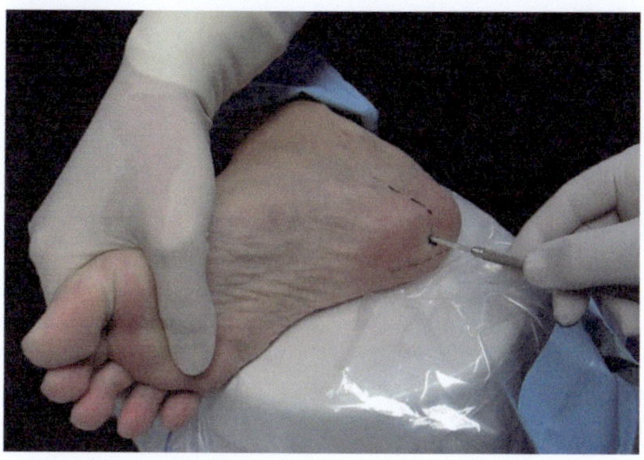

Fig. 31.10 Pressing under metatarsal heads to tension the plantar fascia.

A 2-mm-long incision is made with the Beaver blade, parallel to the plantar side of the calcaneus under the tensioned plantar fascia. The scalpel is placed at the insertion of the aponeurosis or the calcaneal spur, parallel to the calcaneus cortex. This parallel configuration between the instrument and plantar cortex is crucial.

Once the entry point is confirmed, the scalpel blade is pushed in to perform the complete fasciotomy in a single motion, from medial to lateral (Fig. 31.11). Once finished, the surgeon will feel the aponeurosis loosen.

The next step is to excise the calcaneal spur. This is done by inserting a rasp to remove its fibrous layer (Fig. 31.12). Next, the long Shannon No. 44 burr is inserted, which must rest against the lateral side of the tip of the spur. The excision starts by making small sweeping motions under fluoroscopy control, until the spur is no longer visible (Fig. 31.13). One must be careful not to damage the plantar cortex of the calcaneus. This can be accomplished by making sure the burr never becomes perpendicular to the calcaneus. The bone debris is removed with the rasp; the teeth of the rasp must face the soft tissues, not away from them (Fig. 31.14).

The incision is closed with 4/0 monofilament suture (Fig. 31.15) and then a dressing applied on the heel (Fig. 31.16).

31.5.4.6 Postoperative Course

Full weight-bearing in running shoes is allowed immediately after surgery. A clinical follow-up examination is done 7 days later and the suture removed. We recommend that patients wear insoles with rigid arch support for 6–9 months in order to minimize the loss of stability in the longitudinal arch after plantar fasciotomy.

31.5.4.7 Complications

The complication rate for this technique, particularly skin-related and infections, is very low. In the immediate postoperative phase, about

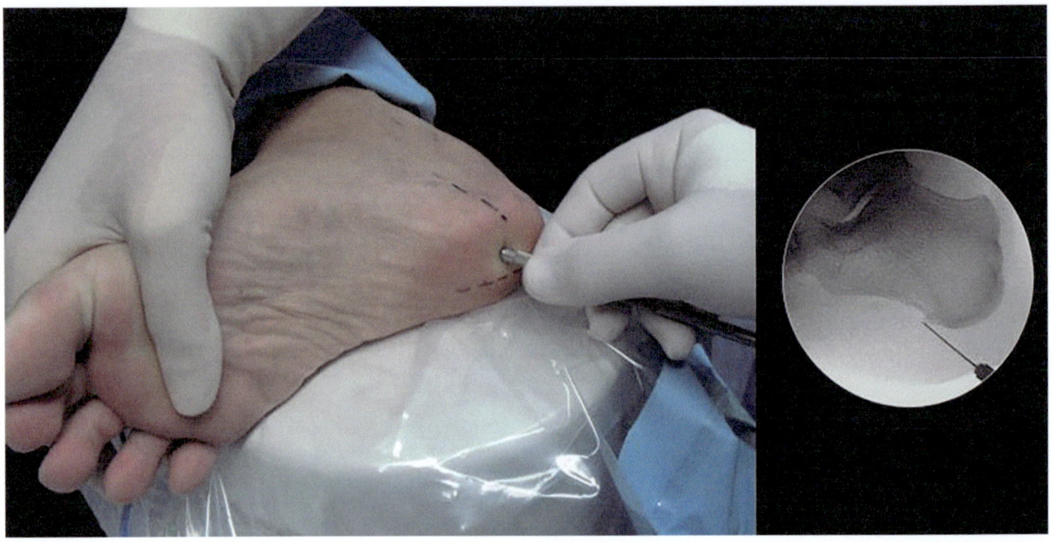

Fig. 31.11 Complete fasciotomy performed with a single motion of the scalpel.

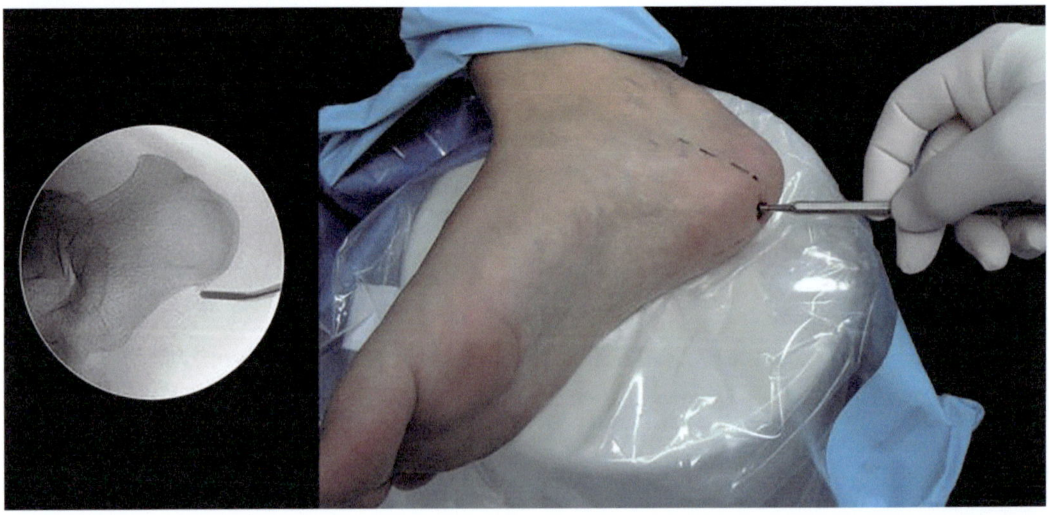

Fig. 31.12 Rasp used to remove fibrous layer on calcaneal spur.

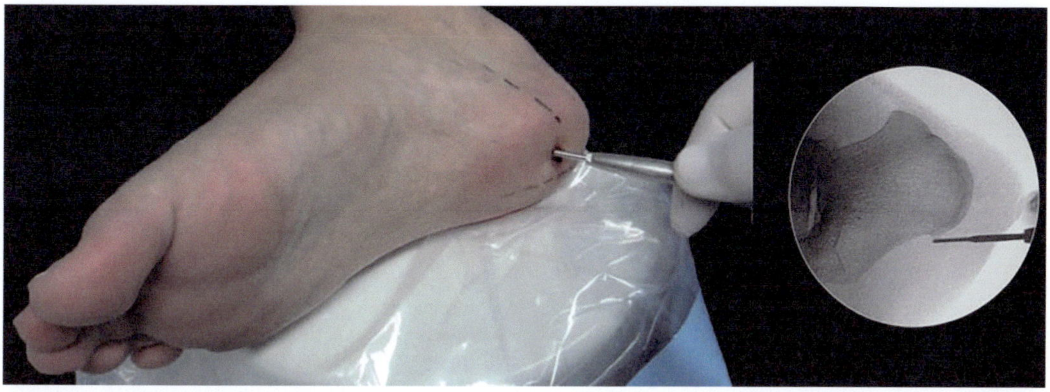

Fig. 31.13 Shannon burr inserted against the lateral side of the spur's tip.

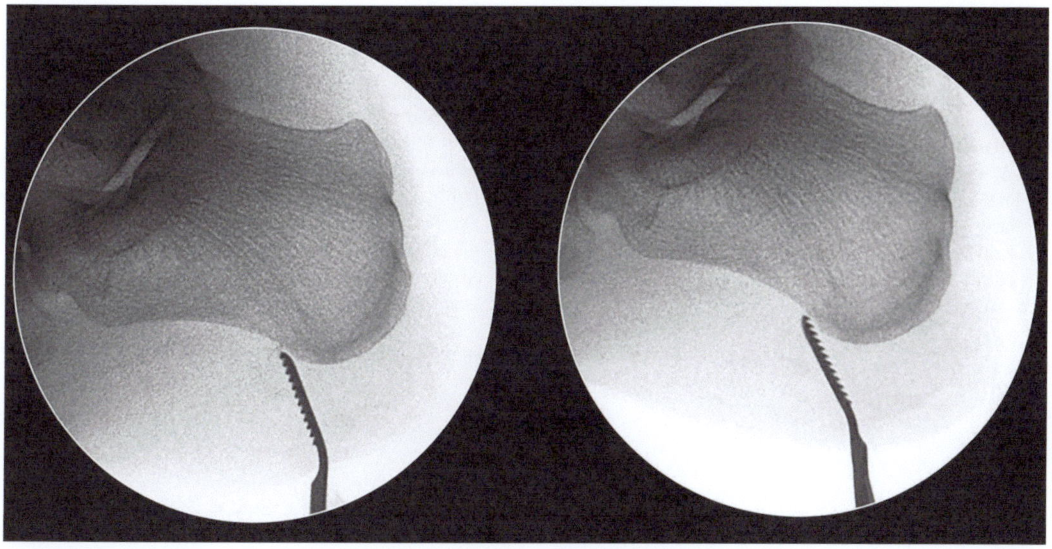

Fig. 31.14 Rasp used to remove bone debris.

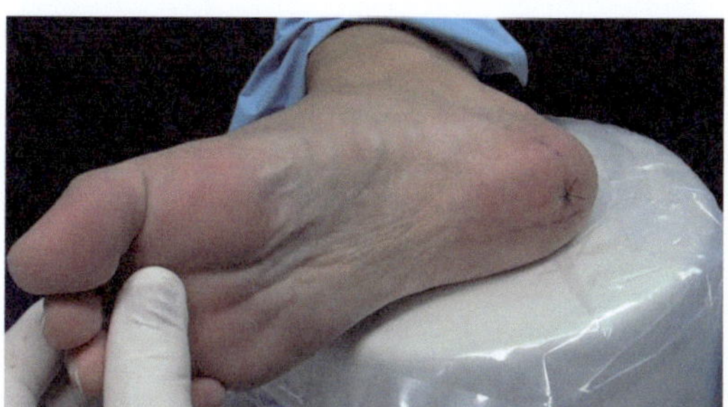

Fig. 31.15 Incision closed with single suture point.

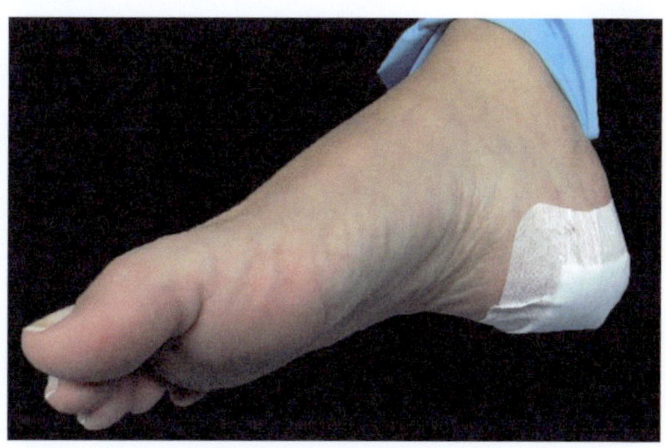

Fig. 31.16 Dressing applied over incision.

30% of patients have pain on the lateral side of their foot, which resolves by itself within the first 3 months. Calcifications may be visible on radiographs; they are without clinical consequence as long as the bone debris was completely removed with the rasp.

Editors' Point of View

This is a difficult technique given the possibility of damaging the posterior tibial neurovascular bundle. It must not be done early in one's learning curve.

References

1. Tong KB, Furia J. Economic burden of plantar fasciitis treatment in the United States. Am J Orthop. 2010;39:227–31.
2. Wilkinson AN, Kilmartin TE. A review of the minimal incision plantar fasciotomy in the treatment of heel pain. Br J Podiat. 2000;3:76–80.
3. Faghihnia N, Clark GD. Percutaneous plantar fasciotomy for recalcitrant plantar fasciitis. The Podiatry Institute Update. 2010. 278–286.
4. Othman AM, Ragag EM. Endoscopic plantar fasciotomy versus extracorporeal shock wave therapy for treatment of chronic plantar fasciitis. Arch Orthop Trauma Surg. 2010;130:1343–7.
5. Barrett SJ, O'Malley R. Plantar fasciitis and other causes of heel pain. Am Fam Physician. 1999;59:2200–6.
6. Perelman GK, Figura MA, Sandberg NS. The medial instep plantar fasciotomy. J Foot Ankle Surg. 1995;34:447–57.
7. Borrelli A. Percutaneous plantar fasciotomy for the surgical treatment of refractive plantar fasciitis. Tech Foot Ankle Surg. 2011;10:49–55.
8. Bordelon RL. Heel Pain. In: Mann RA, Coughlin MJ, editors. Surgery of the foot and ankle. St-Louis: Mosby; 1993. p. 837–47.
9. Pilzer HP, Berlin MJ. Percutaneous plantar fasciotomy–a new approach. Current Podiatry. 1983:32–6.
10. Erdemir A, Piazza SJ. Changes in foot loading following plantar fasciotomy: a computer modeling study. J Biomech Eng. 2004;126:237–43.
11. Crary JL, Hollis JM, Manoli A 2nd. The effect of plantar fascia release on strain in the spring and long plantar ligaments. Foot Ankle Int. 2003;24:245–50.
12. De Prado M, Ripoli PL, Golano P. Minimally invasive foot surgery: surgical techniques, indications, anatomical basis. Barcelona: About Your Health Publishers; 2009.
13. De Prado M. Minimally invasive foot surgery: a paradigm shift. In: Maffulli N, Easley M, editors. Minimally invasive surgery of the foot and ankle. London: Springer; 2011. p. 3–11.

Morton's Neuroma

32

Mariano De Prado and Manuel Cuervas-Mons

32.1 Introduction

The clinical disorder known as Morton's neuroma is a compressive neuropathy of the common plantar digital nerve in the third intermetatarsal space, between the third and fourth metatarsal heads. This condition manifests itself as metatarsalgia, combined with interdigital neurological symptoms such as numbness, dysesthesia, or cramping. It is bilateral in 10% of cases.

The term *Morton's neuroma* is somewhat of a misnomer. A neuroma is a nerve tumor [1]; it must not be confused with nerve thickening that can appear in the context of compression neuropathy, as is the case here [2, 3]. Furthermore, Morton [4] was not the first one to describe this disorder in 1876; instead it was Durlacher [5] who described it first in 1845 and had a better description of the true cause of the symptoms. However, we will use this term here, since it is universally accepted in orthopedic surgery circles.

32.2 Etiology

Various pathophysiological theories have been advanced to explain the origin of Morton's neuroma: tumoral, vascular, inflammatory, etc. The mechanical origin of this compression neuropathy in the intermetatarsal space was demonstrated by Gauthier through anatomical pathology and electromyography studies of the common plantar digital nerve (Fig. 32.1) [6]. The tunnel is made up, from back to front and superficial to deep, of the deep transverse metatarsal ligament (DTML), the metatarsal heads, and the superficial transverse metatarsal ligament.

32.2.1 Anatomy

The third common plantar digital nerve is a branch of the medial plantar nerve stemming from the tibial nerve. This nerve is thicker than the digital nerves because, contrary to the first two digital nerves, it receives fibers from a

M. De Prado (✉) · M. Cuervas-Mons
Hospital Quirón, Murcia, Spain

C. Cazeau, Y. Stiglitz (eds.), *Percutaneous and Minimally Invasive Foot Surgery*,
https://doi.org/10.1007/978-3-030-98791-6_32

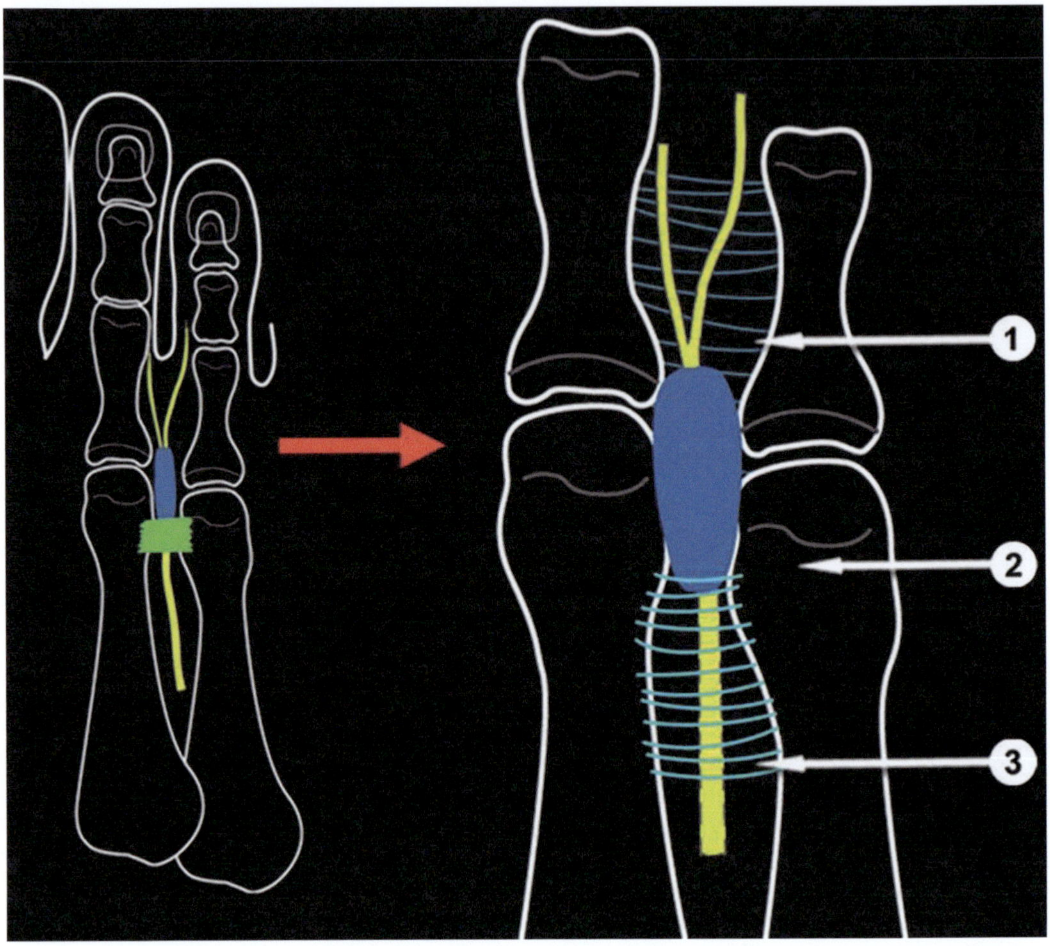

Fig. 32.1 Compressive etiology of Morton's neuroma. Dorsal view (left). Plantar view (right). © Mariano De Prado 2015. All Rights Reserved

branch of the lateral plantar nerve. The plantar digital nerve is accompanied in its course by deep intermetatarsal vascular structures and the lumbrical tendon.

The DTML lines the plantar side of the intermetatarsal space. At the metatarsal heads, on the distal edge of the ligament, the nerve is angled dorsally 45° and divided into two plantar digital nerves. On the dorsal side of the transverse metatarsal ligament (longitudinal fibers from the plantar aponeurosis), it is over the metatarsophalangeal joints and the fibrous expansions of the plantar fascia.

32.2.2 Etiology

During walking, compressive forces alter the relationships of nerve structures with their containers. During the stance phase, the terminal portion of the common plantar digital nerve does not impinge with its anatomical neighbors (Fig. 32.2). When the metatarsophalangeal joint starts its extension, several phenomena occur at the same time: increase in the nerve's dorsal inclination against the intermetatarsal ligament, increase in this structure's tension due to very high pressure under the metatarsal heads, and

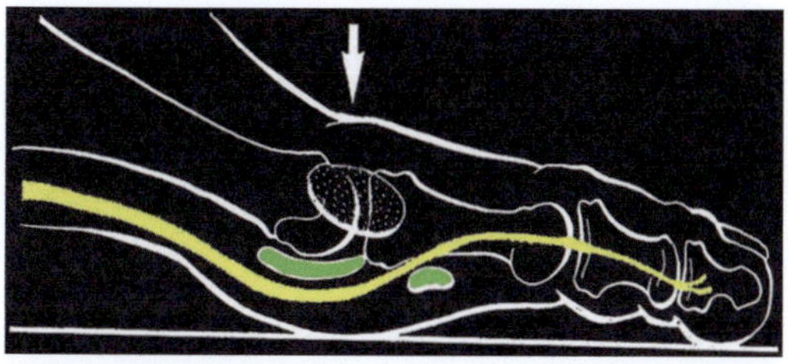

Fig. 32.2 Common plantar digital nerve is *not* compressed during stance phase.

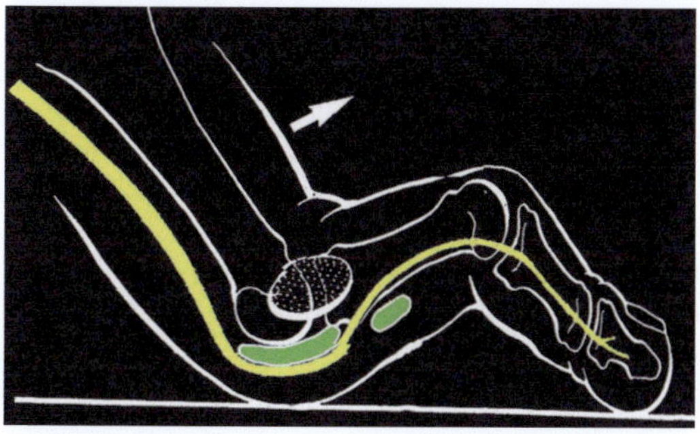

Fig. 32.3 Common plantar digital nerve is compressed during push-off.

reduction in tunnel volume due to direct pressure of the ground on the plantar fascia (Fig. 32.3).

The third common plantar digital nerve is thicker because of its dual origin (medial and lateral plantar nerves), making it less mobile and more sensitive to compression. Anatomical factors (low position of metatarsal heads, forefoot pronation, hammer toes, etc.) and mechanical factors (type of shoes, repeated microtrauma, etc.) also contribute to compression.

32.3 Clinical Findings

The main clinical feature is intermittent forefoot pain that is very intense and occurs suddenly during walking. The patient feels like they suffered a knife wound or a burn in the intermetatarsal space, generally associated with a cramping sensation that radiates between the toes. The pain disappears when the person stops, forcing her to remove her shoes, manipulate her forefoot, and move her toes.

Less often, the patient presents with dull pain, burning, and numbness of the third and fourth toes, which increases during walking and is made worse by wearing narrow shoes. Some patients have pain continually, even when not wearing shoes, and they cannot bear any toe contact at night.

32.4 Diagnosis

The diagnosis of Morton's neuroma is mainly clinical, based on the patient's history and a physical examination to reproduce the symptoms.

32.4.1 History

It is important to ask the patient for details about the pain, how it appeared, its location, intensity, features, radiation, and associated symptoms. One must also determine whether it is isolated or occurs in combination with arthralgia and whether other diseases are present (diabetes, gout, etc.). The type of shoes worn and the nature of athletic and occupational activities must be documented.

32.4.2 Physical Examination

Nothing will appear abnormal—such as associated plantar hyperkeratosis—when looking at the foot. Some patients may have flat feet or other foot deformities that are irrelevant.

Direct palpation of the third intermetatarsal space (Fig. 32.4) will reproduce the signs described above, sometimes associated with electric discharge when pressure is applied on the metatarsal heads.

The Mulder sign is disease specific [7]. This test consists of compressing the intermetatarsal space by applying lateral compression to the heads of the first and fifth metatarsals, combined with dorsiflexion of the toes. It is positive when paresthesia appears in the suspect area, accompanied by an audible click. Other clinical tests exist such as the one described by Gauthier [6] (compression of

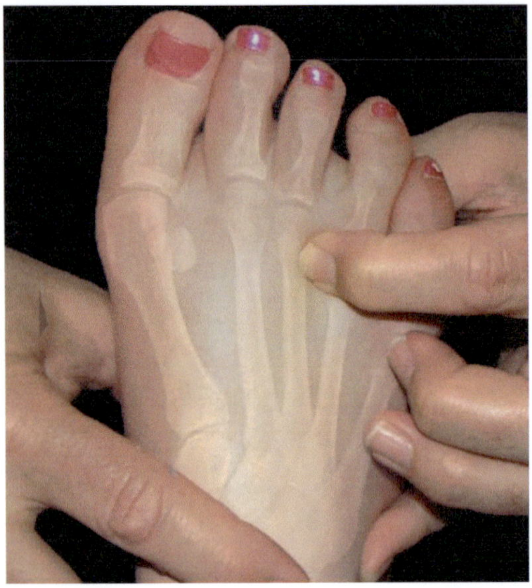

Fig. 32.4 Direct palpation of third intermetatarsal space. © Mariano De Prado 2015. All Rights Reserved

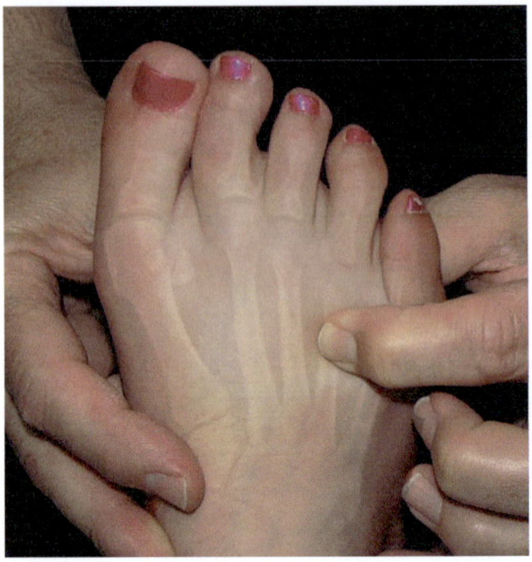

Fig. 32.5 Pain can be elicited by pressing on shaft of third and fourth metatarsals. © Mariano De Prado 2015. All Rights Reserved

metatarsal area with alternative flexion-extension movements of the toes), the Bratkowski test (feeling of a mass or swelling in the intermetatarsal space during plantar compression combined with toe extension), or even the classical Lasègue's sign.

Most patients have pain when the examiner presses on the bone shaft of the third and fourth metatarsals, not inside the intermetatarsal space. For us, this is a very important clinical sign (Fig. 32.5).

32.4.3 Additional Examinations

Standard radiographs are normal but must still be made to rule out differential diagnoses. In some patients, the diaphyseal cortex of the third and/or fourth metatarsals is thickened, indicative of increased loading (Fig. 32.6).

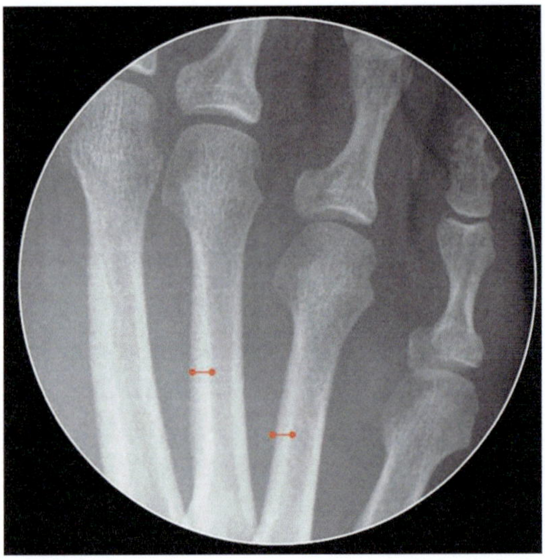

Fig. 32.6 Thickening of diaphyseal cortex of third and/or fourth metatarsals. © Mariano De Prado 2015. All Rights Reserved

Ultrasonography is used to confirm the diagnosis and to rule out other causes. A positive Mulder sonographic sign reproducing the pain [8] increases the sensitivity; the nerve is visibly thickened, and the differential diagnosis is established (vascular tumor, etc.). If there are suggestive clinical signs but the ultrasonography is negative, magnetic resonance imaging can be requested [9]. EMG can be useful to precisely evaluate the condition of the nerve.

32.5 Treatment

The treatment strategy is controversial. It should initially be conservative, with surgical treatment reserved for nonresponders, although some authors recommend performing surgery right away [10].

32.5.1 Conservative Treatment

Conservative treatment consists of postural training and of wearing wide shoes, without heels. It is recommended to combine this treatment with foot orthotics, which help to unload the retrocapital area, and medial posts on the rear foot to control forefoot pronation.

Other treatments have been used such as ultrasound, electrical stimulation, hydrotherapy, and physical therapy, with variable results [11, 12].

Injections can provide transient pain relief. Local anesthetic and corticosteroids are injected most frequently, although recent studies have reported mixed results with other agents such as formaldehyde, phenol, alcohol [13], and vitamin B12 [14].

32.5.2 Surgical Treatment

If conservative treatment fails, surgical treatment is indicated and provides satisfactory outcomes in 80–96% of cases, depending on the technique used [15]. The standard technique consists of neurectomy with nerve release and DTML release.

Open neurectomy through a dorsal approach is the most used method and provides good functional outcomes. New minimally invasive surgical techniques have been described such as neurectomy, electrocoagulation [16], radiofrequency ablation [17], carbon dioxide laser [18], or cryogenic denervation [19].

However, despite these innovations, complete resection in an open procedure remains one of the most frequently used methods [15]. This happens to be the only scenario in human disease where nerve compression is treated by resection, with its inevitable consequences [20].

We believe that Morton's neuroma is a dynamic compression neuropathy, not a nerve tumor, as confirmed by various anatomical pathology studies [2, 3]. For this reason, removing the nerve is not justified.

Plantar nerve release with decompression—not resection—must be considered. In 1979, Gautier [6] described open decompression. This treatment is a good alternative and offers better functional outcomes than neurectomy with lower complication rates [20]. We have described various nerve release techniques that involve cutting the DTML, which reduces the surgery's invasiveness, whether performed by endoscopy [21] or percutaneously [22–24]. Endoscopic nerve release has been described by Barrett and Pignetti [21]. It consists in using a scalpel to transect the DTML attachment under endoscopy guidance through two small incisions [25].

32.5.3 Percutaneous Nerve Release Technique

Instrumentation (Fig. 32.7)

- No. 64 Beaver-type scalpel blade
- Long Shannon No. 44 burr
- Small and large rasps
- Fluoroscopy system

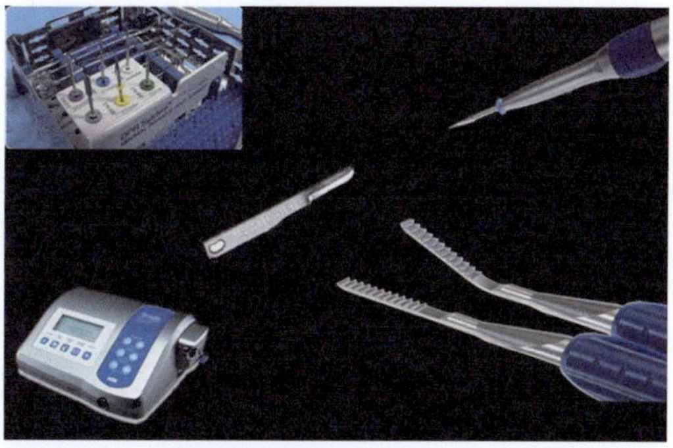

Fig. 32.7 Instrumentation.

Patient Setup (Fig. 32.8)
The patient is positioned supine with the foot over the end of the table resting on the image intensifier; no tourniquet is used.

Anesthesia (Fig. 32.9)
Regional anesthesia targets the medial tibial nerve in the medial retromalleolar area, sural nerve in the lateral retromalleolar area, the sensory branches of the superficial peroneal nerve subcutaneously on the anterior side of the foot, and the deep peroneal nerve on the anterior side of the talonavicular joint.

32.5.4 Isolated Nerve Release

The entry point is located in the third intermetatarsal space, 20 mm proximal to the fourth metatarsophalangeal joint and 2 mm inside the neck of the fourth metatarsal (Fig. 32.10).

A 2-mm longitudinal incision is made with a Beaver blade in the intermetatarsal space. The blade is angled 45° downward and forward (Fig. 32.11). It penetrates the intermetatarsal space while using the cortex of the fourth metatarsal as a guide. The motion is made from plantar to dorsal to transect the DTML (Fig. 32.12). To confirm the procedure was successful, a rasp is inserted under fluoroscopy guidance to verify the absence of resistance.

32.5.5 Nerve Release + DMMO

In our clinical experience, isolated percutaneous nerve release has not always been satisfactory. Given the notion of dynamic compressive neu-

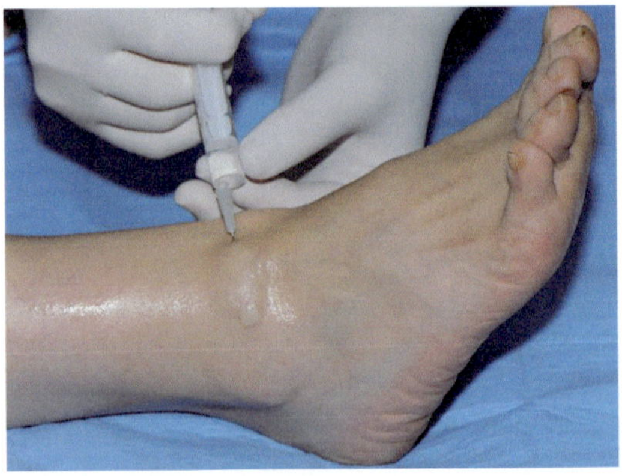

Fig. 32.9 Regional anesthesia.

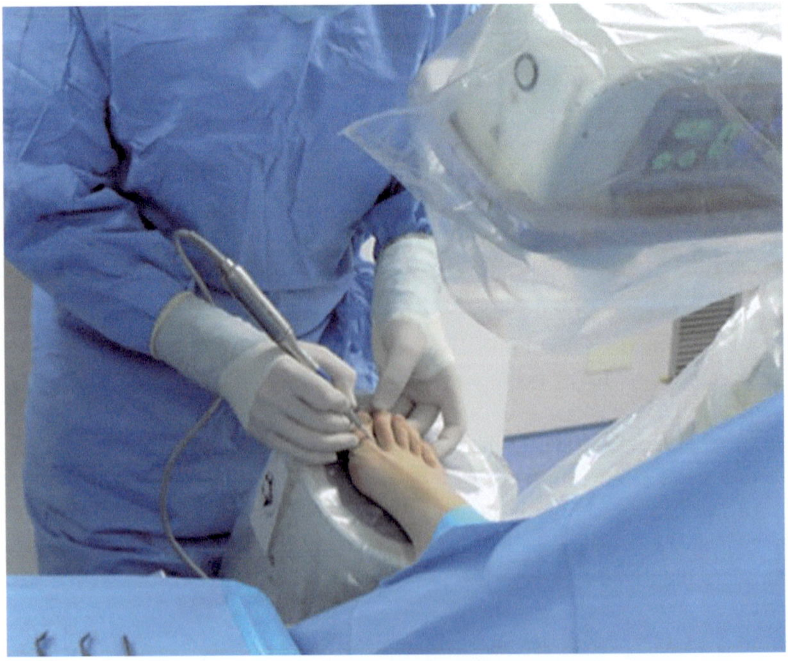

Fig. 32.8 Patient setup.

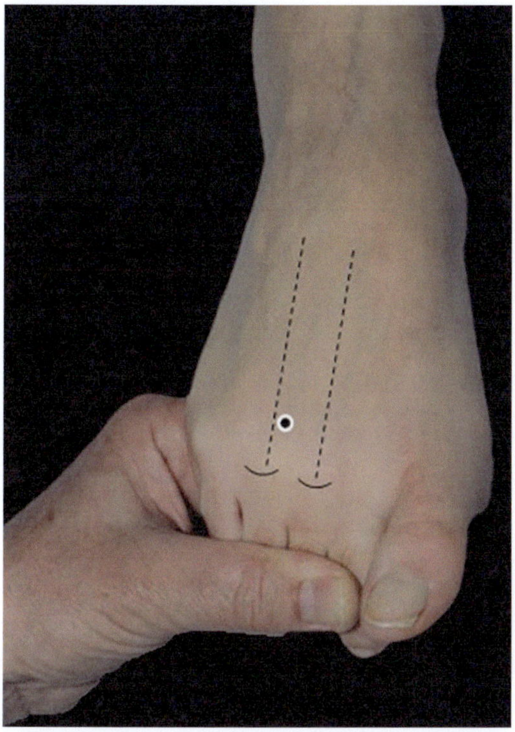

Fig. 32.10 Entry point.

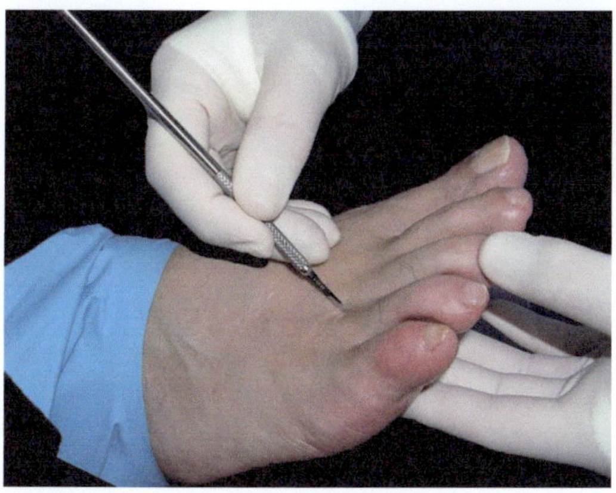

Fig. 32.11 Incision made with Beaver blade.

ropathy when the foot pushes off causing thickening and irritation of the intermetatarsal nerve, we decided to combined nerve release with distal minimally invasive osteotomy (DMMO) of the third and fourth metatarsals. By shortening and

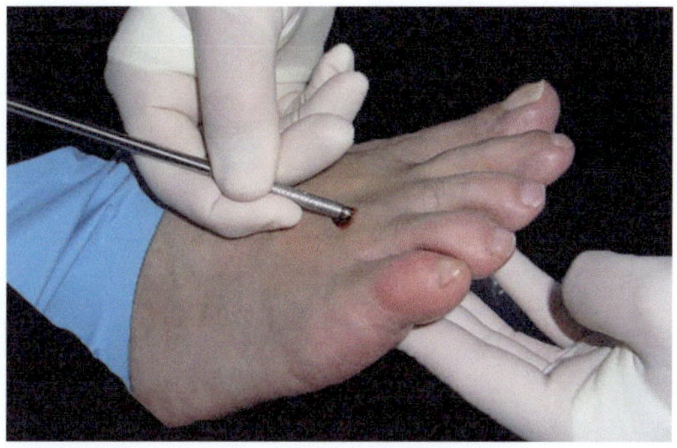

Fig. 32.12 Transection of deep transverse metatarsal ligament.

elevating the metatarsal heads, complete decompression of the common plantar digital nerve is ensured. This double procedure has led to excellent outcomes with normalization of the EMG in the third month and no transfer metatarsalgia.

After performing percutaneous DTML transection, we carry out DMMO [26] of the third and fourth metatarsals. The entry point is in the intermetatarsal space, 2 mm proximal to the metatarsophalangeal joint on the lateral edge of the metatarsal (Fig. 32.13).

A longitudinal 5-mm incision is made with the Beaver blade parallel to the extensor tendon and angled 45° to the dorsal face of the metatarsal. The rasp is used to free up the periosteum. A Shannon burr is inserted and set on the dorsal side of the proximal end of the metatarsal head under fluoroscopy guidance (Fig. 32.14).

An osteotomy is done at a 45° angle relative to the metatarsal axis using a distal to proximal and dorsal to plantar movement. Once started, the direction of the osteotomy cannot be altered without breaking the burr; thus a slight rotational movement is needed at the incision. The osteotomy is started on the lateral cortex and then the plantar one and finally the dorsal and medial ones. During the procedure, the forefoot is held in the opposite hand, placing the thumb on the dorsal side of the metatarsal heads and the fingers along the plantar side (Figs. 32.15 and 32.16).

When the osteotomy is finished, the surgeon will feel less resistance and will feel the head move. The outcome is checked with fluoroscopy.

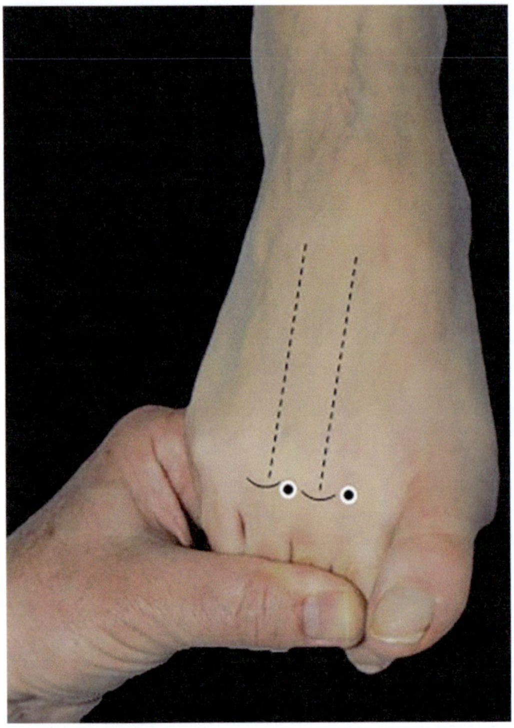

Fig. 32.13 Entry points for DMMO. © Mariano De Prado 2015. All Rights Reserved

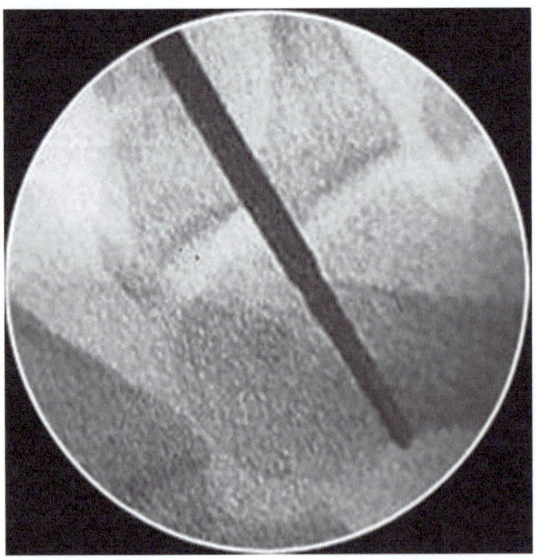

Fig. 32.14 Shannon burr. © Mariano De Prado 2015. All Rights Reserved

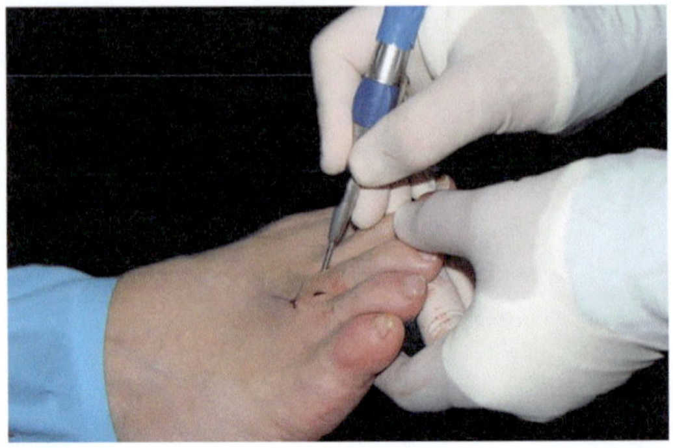

Fig. 32.15 DMMO of third metatarsal: hand and burr positions at the beginning of osteotomy. © Mariano De Prado 2015. All Rights Reserved

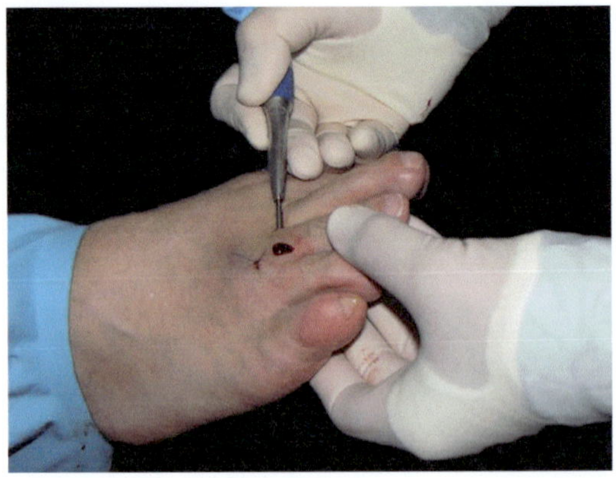

Fig. 32.16 DMMO of third metatarsal: hand and burr positions at the end of osteotomy. © Mariano De Prado 2015. All Rights Reserved

32.5.6 Closure and Dressing

The incision is closed with 4/0 monofilament suture. A dressing is configured to hold the metatarsals. A postoperative shoe is added.

32.5.7 Postoperative Course

Immediate full weight-bearing is allowed using a postoperative shoe. A follow-up visit is scheduled on day 7 to remove the sutures. A new dressing is configured like webbing with 3 M™ Coban™ Self-Adherent Wrap to hold the metatarsals. The patient is taught how to wrap her foot so she can redo it every day.

During the first 4 weeks, walking with full weight-bearing is allowed while wearing an orthopedic shoe. After 1 month, another radiological and clinical follow-up is done; at this point, the patient can start wearing shoes with a rigid sole depending on the amount of swelling.

32.6 Outcomes

We reviewed 68 patients (59 women, 9 men) who underwent percutaneous surgical treatment of a Morton's neuroma between February 1996 and October 2002. Their mean age was 46 years (range 27–69); the follow-up time was 31 months (range 15–84). The left foot had been operated on in 28 cases and the left one in 40 cases. The compression was in the second intermetatarsal space in three cases. In every case, the procedure consisted of percutaneous nerve release and DMMO in the third and fourth metatarsals. In the three patients who had pain in the second space, DMMO was also performed on the second metatarsal.

The patient satisfaction rate was 90% (62 cases): very good 70% (50 cases) and good 18% (12 cases). One patient had a poor result (3%) with persistent pain and paresthesia; this patient did not want to undergo revision surgery. In six patients (9%), the outcome was satisfactory, but three of them (4%) had load transfer metatarsalgia (two on the second metatarsal and one on the fifth metatarsal) leading to revision DMMO. In the three other cases, the patients had diffuse pain with discomfort, but no specific cause could be identified. An EMG was performed before and after the surgery in 37 patients. The EMG had normalized in 29 patients (78%) and was persistently abnormal in the other 8 patients (22%). Of these patients, seven had no clinical signs, and one had persistence of the preoperative neurological symptoms.

While this was only a retrospective study, percutaneous treatment for Morton's neuroma by nerve release and DMMO provides encouraging results. Other teams have reported the same results with this technique [11, 12, 29]. Prospective randomized studies are needed to confirm these initial findings.

Appendix 1 (Dr. Cyrille Cazeau)

It is feasible to carry out the nerve release percutaneously using long thin scissors such as Metzenbaum scissors. A distal cutaneous buttonhole is made in the target interdigital space, and then the scissors or Kelly clamp inserted closed to locate the inferior and superior sides of the DTML (Fig. 32.17). The instrument is then introduced on the inferior side; the foot is lifted off the table, which allows the instrument to press on the plantar side of the DTML. The foot is set back on the table, and the surgeon gradually withdraws it while holding tension. The anterior edge of the DTML is located when one perceives a crack and a dropping motion of the scissors, which is no longer hindered by the ligament. At this point, the scissors are rotated 90° to place the blades in the sagittal plane. They are pushed slightly open from front to back, like one would do when releasing the carpal tunnel proximally. When it is no long possible to lift the foot, the ligament has been cut.

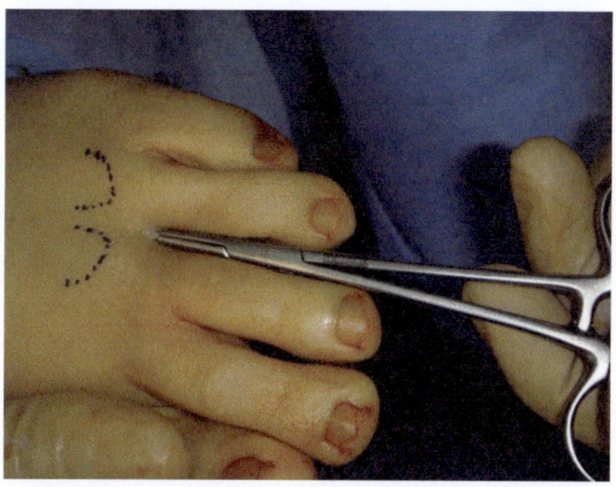

Fig. 32.17 Percutaneous nerve release with Metzenbaum scissors. © Cyrille Cazeau. All Rights Reserved

Appendix 2

It is likely that certain cases of Morton's neuroma are not seen as a foot disorder itself but incorporated into various signs of excessive pressure on the forefoot. These are generally small neuroma-like reactions (5–6 mm) associated with bursitis, and depending on the case, to other typical signs of excess pressure. This explains the effectiveness of the method proposed by Dr. de Prado, who combines DMMO with nerve release.

Editor' Point of View

The DMMO technique applied to Morton's neuroma is intellectually appealing. Historically, Thomas Morton did a resection of the M4 head to decompress the neuroma. The advantage of DMMO is that it reduces compression and removes the excess load on the lateral rays, since these two diagnoses often co-exist and can both be cured if the wrong diagnosis is made. Percutaneous DTML transection between the toes is an elegant technique and much simpler to carry out percutaneously than by arthroscopy.

References

1. Vernadakis AJ, Koch H, MacKinnon SE. Management of neuromas. Clin Plast Surg. 2003;30:247–68.
2. Graham CE, Graham DM. Morton's neuroma: a microscopic evaluation. Foot Ankle Int. 1984;5:150–3.
3. Giannini S, Bacchini P, Ceccarelli F, Vannini F. Interdigital neuroma: clinical examination and histopathologic results in 63 cases treated with excision. Foot Ankle Int. 2004;25:79–84.
4. Morton TG. The Classic. A peculiar and painful affection of the fourth metatarso-phalangeal articulation. Clin Orthop Relat Res. 1979:4–9.
5. Durlacher L. A treatise on corns, bunions, the diseases of nail and the general management of the feet. London: Simkin Marshall; 1845.
6. Gauthier G. Thomas Morton's disease: a nerve entrapment syndrome. A new surgical technique. Clin Orthop Relat Res. 1979:90–2.
7. Mulder JD. The causative mechanism in Morton's metatarsalgia. J Bone Joint Surg Br. 1951;33B:94–5.
8. Barousse R. Signo de Mulder ecográfico. Rev Arg Radiol. 2012;76:71–2.
9. Ashman CJ, Klecker RJ, Yu JS. Forefoot pain involving the metatarsal region: differential diagnosis with MR imaging. Radiographics. 2001;21:1425–40.
10. Gaynor R, Hake D, Spinner SM, Tomczak RL. A comparative analysis of conservative versus surgical treatment of Morton's neuroma. J Am Podiatr Med Assoc. 1989;79:27–30.
11. Cashley D. Manipulative therapy in the treatment of plantar digital neuritis (Morton's neuroma). Br J Podiatry. 2000;3:67–9.
12. Nunan PJ, Giesy BD. Management of Morton's neuroma in athletes. Clin Podiatr Med Surg. 1997;14:489–501.
13. Steinberg MD. The use of vitamin B12 in Morton's neuralgia. 1955. J Am Podiatr Med Assoc. 2007;97:293–5.
14. Thomson CE, Gibson JN, Martin D. Interventions for the treatment of Morton's neuroma. Cochrane Database Syst Rev. 2004:CD003118.
15. Finney W, Wiener SN, Catanzariti F. Treatment of Morton's neuroma using percutaneous electrocoagulation. J Am Podiatr Med Assoc. 1989;79:615–8.
16. Rahimi F, Muehleman C. Epineurial capping via Surgitron and the reduction of stump neuromas in the rat. J Foot Ankle Surg. 1992;31:124–8.
17. Wasserman G. Treatment of Morton's neuroma with the carbon dioxide laser. Clin Podiatr Med Surg. 1992;9:671–86.
18. Hodor L, Barkal K, Hatch-Fox LD. Cryogenic denervation of the intermetatarsal space neuroma. J Foot Ankle Surg. 1997;36:311–4.
19. Dellon AL. Treatment of recurrent metatarsalgia by neuroma resection and muscle implantation: case report and proposed algorithm of management for Morton's "neuroma". Microsurgery. 1989;10:256–9.
20. Barrett SL, Pignetti TT. Endoscopic decompression for intermetatarsal nerve entrapment-the EDIN technique: preliminary study with cadaveric specimens; early clinical results. J Foot Ankle Surg. 1994;33:503–8.
21. De Prado M, Ripoll PL, Golano P. Neuroma de Morton. In: Cirugía percutánea del pie. Técnicas quirúrgicas. Indicaciones, Bases anatómicas. Barcelona: Elsevier-Masson; 2003. 183–192.
22. De Prado M, Ripoll PL, Golano P. Morton Neuroma. In: De Prado M, Ripoll PL, Golano P, editors. Minimally invasive foot surgery: surgical techniques, indications, anatomical basis. Barcelona: About your health publishers; 2009. p. 197–207.
23. Zelent ME, Kane RM, Neese DJ, Lockner WB. Minimally invasive Morton's intermetatarsal neuroma decompression. Foot Ankle Int. 2007;28(2):263–5.
24. Miller S, Nakra A. Morton's Neuroma. In: Banks A, Downey M, et al., editors. McGlamry's comprehensive textbook of foot and ankle surgery. Philadelphia: Lippincott Williams & Willkings; 2001. p. 231–52.

25. De Prado M, Cuervas-Mons M, Golano P, Vaquero J. Distal metatarsal minimal invasive osteotomy (DMMO) for the treatment of Metatarsalgia. Tech Foot Ankle Surg. 2015;0(0):1–7.
26. Bauer T, Gaumetou E, Klouche S, Hardy P, Maffulli N. Metatarsalgia and Morton's disease: comparison of outcomes between open procedure and neurectomy versus percutaneous metatarsal osteotomies and ligament release with a minimum of 2 years of follow-up. J Foot Ankle Surg. 2015;54:373–7.

33 Technique, Indications, and Outcomes of Proximal Medial Gastrocnemius Lengthening

Pierre Barouk

33.1 Introduction

33.1.1 History

Starting in 1970, L.S. Barouk performed Silverskiold's original gastrocnemius-lengthening technique in cerebral palsy patients. From 1997 to 2005, we (L.S. Barouk, P. Barouk, E. Toullec) released the fascia of the medial and lateral gastrocnemius (while preserving the muscle fibers) in patients with static postural problems, mainly related to the forefoot (Fig. 33.1). Matt Solan joined our team in 2004 and performed this procedure also [1].

Since 2005, we only transect the fascia overlying the medial head of the gastrocnemius muscle (Fig. 33.2) for reasons that we will discuss later. J.A. Colombier had been doing it since 2003 [2].

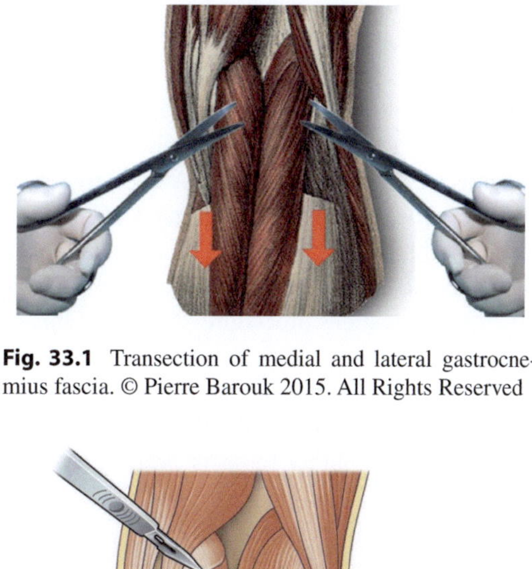

Fig. 33.1 Transection of medial and lateral gastrocnemius fascia. © Pierre Barouk 2015. All Rights Reserved

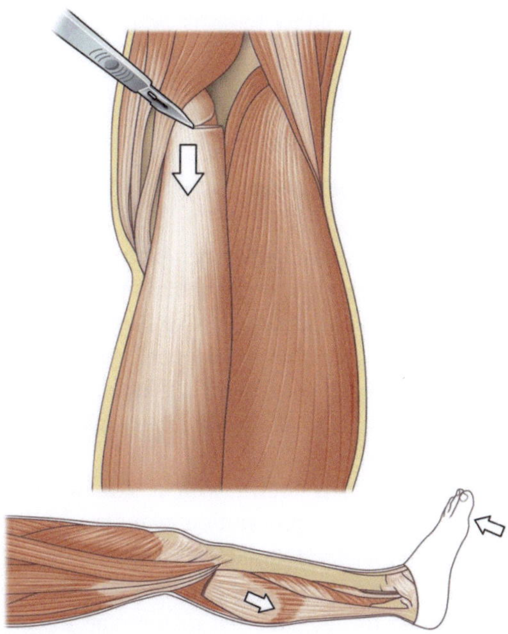

Fig. 33.2 Transection of fascia overlying medial gastrocnemius. © Pierre Barouk 2015. All Rights Reserved

33.1.2 Indications

Our indications are based on isolated gastrocnemius contracture (Silfverskiold's sign), given that this contracture has a negative impact in the ailment for which the patient is seeking care, and also on the presence of secondary signs (cramps,

P. Barouk (✉)
Centre de Chirurgie Orthopédique et Sportive, Merignac, France

C. Cazeau, Y. Stiglitz (eds.), *Percutaneous and Minimally Invasive Foot Surgery*,
https://doi.org/10.1007/978-3-030-98791-6_33

calf tension, difficulty walking in flat shoes, low back pain, instability, etc.).

33.2 Surgical Technique

Other than a few minor variations, L.S. Barouk and P. Barouk, J.A. Colombier, M. Solan, and E. Toullec all use the same surgical technique.

33.2.1 Anesthesia

While general anesthesia can be used, we prefer using peripheral regional anesthesia. Our anesthesiologists perform a sciatic nerve block through an ultrasound-guided lateral subgluteal approach. The choice of local anesthetic agent depends on the duration of the postoperative stay. At our facility, we use Mepivacaine 15 mg/mL for an outpatient procedure or a combination of Mepivacaine 20 mg/mL and Ropivacaine 7.5 mg/mL for an inpatient procedure. About 20 mL is injected per side.

Since this block does not anesthetize the skin (posterior femoral cutaneous nerve), local anesthesia of the popliteal fossa is performed with 20 mg/mL lidocaine plus epinephrine, immediately before the incision is made.

33.2.2 Patient Setup

The patient is installed prone, with a cushion under the anterior side of the ankles to release the gastrocnemius complex. We have tried performing this procedure with the patient supine, but it required two surgical assistants, a larger incision, and more traction on the tissues. Thus, we do not recommend it.

The incision is drawn with a skin marker. After standard skin preparation, two drapes with holes are applied. A tourniquet is not necessary. It is better to have two sets of Farabeuf retractors, a narrow one for the start and a large one for the deep layer.

33.2.3 Procedure

An incision about 3-cm in length is made on the flexion fold, 1 cm from the medial fossa (Fig. 33.3). The subcutaneous fat layer is dissected to expose the posterior leg fascia. The fascia is opened in the leg's axis. Just below this, surrounded by variable amounts of fatty tissue, is the fleshy part of the medial gastrocnemius, covered by a thin fascia. On the medial side of the muscle is the tendon, which extends to the anterior side (Fig. 33.4). All the fascia fibers are transected using Mayo scissors (Fig. 33.5). A finger is used to verify that no tension remains in the muscle when the ankle is dorsiflexed.

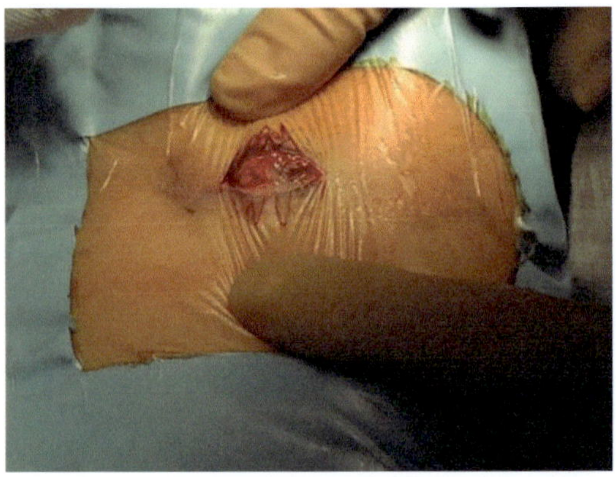

Fig. 33.3 Incision.

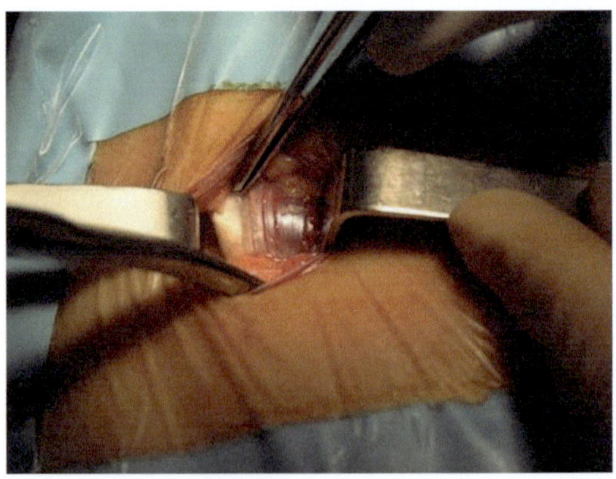

Fig. 33.4 Medial tendon, lateral fascia.

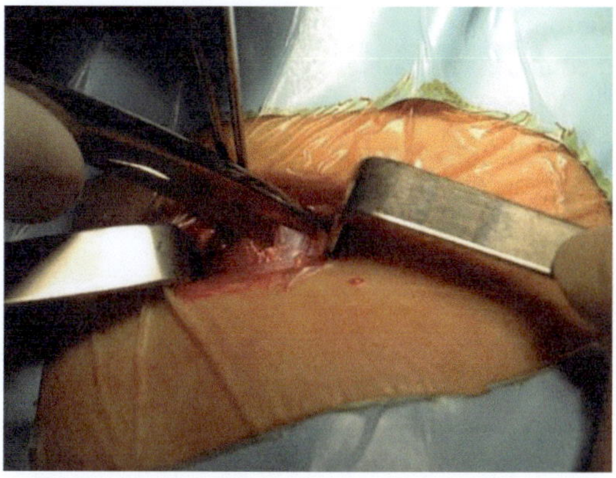

Fig. 33.5 Tendon fibers have been transected and fascia fibers are being cut.

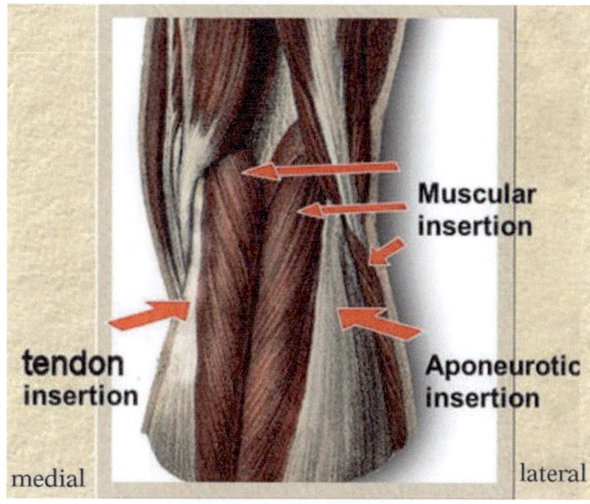

Fig. 33.6 Proximal gastrocnemius insertion.

In a variation described by de Los Santos [3], which is also used by E. Maceira, the medial gastrocnemius tendon is exteriorized before cutting the same tendon fibers. His techniques and its results are described after this section.

Transection of Lateral Gastrocnemius Tendon Fibers

While the indications are limited, it may be useful to transect the tendon fibers of the lateral gastrocnemius in some cases. We did this in every patient for many years. In this scenario, the incision is extended laterally. The lateral gastrocnemius is located by palpation to ensure the incision is not too central (popliteal artery). The posterior leg fascia is opened carefully since the deep fibular nerve trunk is located very close to it. This will expose the fleshy part of the lateral gastrocnemius. Its tendon fibers consist of a narrow fascial strip (Fig. 33.6). Here also, the deep fibular nerve is nearby and must be identified before transecting the tendon fibers.

Hemostasis is verified and the incision closed with two subcutaneous throws and a running intradermal absorbable suture. Wound drainage is not necessary.

The operative time is 3 min per side. The learning curve is relatively fast (ten cases).

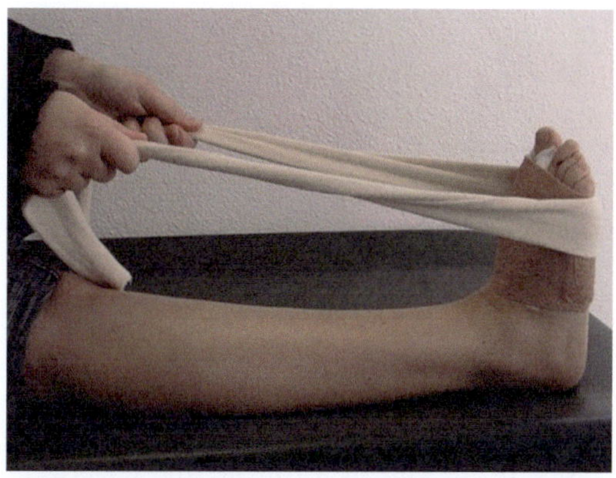

Fig. 33.7 Self-directed rehabilitation.

33.2.4 Postoperative Course

We no longer apply a cast or brace to the patient's foot.

Walking is allowed once the anesthetic has worn off in the legs. A self-directed rehabilitation program is implemented by the clinic's physical therapist. It consists of performing passive ankle dorsiflexion with the knee extended (Fig. 33.7). Walking in flat shoes is recommended along with wearing shoes with heel lift (Type 1) that hold the ankle in dorsal flexion (Fig. 33.8).

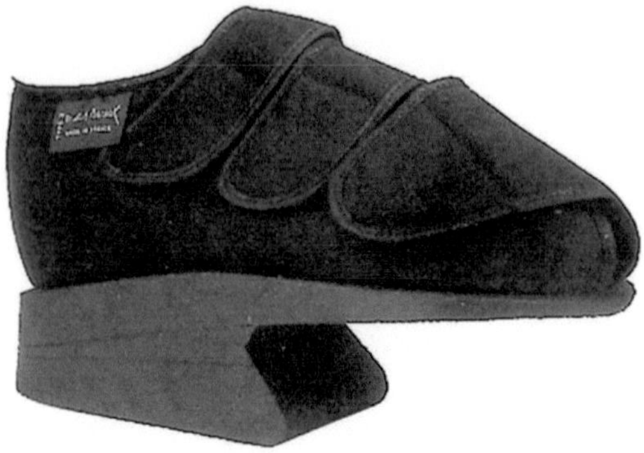

Fig. 33.8 Type 1 postoperative shoe.

33.3 Complications

The following complications were documented in the 354 procedures that we performed:

- Four cases of moderate calf pain, three of which resolved after 1 year; one patient continued to have unexplained pain in the popliteal fossa.
- One case of superficial venous thrombosis (patient also underwent hallux valgus correction).
- One case of tension development in the lateral side of the calf in a patient who underwent medial-only release.
- Two cases of transient dysesthesia on the lateral side of the leg in patients who underwent medial and lateral gastrocnemius lengthening.
- Ten cases of keloid scars; all patients had undergone medial and lateral gastrocnemius lengthening, a procedure that has a longer scar.
- Ten cases of reduced calf strength (subjective finding by the patient), all in patients who had undergone medial and lateral gastrocnemius lengthening; of these ten cases, there was one case of excessive lengthening with ankle dorsal flexion which caused discomfort during sports activities.

These observations showed that releasing the medial tendon only is associated with practically no complications. This, along with the fact that the outcomes were the same, led us to perform medial-only release going forward.

Since that study, we have performed 368 additional procedures (99% medial gastrocnemius lengthening only) during which the following complications were observed:

- Four cases of hematoma—two regressed spontaneously and two had to be drained; this was due to the implementation of a preventative dose of a new anticoagulant, which we subsequently stopped using;
- Two cases of superficial venous thrombosis (patients also underwent hallux valgus correction).
- No cases of dysesthesia, keloid scar, or loss of calf strength.

These observations led us to conclude that complications are very rare and without significant consequences following transection of the medial tendon only.

33.4 Results

33.4.1 Ankle Dorsiflexion with Knee Extended

Whether medial-only (80 cases) or medial + lateral lengthening (274 cases) was done, ankle dorsiflexion with the knee extended improved in every case.

But this outcome depends on how the gastrocnemius is evaluated. We used the following method to test ankle Equinus: subtalar joint held in varus and then moderate load (1.7 kg) applied to the foot to induce ankle dorsiflexion. We strongly believe the examination must be reproducible from one patient to another and from preoperative to postoperative.

Preoperatively, 69% of patients had less than 15° ankle dorsiflexion, which is considered a significant Equinus. Only 4% of patients still had this limitation postoperatively. We found that 22% of patient had 0° to −15° dorsiflexion preoperatively (moderate Equinus) versus 19% postoperatively. Positive dorsiflexion of the ankle was

Table 33.1 Ankle dorsiflexion with knee extended after gastrocnemius lengthening

More than 1°		Between 0° and – 15°		Less than – 15°	
Preop	Postop	Preop	Postop	Preop	Postop
9%	77%	22%	19%	69%	4%

found in 9% of patients preoperatively and 77% postoperatively (Table 33.1).

In a blinded 30-patient study comparing lengthening of both gastrocnemius to the medial-only lengthening, we found no difference in the improvement of ankle dorsiflexion between groups. Colombier reported that 95% of his patients had better ankle dorsiflexion.

33.4.2 Other Effects of Gastrocnemius Contracture

On the Feet

Proximal gastrocnemius lengthening may be enough in certain cases such that another local surgical procedure is not necessary for the following conditions: ankle instability, osteoarthritis in Lisfranc joint, hallux limitus, and metatarsalgia (Biomechanical studies by Dr. Cyrille Cazeau [4]). But in most cases, in all locations, it can reduce the need for a local surgical procedure or supplement it.

Direct Signs

It significantly reduces cramps and tension in the calf muscles (87% of cases) and makes it easier to walk in flat shoes (96% of cases).

Secondary Signs

Significant reduction in low back pain (87% of cases) and feelings of leg instability (98% of cases).

33.4.3 Complications

The complication rate is also very low, particularly in cases of medial-only lengthening. The surgical approach for proximal medial gastrocnemius lengthening has no nerve and vascular structures in the area that could be damaged during the surgery [5].

33.5 Discussion

33.5.1 Outcomes

There are few studies on the outcomes of proximal gastrocnemius release. One of the studies was presented during the *Symposium des Sociétés Françaises de Chirurgie du Pied* at Toulouse in 2006 and subsequently published, in collaboration with J.A. Colombier and E. Toullec [2, 6], another one by M. Solan's team in Great Britain [1], and more recently, the study by R. Dos Santos and Maceira. In fact, very few surgical teams currently use this procedure. To lengthen the gastrocnemius, the most popular technique is the one described by Strayer [7].

Our procedure's effectiveness is like we would expect; the Silfverskiold's sign disappears, and passive ankle dorsiflexion (knee extended) returns to normal in 79% of cases. The 19% of cases with moderate postoperative Equinus (−1 to −15°) correspond to patients who had notable Equinus of more than −15° preoperatively. They also improved after this procedure, even though minor Equinus persisted.

The improvement is likely less than the one achieved with the traditional distal lengthening procedure (Strayer) of +25° [5]. Rabat reported achieving 12° dorsiflexion with endoscopic transection. However, distal lengthening, no matter which technique is used, most often impacts the soleus fascia, not only the gastrocnemius fascia [5, 7].

33.5.2 Bilateral Procedure

Another advantage of this procedure is that it can be performed bilaterally. This is important because the contracture is generally bilateral. It is logical to perform it bilaterally if one wants to eliminate low back pain or cramps that are bilateral. The same goes for problems with walking in flat shoes: it would be useless to allow the patient to walk in flat shoes only on one foot.

33.5.3 Reasons to Lengthen the Medial Gastrocnemius Only

We prefer simple medial gastrocnemius lengthening for the following reasons:

1. The medial tendon is powerful, while the lateral one is very thin (Fig. 33.9).
2. "Tennis leg" always occurs medially, which suggests the tension is higher on the medial side.
3. There are fewer complications, especially lateral dysesthesia, keloid scars, and postoperative pain (Fig. 33.10).
4. This is truly a minimally invasive procedure that is virtually free of complications and has a very short operative time.

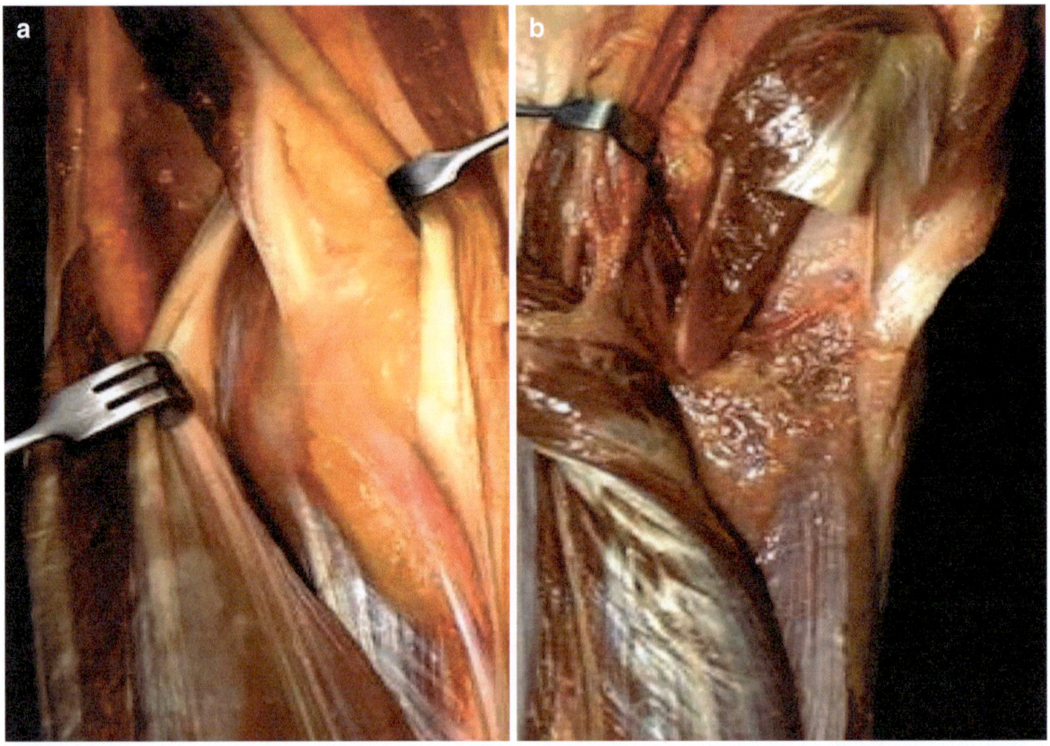

Fig. 33.9 Medial gastrocnemius (**a**). Lateral gastrocnemius (**b**), © Pierre Barouk 2015. All Rights Reserved

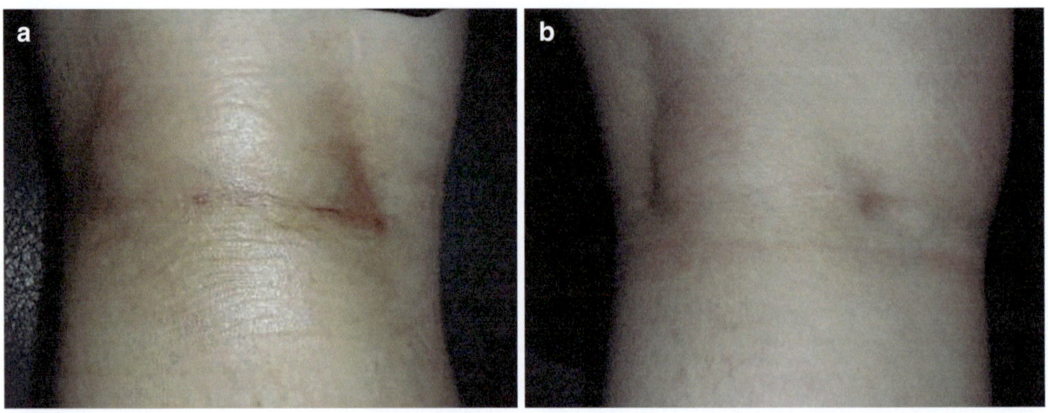

Fig. 33.10 Scar at 1 month postoperative (**a**) and at 1 year postoperative (**b**). © Pierre Barouk 2015. All Rights Reserved

5. Lastly, isolated medial gastrocnemius lengthening has comparable effectiveness to combined medial/lateral lengthening (comparative study).

33.5.4 Reasons Why Proximal Lengthening Is Preferred to Distal

We have found that proximal lengthening is more effective than distal lengthening:

1. Distal release involves the gastrocnemius and very often the soleus fascia because the plane between these two structures cannot always be identified. The junction between these two structures is often lengthy (Fig. 33.11).
2. Distal release interrupts muscle continuity and may contribute to lower strength [8]. However, this reduction has not been reported in recent studies [9, 10].
3. Distal release leaves the sagittal slip of the soleus intact (Fig. 33.12) which, since it is the only remaining soleus tendon structure, is likely to rupture secondarily. The latter two scenarios mean that postoperative immobilization is needed.
4. Bilateral lengthening is difficult when distal release is performed.
5. The scar on the medial side and middle third of the calf, which is made on the distal portion, is less attractive than when it is placed in the popliteal fossa. For this reason, the endoscopic method is superior to the open method.
6. The complications related to distal lengthening are not insignificant [11].

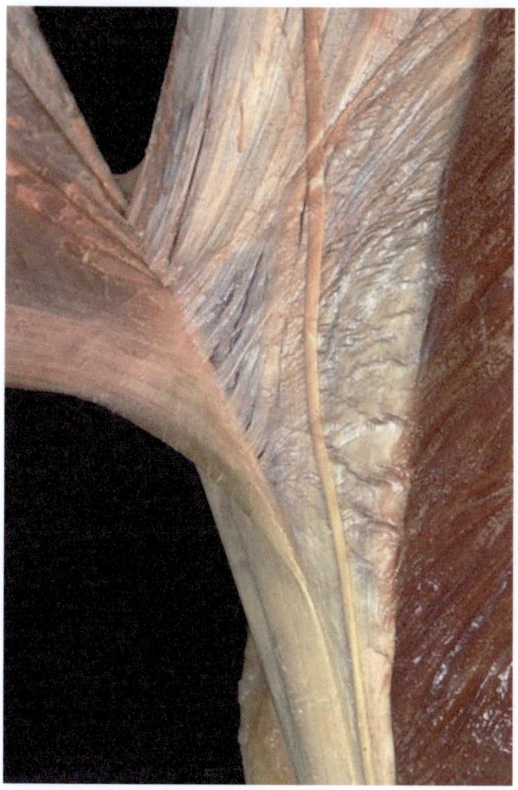

Fig. 33.11 Gastrocnemius-soleus junction. © Pierre Barouk 2015. All Rights Reserved

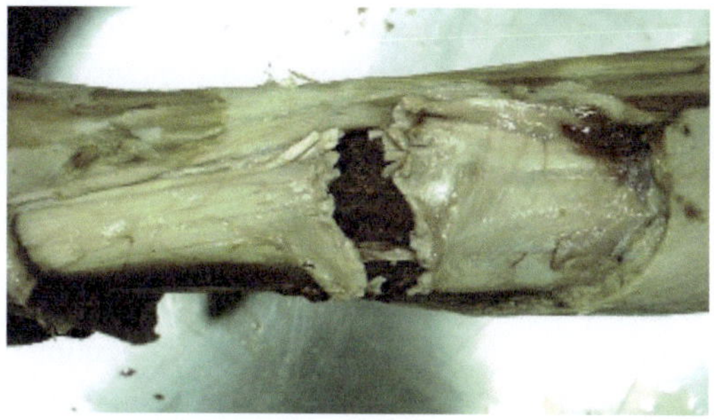

Fig. 33.12 Soleus sagittal slip. © Pierre Barouk 2015. All Rights Reserved

Nevertheless, we have retained some indications for distal lengthening (as described by Strayer): cases in which immobilization is required for another procedure done on the foot (e.g., hindfoot osteotomy), and when we do not want to change the patient's position during surgery. Another scenario is when gastrocnemius contracture occurs in addition to that of the soleus. In this situation, distal release results in better dorsiflexion. The endoscopy technique appears to be effective, reliable, and less invasive.

33.5.5 Other Thoughts

Proximal medial gastrocnemius lengthening is a simple, fast technique to carry out. The postoperative course is also simple, with immediate return to walking, without immobilization. Complications are very rare, resolve themselves, and have no lingering effects.

Reduced strength has only been observed in one patient who underwent medial lengthening. While calf strength has not been quantified (KT 1000), no patient has complained of loss of strength (except one who had an overcorrection). But it is important to note that most of our patients were not athletes.

This leads us to suggesting this procedure in cases of gastrocnemius contracture in foot pathologies, especially when there are also direct and indirect signs. We also suggest a stretching regimen—but less often than surgical procedures—as we are aware of the low patient compliance with stretching and how difficult it can be. Also, some studies have shown that stretching is not very effective and may be harmful.

33.6 Sequencing

This gastrocnemius procedure must be done before any other procedures on the foot for three reasons:

1. To reduce it. For example, hallux valgus with metatarsalgia due mainly to gastrocnemius contracture. No bone procedures will be needed on the lateral metatarsals since hallux valgus correction and gastrocnemius lengthening are sufficient.
2. To cancel it. In cases of metatarsalgia (without apparent reason) where the procedure on the gastrocnemius replaces the need for multiple metatarsal osteotomies (which will not solve the associated signs). In fact, this simple procedure can be performed first. At a certain stage, it is more logical to address the cause than the consequences.

   Figures 33.13 and 33.14 illustrates the first two advantages.
3. And, no matter what, to safeguard it.

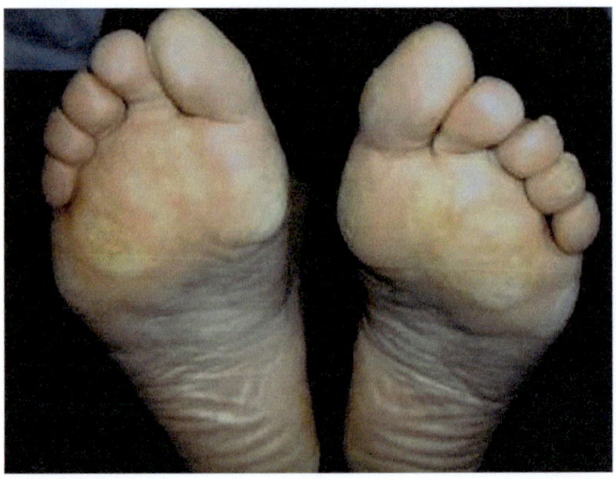

Fig. 33.13 Patient with bilateral metatarsalgia.

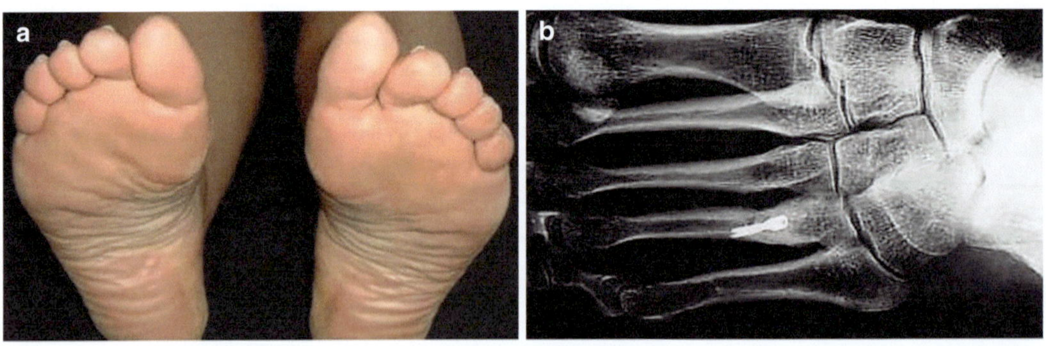

Fig. 33.14 Clinical result 6 months after gastrocnemius lengthening and isolated M4 elevation in the same patient as Fig. 33.13 (**a**). Barouk-Rippstein-Toullec osteotomy (**b**).

33.7 Patient Information

Performing this procedure means that the patient must be aware of his/her pathology sufficiently to understand the reasons why a procedure is being done behind the knee—direct signs (cramps, calf tension), low back pain, problems walking in flat shoes, and instability—which will contribute to the decision to undergo surgery. The verbal information is supplemented by a patient brochure and a website about the condition and procedure. The goal is for the patient to agree to this procedure, even though it is not being done at the foot.

33.8 Conclusion

For us, proximal medial gastrocnemius lengthening is a simple, effective, and logical procedure for patients who have a foot and ankle problems related to gastrocnemius contracture. It is important to know how to identify this contracture and to explain to the patient how it contributes to his/her pathology and the associated signs.

Over a 12-year period, we have lengthened more than 1000 gastrocnemius muscle-tendon units proximally. The reliability of the outcome and the near complete absence of complications have encouraged us to continue down this path.

Editors' Point of View

Tenotomy of the medial gastrocnemius is easy to carry out without a tourniquet or drain. This bi-articular muscle is immediately placed under tension by the automated nature of walking, especially the ankle dorsiflexion that occurs during the push-off phase.

References

1. Kohls-Gatzoulis JA, Solan M. Results of proximal medial gastrocnemius release. J Bone Joint Surg Br. 2009;91(Supp II):361.
2. Colombier JA. Libération proximale pure dans la prise en charge thérapeutique des Gastrocnémiens. Med Chir Pied. 2006;22:156–7.
3. De Los Santos Real R, Morales-Muñoz P, Payo Rodriguez J, Escalera Alonso J. Liberación proximal del gemelo medial por mínima incision [Medial Gastrocnemius release with minimal incision]. Rev Pie y Tobillo. 2011;25:37–41.
4. Cazeau C, Stiglitz Y. Effects of gastrocnemius tightness on forefoot during gait. Foot Ankle Clin. 2014;19:649–57.
5. Hamilton PD, Brown M, Ferguson N, Adebibe M, Maggs J, Solan M. Surgical anatomy of the proximal release of the gastrocnemius: a cadaveric study. Foot Ankle Int. 2009;30:1202–6.
6. Barouk LS, Barouk P, Toulec E. Résultats de la libération proximale des gastrocnémiens. Med Chir Pied. 2006;22:151–6.
7. Strayer LM. Gastrocnemius recession. J Bone Joint Surg Am. 1958;40:1019–30.
8. Pinney SJ, Hansen ST Jr, Sangeorzan BJ. The effect on ankle dorsiflexion of gastrocnemius recession. Foot Ankle Int. 2002;23(1):26–9.
9. Mann RA. Re: the effect on ankle dorsiflexion of gastrocnemius recession. Foot Ankle Int. 2003;24:726–7.
10. Maskill JD, Bohay DR, Anderson JG. Gastrocnemius recession to treat isolated foot pain. Foot Ankle Int. 2010;31:19–23.
11. Rush SM, Ford LA, Hamilton GA. Morbidity associated with high gastrocnemius recession: retrospective review of 126 cases. J Foot Ankle Surg. 2006;45:156–60.

34 Postoperative Dressings and Supports for Minimally Invasive Foot Surgery

Julien Beldame and Cyrille Cazeau

34.1 Introduction

Dressings have several functions ranging from simple postoperative antiseptic wound coverage to more complex ones.

34.1.1 Antiseptic Function

The initial dressing applied by the surgeon in the operating room will be the most sterile of all the subsequent dressings. For this reason, redoing it is not urgent. Some have proposed waiting 3 weeks after the surgery before redoing it, except if postoperative bleeding causes maceration.

34.1.2 Psychological Function

Isolating the surgically impacted zone allows the patient's psychological repair mechanism to kick in during the first few days, especially since pain is suppressed by the local anesthetic's prolonged action. The dressing's bulk, along with the fact that it looks like a sock, allows the patient to immediately use their foot when they get home, which contributes to the demedicalization process. It is important to preserve the automatic nature of walking and pushing off. But if the patient sees even a speck of blood, this progress could be negated!

34.1.3 Compliance Function

The volume of the initial dressing prevents the patient from wearing shoes initially and requires him/her to stay home for 2 or 3 days. This increases their confident enough to start putting weight on their foot in a controlled setting. The low bulk of the later dressings allows the patient to wear wide sneakers or orthopedic shoes for activities around the house.

34.2 Selecting the Dressing Type

34.2.1 Based on Goals

Minimally invasive and percutaneous surgery may or may not be supplemented by internal fixation. While this is not a required combination, applying these new techniques does not mean that fixation is not used.

To achieve good functional outcomes, the operated organ must be placed in its usual functional setting as quickly as possible. Allowing full weight-bearing and moving the MTP joints immediately after the surgical procedure, even

J. Beldame (✉)
Clinique Blomet, Paris, France

C. Cazeau
Clinique Victor Hugo, Paris, France

C. Cazeau, Y. Stiglitz (eds.), *Percutaneous and Minimally Invasive Foot Surgery*,
https://doi.org/10.1007/978-3-030-98791-6_34

before bone union has been achieved, yield the best results. But to achieve this, primary mechanical stability is needed. This key point requires prior agreement. This stability depends on both the geometry and location of the osteotomies and the presence of internal fixation. Depending on the construct's stability, the dressing may or may not have a support function.

34.2.2 Based on Procedures Performed

34.2.2.1 M1 Osteotomy

Certain techniques are mechanically stable right away and do not require additional support in the form of a dressing, e.g., a chevron osteotomy in dense epiphysio-metaphyseal cancellous bone where the two 60° cuts result in a geometric fit and the moments are low. Additional stability is ensured by internal fixation using a compression screw. For unstable osteotomies, the gauzes are fashioned to maintain reduction; the dressing will be changed under medical supervision.

34.2.2.2 P1 Osteotomy

Some techniques can achieve good stability right away, e.g., a proximal varus-inducing metaphyseal osteotomy that preserves the lateral cortex to act as a hinge and is supplemented with internal fixation. For unstable osteotomies, the construct is stabilized with a silicone spacer made by the surgeon, which is placed inside the dressing and kept for 3 weeks.

34.2.2.3 DMMO

DMMOs are stabilized by a force couple: the ground reaction force of the weight transferred by weightbearing and the front to back shortening force applied by the dorsal tendon, capsule, and ligament structures. There may also be associated deformities such as lateral or medial deviation or overlap of the second toe. In this scenario, gauzes are placed in an angled overlap configuration around the toes to immobilize them in the opposite direction to the initial deformity.

34.2.2.4 Tailor's Bunion and Fifth Toe Varus

A fifth toe varus-inducing osteotomy can be held by a K-wire and does not require any specific dressings. If no K-wire is used, angled overlapping dressings are placed around the toe to hold its reduction. Tailor's bunion may benefit from console pinning; a K-wire placed in the intramedullary canal of the diaphysis prevents the M5 head from shifting laterally. Here also, no specific dressings are needed. If no K-wire is used, a transverse bandage is placed over the M5 head to maintain its lateralized position.

34.2.2.5 Claw Toe Deformity

The dressing is simple for cases of fusion or osteotomy with fixation. When no fixation is used, the situation resembles that of isolated tenotomies. The phalanges must be immobilized in a position opposite to the deformity. If P1 is in an erect position (MTP2, 3, 4 hyperextension), it will be held by gauzes acting as a collar on its dorsal side in MTP plantar flexion. When correcting PIP flexion deformity, the joint is held straight by collaring P2 by its plantar side. The same principle applies to the DIP joint.

34.3 Dressing Application

34.3.1 Materials

The materials needed are woven gauze dressings, crepe bandages, and elastic adhesive bandages; the latter is the only non-sterile component and is used last (Fig. 34.1).

- The gauze dressings should be at least 15 cm long (to wrap the foot effectively and have a mechanical action for clinical correction) and be about 2 cm wide.
- The crepe bandages will be about 10 cm wide and are used to wrap the ankle and forefoot several times.
- The elastic adhesive bandages that will go between the toes are about 15 cm long but

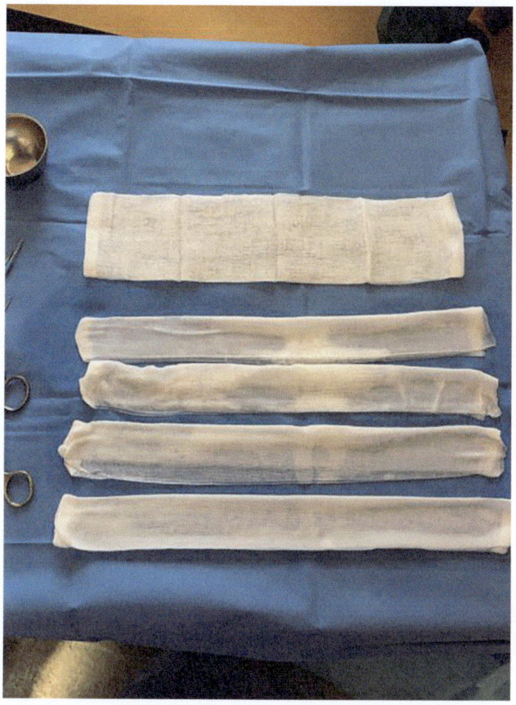

Fig. 34.1 Materials used for postoperative dressings.

fairly narrow (1 cm approximately). Wider bands (10 cm) will be placed over the prior dressings and the crepe bandages to hold everything together, while going around the ankle and forefoot.

When the dressings are changed (once bleeding has stopped), some practitioners use self-adhesive cohesive bandages instead of the crepe bandages and wide elastic bandages.

34.3.2 Principles

The first dressing made at the end of the procedure is preferably moistened or wetted with sterile saline (or antiseptic solutions in some cases). Since the gauzes are moist, the heat emanating from the foot hardens them and produces a cast effect that improves support. This moistness also provides a blotting paper effect on the bleeding. This postoperative support will help to reduce the inflammatory phenomena, pain, and to get through the edema phase, which peaks on postoperative day 4 (Gottlieb, 2013).

All dressings have a common base upon which specific configurations are added depending on which ray was operated on and which type of correction is desired. The base consists of passing a long but narrow woven gauze dressing between each toe, finishing at the base of the toes (P1 level). One starts at the first space by making a figure-of-eight configuration on the medial side of the MTP joint of the hallux. The dressings in the neighboring spaces are then passed one after the other (medial to lateral) and will come back to collar the gauze dressing on the ray immediately medial to it. The toes are systematically separated one from the other, even if they were not operated on, to prevent maceration between the toes (Fig. 34.2).

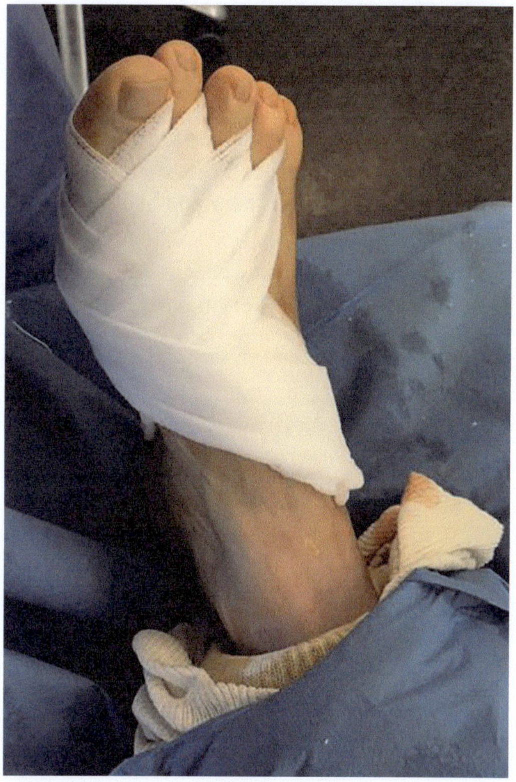

Fig. 34.2 Figure-of-eight configuration of the gauze dressings with toe separation.

Surgical correction of the various joint segments is set by the manner in which the gauze dressing (and elastic bandages) is configured: if the dressing is passed and tightened from dorsal to plantar, this will lower the bone segment on which it is placed. If passed from plantar to dorsal, it will result in elevation. Support for deformities in the horizontal plane (varus/valgus) is managed by the varus-inducing tension on the figure-of-eight dressings, which are brought back on the medial side of the hallux. The scrub nurse (in the operating room) or the patient (office consultation) can be called upon to hold tension on the various gauze dressings, before the crepe bandage is applied over all of it.

The crepe bandage or elastic bandage is then wrapped around the forefoot and midfoot, finishing at the ankle to prevent loosening of the dressing (Fig. 34.3).

Thinner non-sterile elastic adhesive bandages can be added on the toes to adjust the correction (Fig. 34.4). One must be careful when placing the gauze dressings and elastic bandages between the toes. They must not be too narrow and must always sit flat on the skin surface; otherwise they may cause compression, leading to distal ischemia or skin necrosis at the contact points.

Lastly, a wide (10 cm) elastic adhesive bandage is used to cover everything, going around the ankle then over the forefoot (Fig. 34.5).

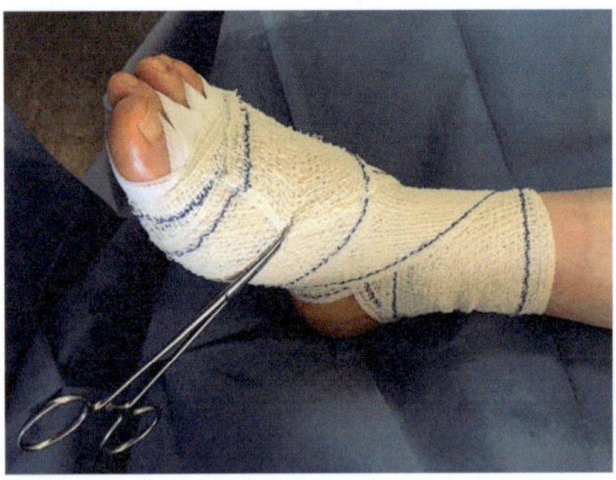

Fig. 34.3 Foot wrapped with crepe bandage.

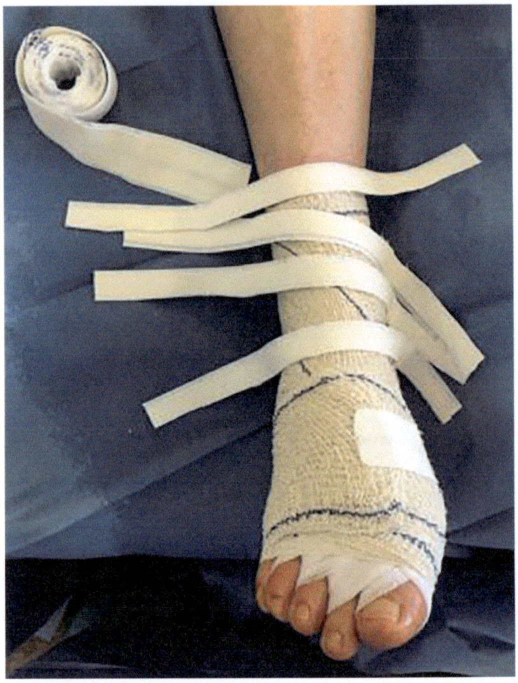

Fig. 34.4 Adjusting the toe correction.

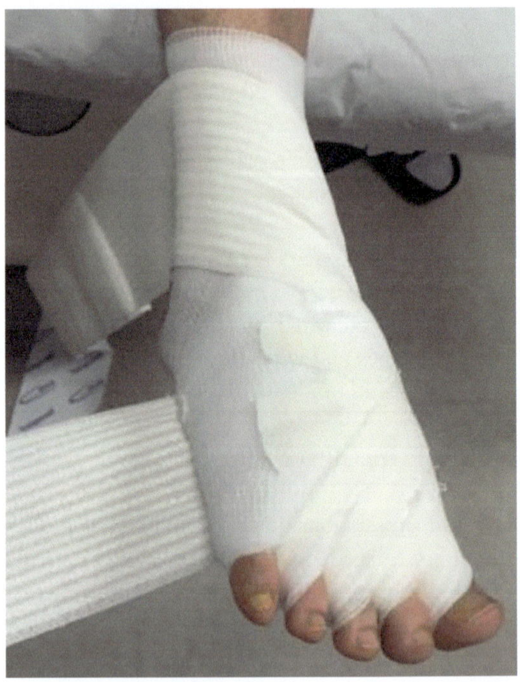

Fig. 34.5 Wide elastic adhesive bandage applied last.

34.3.3 Dressing Changes

The initial dressing is changed sometime between postoperative days 7 and 15, depending on the surgeon's preferences. It is rare for the dressing to be changed before day 7 because of the inflammatory process and edema reaction, which peaks around day 4 (Gottlieb, 2013). If the dressing is changed before day 7, it will provoke pain and reinforce the edema, thereby making the correction more difficult.

These dressings are changed during an office visit, either by the surgeon or a member of the surgical team. They are configured in the same way as the intraoperative dressing but are generally less bulky and are made using dry gauze dressings. The crepe bandage can be thinner also, or even replaced by a self-adhesive cohesive bandage.

These dressings, which are redone every 7 or 15 days, must continue to support the surgical correction for 4–6 weeks, in order to allow development of a bone callus in non-fixed osteotomies or an organized hematoma for surgery on soft tissues. In cases of more stable surgical constructs, the dressing can be removed completely around postoperative day 10. The final dressing changes can be assigned to enthusiastic patients when only very minor corrections are involved.

34.4 Alternatives to Dressings

The need for 4–6 weeks of support (for the least stable constructs) with repeated dressing applications appears time-consuming, even if, as time goes on, these dressings are less and less bulky, amounting to only a few layers of gauze or elastic bandages. There are alternatives to repeated dressing applications, depending on the stability, correction, surgeon preferences, and patient preferences. These alternatives are sometimes used as the second dressing, once the wounds are closed and clean. The main advantage is that they allow the patients to wear fitted shoes and start venous compression stockings, rehabilitation, and personal care, which all accelerate the patients' functional recovery.

34.4.1 Toe Spacers

Toe spacers are removable, silicone inter-toe orthoses that are custom made. In the context of postoperative orthoses, they have the same function as dressings—to hold the surgical correction. But they have the advantage of being removable, which allows the patient to bathe or perform rehabilitation.

They can be made by the surgeon or a chiropodist in the team starting on postoperative day 10 (for the most stable surgical corrections). They are made from two-component silicone rubber (base + curing agent) whose hardness is chosen based on the type of correction needed (Shore hardness of 30–45 for postoperative toe orthoses). Rubbers in paste form (50% base, 50% curing agent) are easy to measure out with measuring spoons without having to calculate the number of liquid-curing agent drops needed.

After mixing the two components until a uniform color is achieved, the paste ball is shaped into a tube that is placed between the toes. The paste tube should be applied as a continuous cylinder (above, below and between the toes, depending on the correction needed) without breaking its continuity, as the paste does not stick to itself easily. Once in position and smoothed out, the clinical correction is held manually until the rubber cures completely (about 5 min). Once hardened, it can be removed to show the patient how to put it into place; an oil-based lubricant can be used to help the device slide on and off.

The most commonly used and easiest devices to make are M1–M2 spacers in the context of hallux valgus, tubes in the context of claw toe deformity, or dividers for surgery on the lateral metatarsals, to combat against lateral translation by binding the toes to each other and to the hallux (Fig. 34.6a, b).

34.4.2 Braces

In recent years, postoperative braces have been introduced that are specific to foot surgery. These are cloth braces, consisting of a band around the forefoot, on which straps are attached (like ties

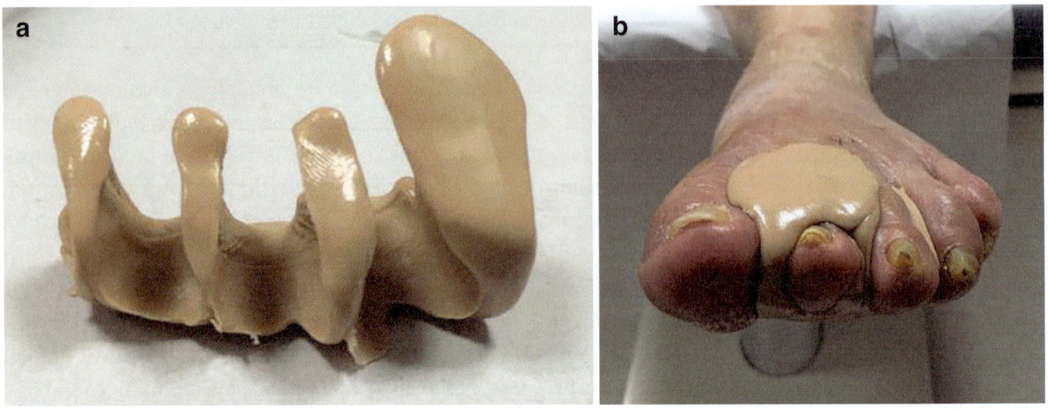

Fig. 34.6 Toe spacer after hardening (**a**) and in place on the operated foot (**b**).

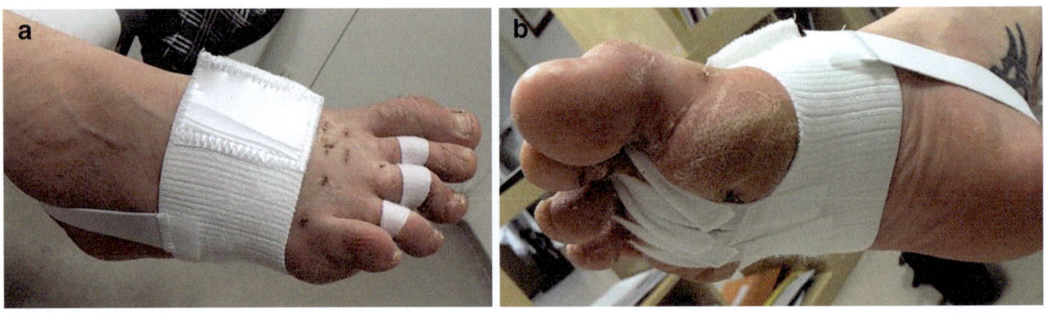

Fig. 34.7 Postoperative foot brace: top view (**a**) bottom view (**b**).

made of gauze dressings or elastic bands) that provide support (Fig. 34.7a, b). They are positioned by the patient or the surgeon. The main drawback is that they loosen over time and must be repositioned in a very specific manner after being taken off, which is difficult for the patient to do (unlike toe spacers that are always in the same position).

34.5 Conclusion

The role of dressings differs depending on how the surgeon designs the minimally invasive or percutaneous surgery. If the goal is solely to make small scars without internal fixation, the dressing must make up for the latter and will change depending on the type of procedure done.

When the surgeon believes that minimally invasive approaches are not an end in themselves but one of the key elements to allow immediate return to function, then the dressings must be viewed differently. They must be combined with other criteria such as immediate mechanical stability before any bone union occurs and with extended postoperative analgesia using local anesthetics.

Percutaneous surgery has its own rules and indications. It requires surgeons to alter their surgical habits, along with their postoperative habits to achieve its full benefits and avoid certain complications. Application of the dressing and its postoperative management are the main stumbling block for this surgery. They are as important as the surgical procedure itself. The time needed to apply the postoperative dressings and the in-office consultations may appear to be longer than the time it took to do the surgery itself. But this careful and attentive management makes this surgical technique reliable and determines the clinical outcome.

Editors' Point of View

Dressings play a key role in percutaneous surgery; they are an integral part of the surgical technique. They are more complex when minimal fixation is used and vary widely depending on surgeon preference.

Suggested Reading

Cazeau C. Chirurgie mini-invasive et percutanée du pied Montpellier : Sauramps médical (2009). 11–24.

De Prado M., Ripoll P.L., Golano P. Hallux valgus. In: Cirurgia percutanea del pie Barcelona: Masson SA (2003). pp. 57–94.

Determe P. Chirurgie mini-invasive et percutanée du pied Montpellier: Sauramps médical (2009), pp. 169–181.

Gottlieb T, Klaue K. The Jones dressing cast for safe aftercare of foot and ankle surgery. A modification of the Jones dressing bandage. Foot Ankle Surg. 2013;19(4):255–60. https://doi.org/10.1016/j.fas.2013.06.015. Epub 2013 Aug 17

Laffenêtre O, Cermolacce C, Coillard JY, et al. Chirurgie mini-invasive de l'hallux valgus Cahiers d'enseignement de la SOFCOT : Chirurgie de l'avant-pied. Paris: Elsevier; 2005. p. 96–104.

Saragas NP. Clinical tip. Postoperative dressing for hallux valgus. Surg Foot Ankle Int. 2005;26(10):899–900.

35 Complications of Percutaneous Forefoot Surgery

Thomas Bauer and Olivier Laffenêtre

35.1 Introduction

Percutaneous surgery is at the same stage as knee arthroscopy was in the 1980s. As with every new technique, it has received tremendous media coverage, and while the medical community has its reservations, it is more often requested by patients than suggested by practitioners.

Of course, every surgical technique has potential complications, and sometimes a new procedure leads to specific problems. For example, arthroscopy was found to have a higher neurological complication rate than conventional surgery. The best way to make progress is to analyze the reasons for failures and complications in order to prevent them and inform our patient about the possibilities beforehand.

There are three types of complications associated with percutaneous forefoot surgery: those related to the learning curve; those that are not really complications but are specific progressions that we must be acutely aware of; and lastly, true complications. We will use this list to frame this review.

T. Bauer (✉) · O. Laffenêtre
Orthopedic Department, Ambroise Paré University Hospital, Boulogne-Billancourt, France

Institut de la Cheville et du Pied, Paris, France
e-mail: thomas.bauer@aphp.fr

35.2 Learning Curve

Hermann Ebbinghaus first used this concept in 1885 by claiming that for each technique, there is a quantifiable graphical relationship between time and the efforts made to acquire it (and of course, its result). Thus, the learning curve is specific to each procedure. For example, in the context of percutaneous surgery, it will be very different between a distal metatarsal mini-invasive osteotomy (DMMO) and the Reverdin-Isham osteotomy to correct hallux valgus. The emphasis is on integrating the specifics of percutaneous techniques, namely, the materials and instrumentation, in the same way as it would be for arthroscopy. Osteotomy procedures are done using rotating burrs, which are completely different than all the other methods used to make bone cuts. Thus, the use of burrs can cause very specific lesions—such as burns—that have no parallel in conventional surgery.

We can identify a certain number of complications, which are very often minor, but are directly related to learning how to use these new tools and that will completely disappear once the surgeon has acquired enough experience.

The main complication related to inappropriate instrumentation use is superficial skin burns. Very often, we notice that colleagues who recently attended a basic percutaneous surgery course are keen to start using their new skills. But very few have the appropriate—and essential—

C. Cazeau, Y. Stiglitz (eds.), *Percutaneous and Minimally Invasive Foot Surgery*,
https://doi.org/10.1007/978-3-030-98791-6_35

materials available in their operating suite. Of all the tools, we feel the powered surgical instrument is the most important. Without the appropriate powered handpiece, percutaneous procedures become extremely dangerous, even in the hands of an expert. The surgical handpiece must have the same axis of rotation as the burr and have a high-torque capacity. The rotation speed should be controllable by a foot pedal and must be on the slow side (maximum of 10,000–15,000 rpm). Some manufacturers offer specific torque reducers, while others have integrated this function in the console. No matter which option is used, insufficient torque does not allow slow-speed work. When the speed is too high, the risk of superficial skin burns (Fig. 35.1), and deeper bone burns increases. In general, they are without consequence and can be treated either by applying a paraffin gauze dressing to direct wound healing or by immediate tissue excision and suture repair.

Damage to critical structures can be prevented by mastering the surgical approaches, which have been shown to be completely safe [1]. The procedure is exactly like in arthroscopy: any deviation—even a slight one—of the insertion point of a blade or burr can cause damage.

At the start, due to lack of experience, surgeons often have flaws or deficiencies in how the procedures are performed (Fig. 35.2). Similarly, mastery of postoperative dressings—some of which are critical to maintaining the position of the osteotomy performed—is very important (Fig. 35.3). Incorrectly performed, it can contribute to various types of secondary displacement and malunion.

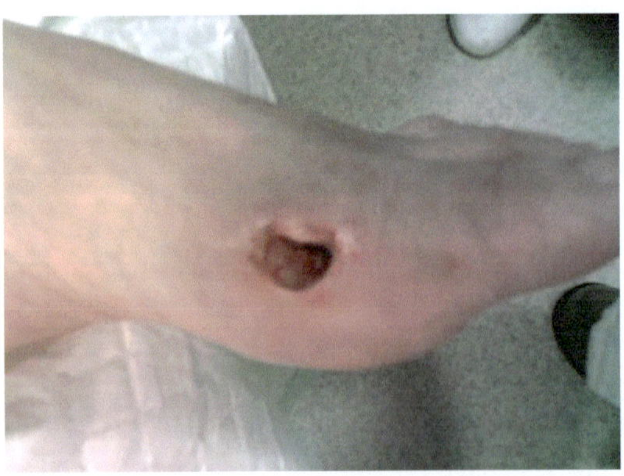

Fig. 35.1 Deep burn after percutaneous surgery of the first ray. © Thomas Bauer 2015. All Rights Reserved

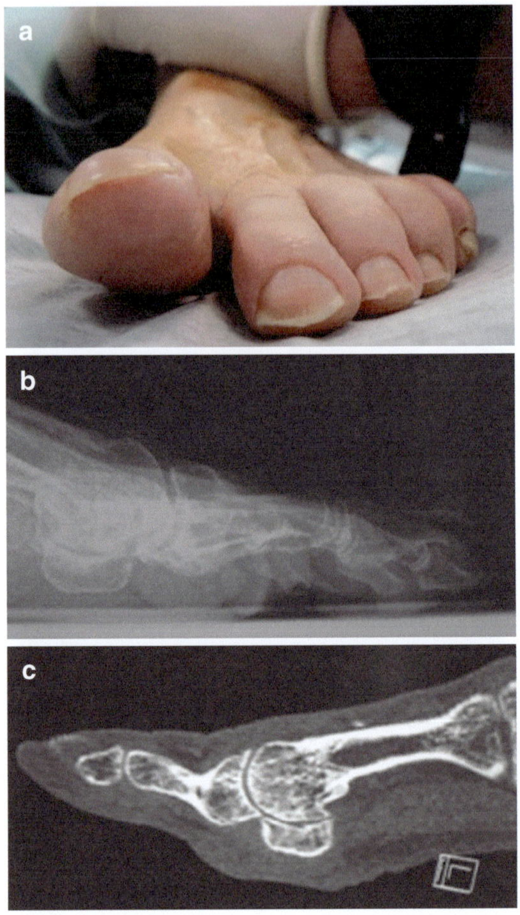

Fig. 35.2 Malunion in erectus after Akin osteotomy without fixation. Clinical appearance (**a**), weight-bearing radiograph (**b**), and CT scan (**c**). © Thomas Bauer 2015. All Rights Reserved

Each technique will have its own learning curve. It is probably wise to integrate them one after the other so that all the inconveniences unavoidably related to their learning are not cumulative.

Rigorous practical and theoretical learning is essential for reducing the impact of this inevitable step by participating in organized courses (Fig. 35.4) in conditions that mimic real practice as much as possible (cadavers, real instrumentation, fluoroscopy), by studying books or scientific publications on this topic, by pairing up with

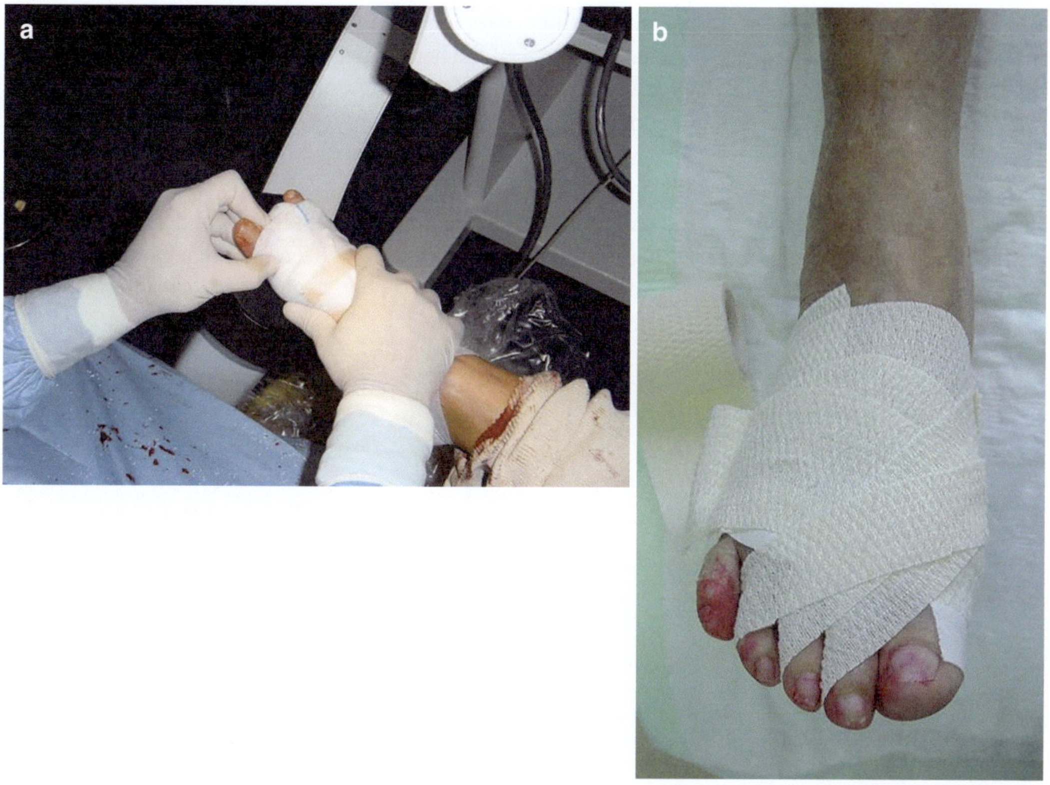

Fig. 35.3 Careful postoperative bandaging performed by the surgeon with fluoroscopy checks (**a**); first postoperative dressing at the 15th day: toes in which the metatarsals underwent DMMO are held by two elastic strips that orient them towards the hallux for two more weeks (**b**).

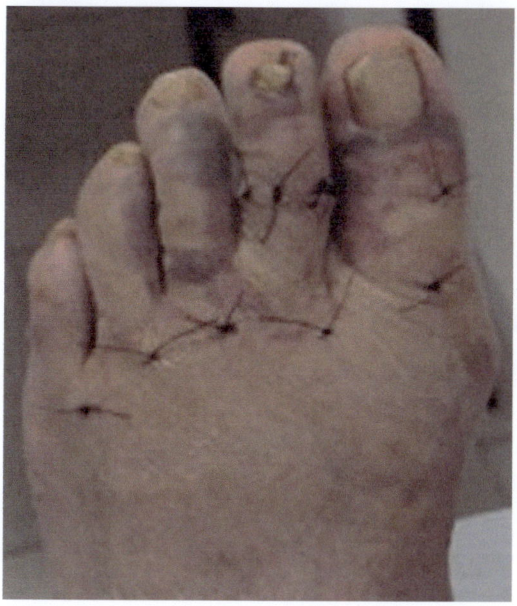

Fig. 35.4 Usual hematoma 8 days after percutaneous surgery.

an expert in the area, and also by having impeccable knowledge of conventional surgery, both its practice and its indications.

35.3 Specific Progressions that Are Not Actual Complications

It is important to know about the expected postoperative progressions so that patients can be made aware of them before the surgery. This will help to reassure the patient, his/her friends, and family and even the general practitioner or radiologist who may be concerned about the postoperative course and the result of a procedure, of which they may know nothing about. Although it is true that the dissemination of these techniques has helped to minimize this aspect, it has caused a lot of grief for some of us in recent years.

Hematoma (Fig. 35.4) is inseparable from percutaneous surgery, because of the innate nature of the technique. It is always present and can be painful if it is too large. It is controlled by carefully fabricating postoperative dressings, by not closing the stab incision and by the patient elevating their foot after the procedure as instructed. In principle, given the importance of the postoperative dressing, icing is not very effective. Not using a tourniquet may reduce the size of the hematoma after lateral ray osteotomy combined with conventional first ray surgery. In principle, when only percutaneous surgery is being done, even with stabilization, the general rule is not to use one.

Edema (Fig. 35.5) is also relatively inseparable from this surgery, even if it often has a multifactorial origin: poor venous predisposition, no skin

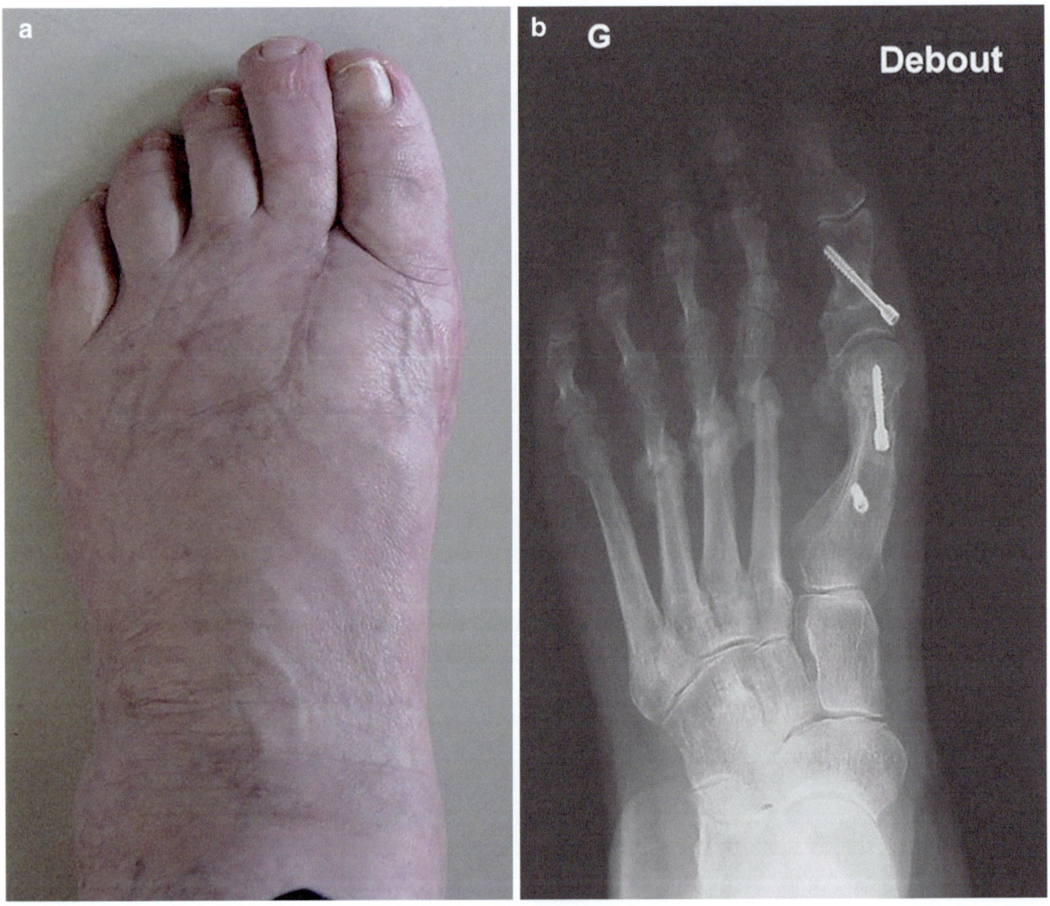

Fig. 35.5 Postoperative edema 2 months after the revision surgery. Clinical appearance (**a**) and radiographic view (**b**).

opening, and bone origin. It can be very noticeable (present in 22% of 241 feet operated using a hybrid technique after 4 months) but is never really a problem from a therapeutic viewpoint [2]. It is less in hallux valgus surgery, with a 2% rate reported by Mouton [3]. It can be prevented by not closing the skin incisions, instructing the patient to keep the foot elevated postoperatively, immediate resumption of walking while using a postoperative shoe, early application of a poultice of green clay paste, and secondarily, for certain cases, lymphatic drainage during rehabilitation. In generally, the edema always resolves after a few months, without any negative consequences.

Type I complex regional pain syndrome (CRPS) is not specific to percutaneous surgery, but it may occur slightly more often when certain osteotomies are performed without fixation and weight-bearing occurs rapidly. The reported rate is 2–6% [2–5]. Since there is no specific treatment for CRPS, various teams have used calcitonin (despite withdrawal of marketing approval for this indication, the response rate is above 50% when used early on), intravenous Fonzylane (Buflomedil) block, bisphosphonate infusion, or regional plexus block through a catheter for 48 h or more. CRPS has a specific progression and generally does not leave any sequelae.

Dysesthesia is fairly specific to the procedure and is truly related to the learning curve: nonoptimal positioning of the entry points and especially, lack of accuracy during the procedure, incomplete mastery of maneuvers, and lack of experience with powered surgical instruments. Mouton reported a 2.8% rate for 264 entry points, and Darcel reported a 0% rate for 693 entry points, with the learning curve having been completed on the first ray [2, 3]. Hypoesthesia occurs more often than hyperesthesia. No permanent anesthesia has been reported in these studies. Prevention requires knowing the local anatomy well, using a meticulous technique (very precise maneuvers, not resting on skin and soft tissues, but on bone instead), and especially, using a very low-speed-powered surgical instruments [1].

Delayed union on radiographs is a progression that must not be ignored, although it is not truly a complication. This mainly occurs in the lateral rays and is not very common. There is generally no abnormal clinical finding except for edema; most importantly, there is no pain or stiffness. But it can throw off a radiologist who is not familiar with the technique and who may induce panic in the patient for no reason (Fig. 35.6). The cause is controversial: it is a given that any bone paste that remains contributes to extensive union (even in cases of very large displacement) is nearly foolproof (nonunion rate of nearly zero) and that this large, plastic callus is much more active than in cases of fixation. It appears difficult to prevent it during percutaneous surgery, as this would cast doubt on the non-fixation principle that is specific to this method, particularly for the lateral rays. The strategy is less clear for the first ray and has led some surgical teams to switch to a different percutaneous technique (chevron), with or without fixation, and in this case, extra-articular sliding osteotomy, leaving very narrow indications for the Isham-Reverdin technique.

Hypertrophic callus is especially common after DMMO. This is a completely normal progression and is often an early sign of good bone union (Fig. 35.7). It is likely triggered by not having removed the bone paste, as it occurs much less often in the first ray, which often undergoes intra-articular lavage. Be that as it may, it is very rarely causes slight pain (discomfort when wearing shoes, compression), and bone remodeling restores the normal architecture most of the time.

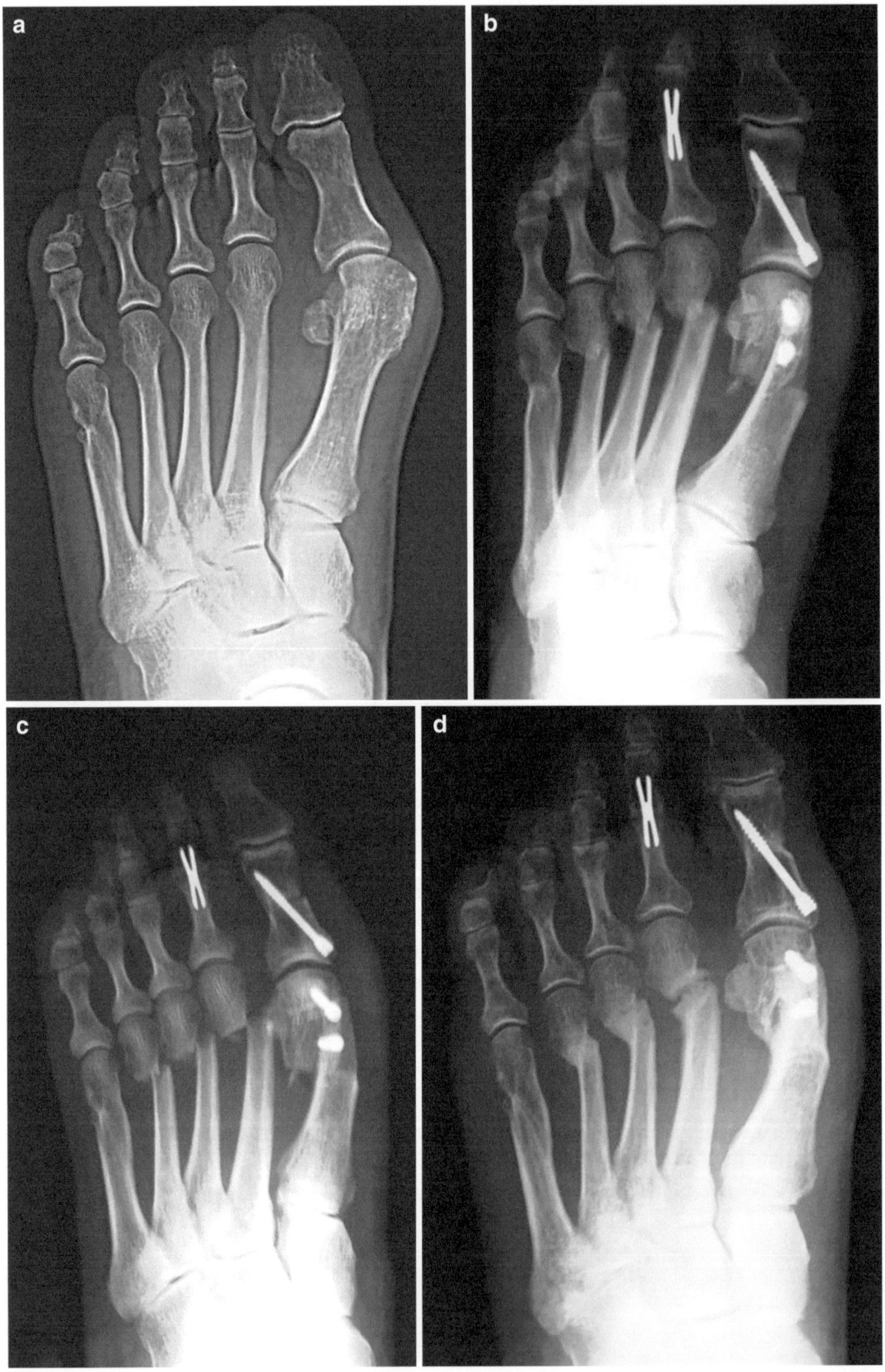

Fig. 35.6 Preoperative (**a**) and immediate postoperative appearance (**b**) of DMMO. Note how healing progresses with bone remodeling at 3 months (**c**) and 6 months (**d**) 12 months (**e**) and 18 months (**f**).

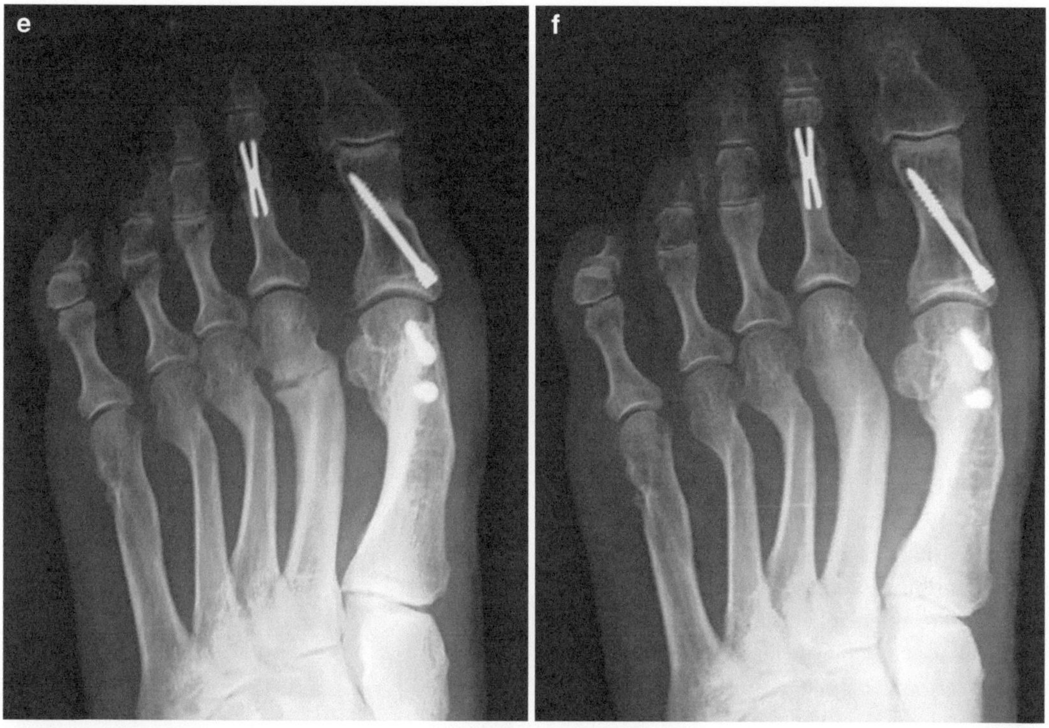

Fig. 35.6 (continued)

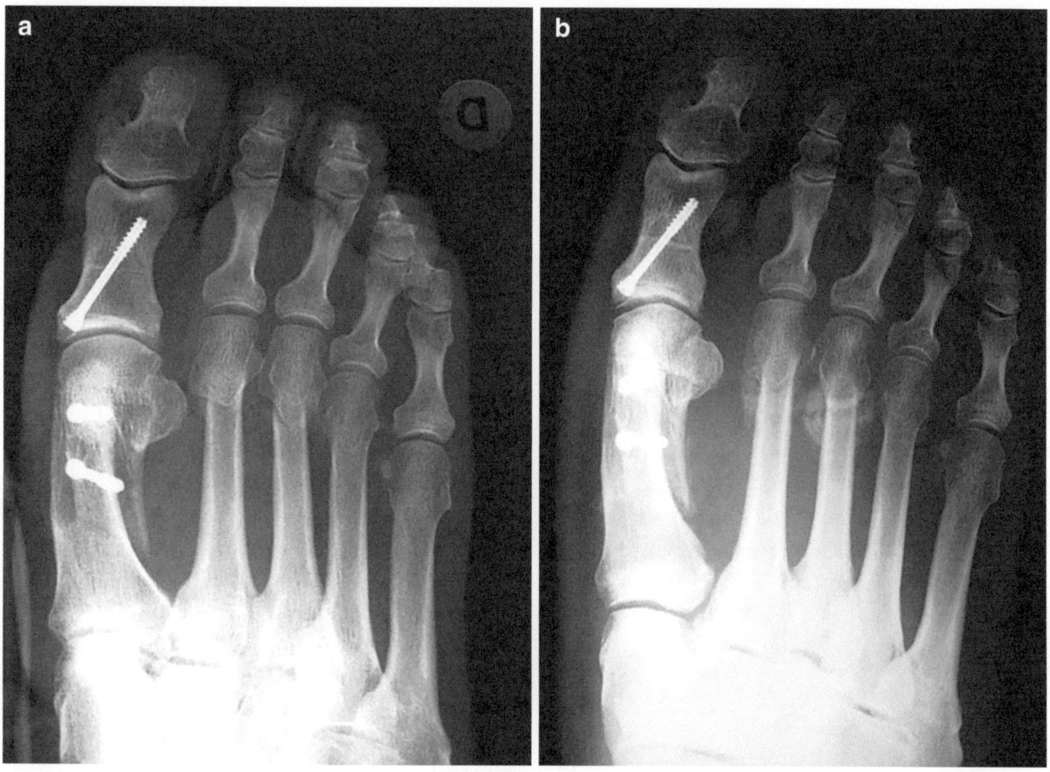

Fig. 35.7 Typical hypertrophic callus after hybrid forefoot surgery. Early postoperative appearance (**a**). Long-term follow-up with hypertrophic calluses after M2 and M3 DMMO (**b**). © Thomas Bauer 2015. All Rights Reserved

35.4 True Complications

Under the umbrella of true complications are all the adverse events that can occur after any forefoot surgery, whether percutaneous or not. The aim of this section is to compile the main complications that occur after percutaneous forefoot surgery, evaluate their incidence, discuss the causes, and propose appropriate treatments for each one.

Surgical site infection is very rare after percutaneous forefoot surgery because of the minimalistic incisions and absence of subcutaneous release. No cases of deep surgical site infection requiring surgical revision have been documented in any GRECMIP study. However, some patients (less than 3%) have inflammation with wound discharge that resolves completely after a few days of antibiotics. These episodes of superficial infection are often related to the learning curve with soft tissue damage (burns) and incomplete removal of bone debris (insufficient lavage) that trigger prolonged inflammation with secondary contamination.

Deep vein thrombosis with percutaneous surgery is very rare, especially when no tourniquet is used (0–1.6%) [2–5]. This complication is most likely to develop in high-risk patients (history of vein thrombosis, embolism, anticoagulant treatment, neoplasia, etc.) and is not specific to percutaneous surgery.

Stiffness in the metatarsophalangeal joint is a known risk factor for every surgical procedure on the forefoot. Reduction of 12–21% in the overall mobility of the MTP1 joint has been reported after percutaneous surgery on the first ray, which is comparable to conventional surgery [3–6]. First and foremost, the preoperative joint mobility determines the postoperative mobility and how fast the joint range of motion is restored [5]. The absence of bone fixation, damage to soft tissues with the burr and insufficient joint lavage may contribute to some stiffening. Only 1% or 2% of patients need surgical revision with arthrolysis after percutaneous surgery. DMMO is an extra-articular procedure, and stiffness is very rare after percutaneous surgery on the lateral rays.

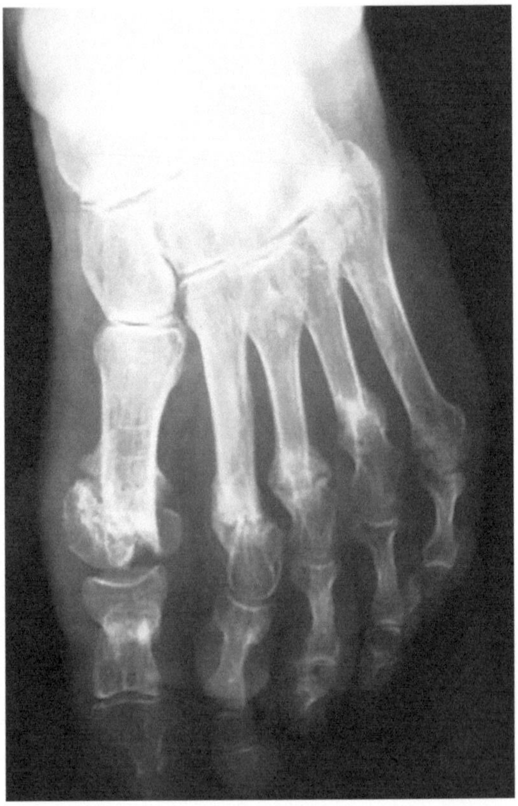

Fig. 35.8 Secondary displacement at 2 months after percutaneous Reverdin-Isham osteotomy in an 82-year-old female patient. At 2 years' follow-up, the MTP1 joint was stiff but not painful; thus no revision was performed.

Secondary displacement can occur due to the absence of fixation, osteoporosis, and the direction of the osteotomy cut (Fig. 35.8). The most worrisome is first metatarsal elevatus. This complication can also be attributed to technical errors. In cases of large secondary displacement (in elevatus, lateral translation, or rotation), open revision may be needed with fixation to better stabilize the osteotomy. The opposite is true for the lateral rays where secondary displacement in elevatus and shortening is not a complication; it is the goal of immediate full

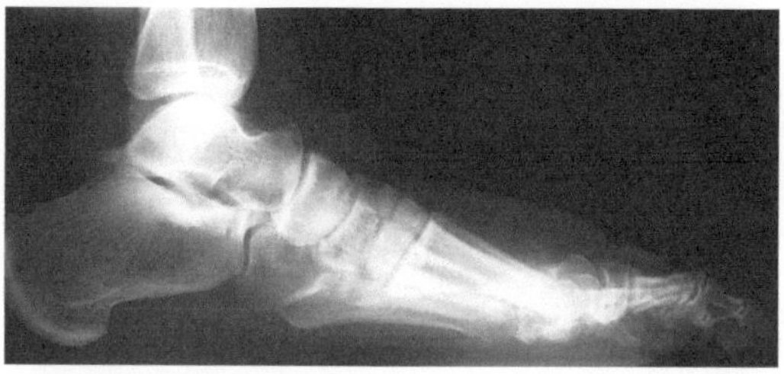

Fig. 35.9 Malunion in elevatus of a percutaneous chevron osteotomy of the first metatarsal with no clinical consequences (DMMO performed at the same time).

weight-bearing; no fixation is required in this scenario.

Certain radiographic findings after lateral metatarsal osteotomy may be worrisome; thus the surgeon must warn his colleagues (family physician and especially radiologist) that this displacement is not a complication and does not require revision surgery.

Malunion of the first metatarsal may cause pain in the first ray or transfer metatarsalgia. Malunion in elevatus (Fig. 35.9) that negatively impacts function will require revision with new osteotomy and bone fixation. Union with excessive shortening of the first metatarsal can lead to transfer metatarsalgia that will require distal metatarsal osteotomies of the lateral rays.

Malunion in rotation of the first metatarsal is definitely the hardest to correct. Overcorrection of the distal metaphyseal articular angle (DMAA) (<0) has been observed in 3–5% of cases of Isham-Reverdin osteotomy with the consequence being joint incongruity (Fig. 35.10) [5, 6].

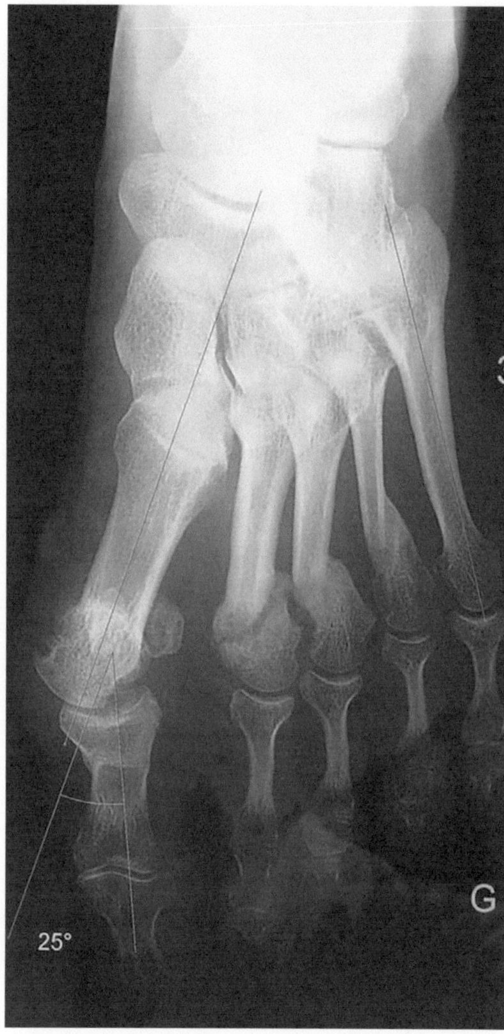

Fig. 35.10 Overcorrection of the DMAA with recurrence of the hallux valgus deformity and joint incongruity.

Malunion of P1 that negatively affects function can be corrected by performing a new osteotomy (percutaneous or not) with or without fixation. In general, this progression can be prevented with impeccable technique and by closely following the postoperative instructions (intraoperative bandaging performed by surgeon, often wet, that hardens when it dries out; it is left in place for 2 weeks and protected by a stiff-soled postoperative shoe that still allows full weight-bearing).

Nonunion of percutaneous distal metatarsal osteotomy is very rare both in the lateral rays (0.1%) and the first metatarsal (no cases reported) (Fig. 35.11) [2–5]. However, the time to union after DMMO varies greatly, ranging from

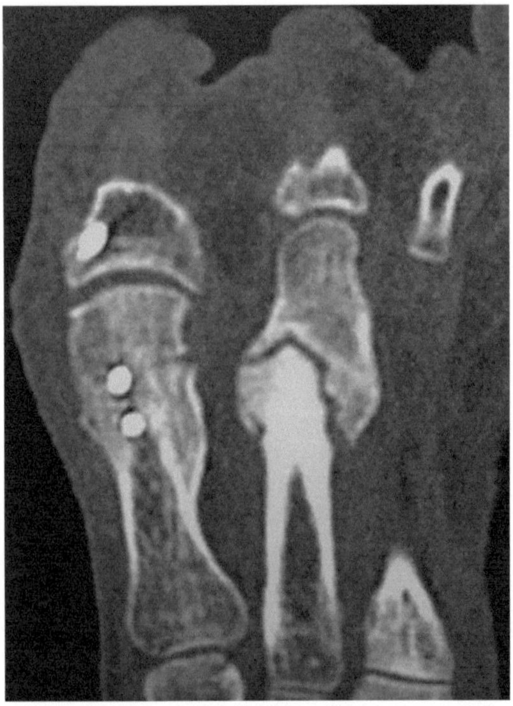

Fig. 35.11 Nonunion of DMMO of the second metatarsal confirmed by CT scan reconstruction.

6 weeks to 18 months. The surgeon must be patient before making the diagnosis of nonunion, especially since delayed union of the lateral metatarsals is asymptomatic.

If the pain persists after sufficient time has elapsed (and never before 18 months), two solutions are possible: reload the unloaded head(s) by making new percutaneous osteotomies around it, or on the contrary, as described by Diebold, link it with the neighboring bones during 6 weeks of protected weight-bearing with a stiff-soled shoe, with trans-metatarsal pinning on either side of the nonunion. This is the strategy that we employed to treat the single case of pain after bone union out of 693 patients 2 years after the osteotomy was performed (Fig. 35.12).

Under- or overcorrection of deformities is a well-known complication of forefoot surgery. Correction of hallux valgus by percutaneous Isham-Reverdin osteotomy will help to reduce the metatarsophalangeal valgus by about 50% in the medium term (2–3 years) with a 2–6% risk of the deformity recurring [3–6]. To date, no cases of hallux varus have reported. For the percutaneous treatment of metatarsalgia, DMMO results in fast, significant improvement, and the risk of persistent hyperkeratosis is 5.8% [2].

Secondary postural disorders after percutaneous forefoot surgery mainly consists of transfer metatarsalgia after hallux valgus surgery (2–5.6%) [3–5]. For surgery on the lateral rays, transfer metatarsalgia has been reported in 2.9% of cases after DMMO [2]. Metatarsalgia of the fourth ray is common and develops rapidly after isolated osteotomy of the second and third rays. It is prudent to perform simultaneous osteotomy of the second, third, and fourth metatarsals to eliminate the possibility of this complication developing.

Metatarsophalangeal arthritis of the first ray has been reported in 4.5% of cases after Isham-Reverdin osteotomy, but it is asymptomatic and does not require surgical revision (Fig. 35.13) [3].

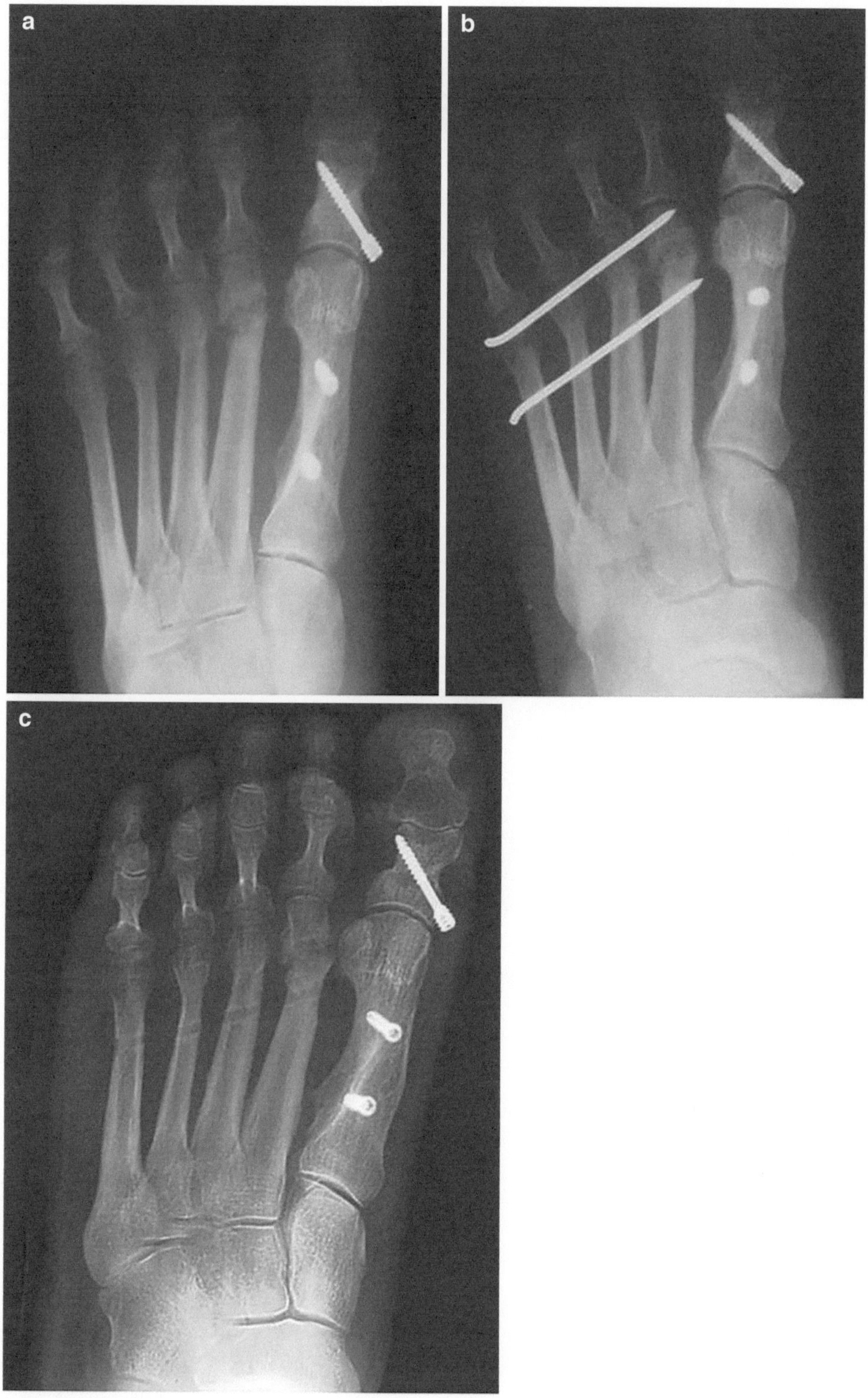

Fig. 35.12 M2 nonunion that was still painful 2 years after hybrid surgery (**a**). M2–M5 intermetatarsal pinning for 6 weeks with protected weight-bearing on a postoperative shoe with no other procedures performed (direct approach, graft, etc.) (**b**). Results 12 weeks after pinning: good progression of the bone union. Pain was completely gone (**c**).

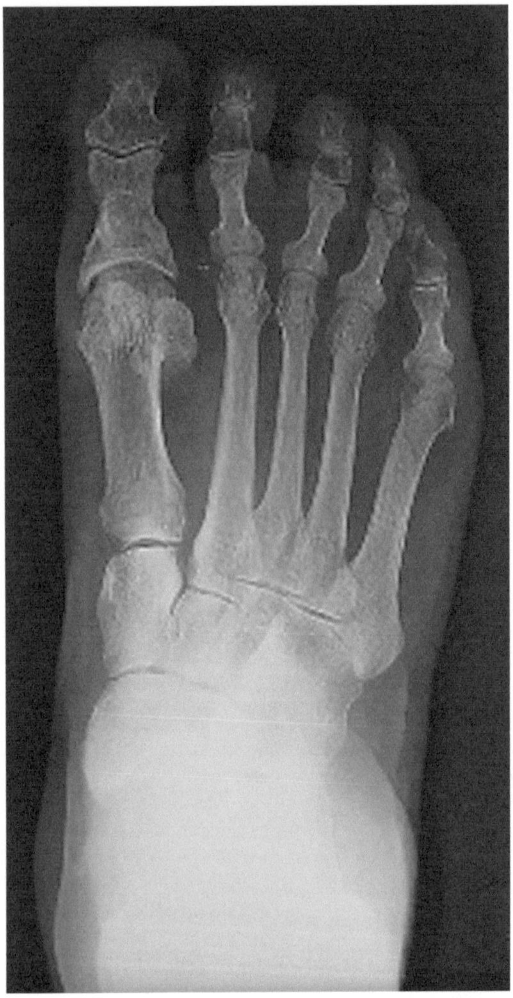

Fig. 35.13 MTP1 arthritis after percutaneous hallux valgus treatment.

Metatarsal osteonecrosis has not been reported in the first ray or the lateral rays after percutaneous surgery in the GRECMIP studies. Some cases have been reported that have a radiological appearance consistent with osteonecrosis but without any symptoms (Fig. 35.14).

Synostosis between the second and third metatarsals have been described after DMMO. If the patient reports discomfort, open revision can be performed (Fig. 35.15).

Tendon transection has not been reported after percutaneous surgery on the first ray. Nevertheless, active plantarflexion of the hallux can be slow to recover.

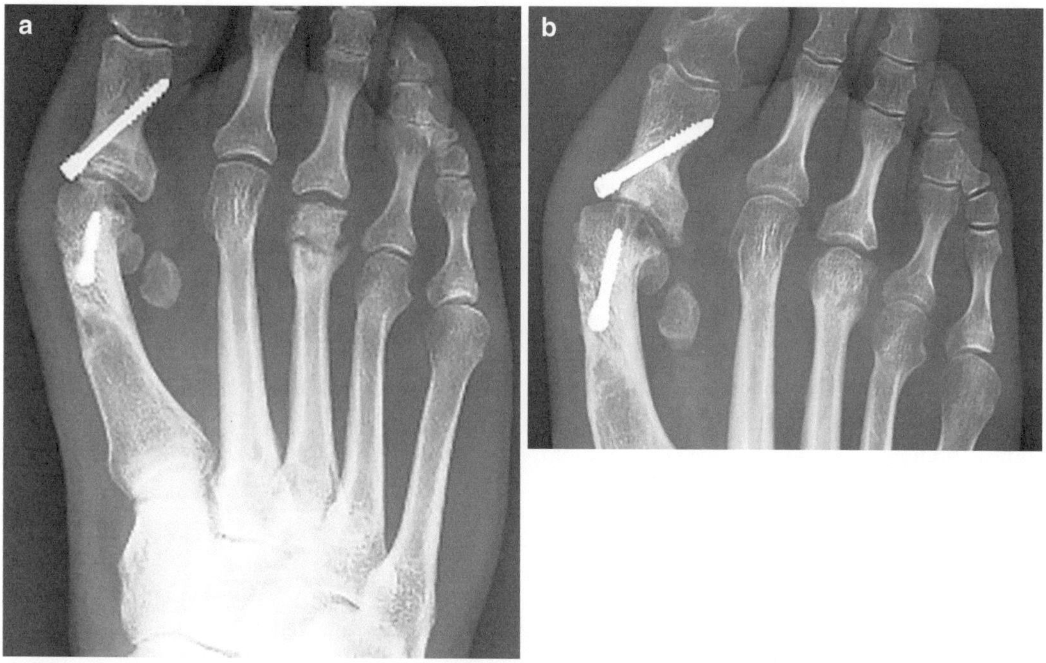

Fig. 35.14 Osteonecrosis of the head of the third metatarsal after DMMO; appearance at 1 year in an asymptomatic patient (**a**); appearance at 2 years after head reconstruction (**b**). © Thomas Bauer 2015. All Rights Reserved

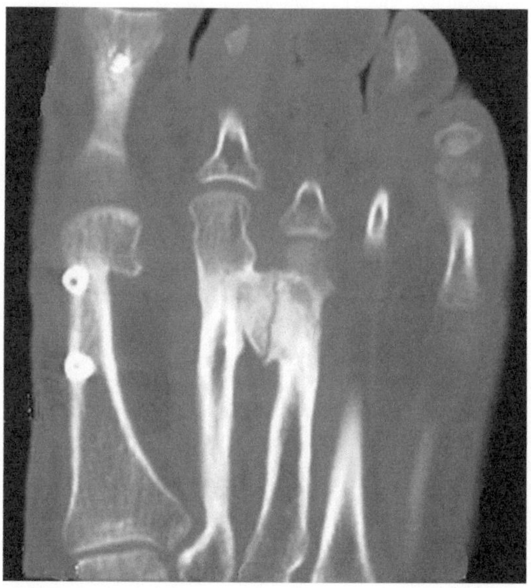

Fig. 35.15 Synostosis between the second and third metatarsal after DMMO. © Thomas Bauer 2015. All Rights Reserved

35.5 Conclusion

Percutaneous surgery has helped to gradually change certain treatment strategies for the corrective surgery in the forefoot, especially the lateral rays. At the same time, certain limitations and complications have emerged.

The biggest error would be to see percutaneous surgery as the only technique that can be used for forefoot surgery. It is impossible to perform percutaneous surgery of the forefoot without first having mastered conventional open procedures. The current trend is toward mixed or hybrid surgery (open or percutaneous), which finds a compromise between the advantages and disadvantages of each technique [7].

Percutaneous surgery requires specific instrumentation and extensive learning in dedicated courses (anatomical bases, surgical approaches, instrumentation use, bandaging) and with experienced surgeons to be able to start without major risks and to make consistent progress. While this technique appears easy at first glance, it actually requires a long learning curve before it can be mastered fully. The postoperative care, monitoring, and bandaging specific to this technique also require organization and adaptation. Some minor complications are inevitable; they are related to the learning curve and disappear with experience.

It is important to know the typical progression of a foot operated percutaneously, as certain clinical findings (bruising, dysesthesia, edema) and especially radiological ones (secondary displacement of certain osteotomies, appearance of callus, delayed union) may needlessly worry some healthcare practitioners and patients. These are not actually complications, but standard progressions after percutaneous surgery; it is important to recognize them in order to reassure the patients and physicians who are not familiar with this type of surgery.

Lastly, there are true complications associated with percutaneous surgery, exactly like the ones associated with conventional forefoot surgery. These complications—infection, phlebitis, secondary displacement, stiffness, malunion, nonunion, osteoarthritis, necrosis, under or overcorrection, and secondary postural disorders—are not specific to percutaneous surgery. The results of prospective studies conducted by the GRECMIP have helped identify these complications and their incidence, which are comparable or lower than the incidence of complications associated with conventional forefoot surgery. The best example is surgery on the lateral rays; here, percutaneous surgery is a leap forward because the procedures are simple and reliable, which quickly leads to very good results with very few complications.

Editors' Point of View

Surgeons must be highly aware of the potential complications of percutaneous and minimally invasive foot surgery. They are difficult to avoid early in one's learning curve. One of the main causes is using inappropriate instrumentation. Hand movements must be highly precise. Surgeons must be familiar with the procedure-specific changes on postoperative radiographs, especially for DMMO, so as to not confuse specific progressions with complications.

References

1. De Prado M, Ripoll PL, Golano P. Minimally invasive foot surgery: surgical techniques, indications, anatomical basis. Bilbao: About Your Health; 2009.
2. Darcel V, Villet L, Chauveaux D, Laffenêtre O. Prise en charge des métatarsalgies statiques par ostéotomies distales percutanées: suivi prospectif de 222 pieds. In: Monographie AFCP. Montpellier: Sauramps Ed. 2009; 5: pp. 229–242.
3. Mouton A, Villet L, Chauveaux D, Laffenêtre O. Chirurgie percutanée de l'hallux: résultats d'une étude prospective continue de 80 interventions. In: Monographie AFCP Montpellier: Sauramps Ed 2009; 219–227.
4. Bauer T, de Lavigne C, Biau D, De Prado M, Isham S, Laffenétre O. Percutaneous hallux valgus surgery: a prospective multicenter study of 189 cases. Orthop Clin N Am. 2009;40:505–14.
5. Bauer T, Biau D, Lortat-Jacob A, Hardy P. Traitement percutané de l'hallux valgus par ostéotomie de Reverdin-Isham: Résultats à 2 ans d'une série monocentrique prospective continue de 104 cas. Rev Chir Orthop Réparatrice Appar Mot. 2010;96:474–84.
6. Laffenêtre O, Cermolacce C, Coillard JY, et al. Chirurgie mini-invasive de l'hallux valgus. In: Valtin B, Leemrijse T, editors. Cahiers d'enseignement de la SOFCOT: chirurgie de l'avant-pied. Paris: Elsevier SAS; 2005. p. 96–104.
7. Laffenêtre O, Solofomalala GD, de Lavigne C, Bauer. Hallux valgus: définition, physiopathologie, études clinique et radiographique, principes du traitement. EMC–Appareil locomoteur. 2009;4:1–9. [article 14–126-A-10].

MIX
Papier aus verantwortungsvollen Quellen
Paper from responsible sources
FSC® C105338
FSC
www.fsc.org

If you have any concerns about our products,
you can contact us on
ProductSafety@springernature.com

In case Publisher is established outside the EU,
the EU authorized representative is:
Springer Nature Customer Service Center GmbH
Europaplatz 3, 69115 Heidelberg, Germany

Printed by Libri Plureos GmbH
in Hamburg, Germany